AF784449

Complications of Organ Transplantation

IMMUNOLOGY SERIES

1. Mechanisms in Allergy: Reagin-Mediated Hypersensitivity
   Edited by Lawrence Goodfriend, Alec Sehon and Robert P. Orange
2. Immunopathology: Methods and Techniques
   Edited by Theodore P. Zacharia and Sidney S. Breese, Jr.
3. Immunity and Cancer in Man: An Introduction
   Edited by Arnold E. Reif
4. *Bordetella pertussis:* Immunological and Other Biological Activities
   J.J. Munoz and R.K. Bergman
5. The Lymphocyte: Structure and Function (in two parts)
   Edited by John J. Marchalonis
6. Immunology of Receptors
   Edited by B. Cinader
7. Immediate Hypersensitivity: Modern Concepts and Development
   Edited by Michael K. Bach
8. Theoretical Immunology
   Edited by George I. Bell, Alan S. Perelson, and George H. Pimbley, Jr.
9. Immunodiagnosis of Cancer (in two parts)
   Edited by Ronald B. Herberman and K. Robert McIntire
10. Immunologically Mediated Renal Diseases: Criteria for Diagnosis and Treatment
    Edited by Robert T. McCluskey and Giuseppe A. Andres
11. Clinical Immunotherapy
    Edited by Albert F. LoBuglio
12. Mechanisms of Immunity to Virus-Induced Tumors
    Edited by John W. Blasecki
13. Manual of Macrophage Methodology: Collection, Characterization, and Function
    Edited by Herbert B. Herscowitz, Howard T. Holden, Joseph A. Bellanti, and Abdul Ghaffar
14. Suppressor Cells in Human Disease
    Edited by James S. Goodwin
15. Immunological Aspects of Aging
    Edited by Diego Segre and Lester Smith

16. Cellular and Molecular Mechanisms of Immunologic Tolerance
Edited by Tomáš Hraba and Milan Hašek

17. Immune Regulation: Evolution and Biological Significance
Edited by Laurens N. Ruben and M. Eric Gershwin

18. Tumor Immunity in Prognosis: The Role of Mononuclear Cell Infiltration
Edited by Stephen Haskill

19. Immunopharmacology and the Regulation of Leukocyte Function
Edited by David R. Webb

20. Pathogenesis and Immunology of Treponemal Infection
Edited by Ronald F. Schell and Daniel M. Musher

21. Macrophage-Mediated Antibody-Dependent Cellular Cytotoxicity
Edited by Hillel S. Koren

22. Molecular Immunology: A Textbook
Edited by M. Zouhair Atassi, Carel J. van Oss, and Darryl R. Absolom

23. Monoclonal Antibodies and Cancer
Edited by George L. Wright, Jr.

24. Stress, Immunity, and Aging
Edited by Edwin L. Cooper

25. Immune Modulation Agents and Their Mechanisms
Edited by Richard L. Fenichel and Michael A. Chirigos

26. Mononuclear Phagocyte Biology
Edited by Alvin Volkman

27. The Lactoperoxidase System: Chemistry and Biological Significance
Edited by Kenneth M. Pruitt and Jorma O. Tenovuo

28. Introduction to Medical Immunology
Edited by Gabriel Virella, Jean-Michel Goust, H. Hugh Fudenberg, and Christian C. Patrick

29. Handbook of Food Allergies
Edited by James C. Breneman

30. Human Hybridomas: Diagnostic and Therapeutic Applications
Edited by Anthony J. Strelkauskas

31. Aging and the Immune Response: Cellular and Humoral Aspects
Edited by Edmond A. Goidl

32. Complications of Organ Transplantation
Edited by Luis H. Toledo-Pereyra

33. Monoclonal Antibodies: Hybridoma Techniques
Edited by Lawrence B. Schook

Additional Volumes in Preparation

Complications of Organ Transplantation

edited by

LUIS H. TOLEDO–PEREYRA
Chief, Transplantation
Director, Research
Department of Surgery
Mount Carmel Mercy Hospital
Detroit, Michigan

MARCEL DEKKER, INC. **New York and Basel**

Library of Congress Cataloging-in-Publication Data

Complications of organ transplantation.

(Immunology series ; v. 32)
Includes bibliographies and index.
1. Transplantation of organs, tissues, etc.--
Complications and sequelae. I. Toledo-Pereyra, Luis H.
II. Series. [DNLM: 1. Postoperative Complications.
2. Transplantation--adverse effects. W1 IM53K v. 32
WO 660 C737]
RD120.7.C64 1987 617'.95 86-24135
ISBN 0-8247-7639-9

MARCEL DEKKER, INC.
270 Madison Avenue, New York, New York 10016

Current printing (last digit):
10 9 8 7 6 5 4 3 2 1

PRINTED IN THE UNITED STATES OF AMERICA

To all my professors and colleagues of the
University of Minnesota Graduate Medical School–
source of knowledge, innovative ideas, and definitive guiding force

Series Introduction

Organ and tissue transplantations have emerged as standard methods for treating many forms of end-organ failure, including those in kidney, liver, heart, pancreatic islet, and bone marrow. Each of these applications has brought untold benefits in the length and quality of life. At the same time, each operation entails significant risks, including those due to the surgical procedure itself, postsurgical problems, infection associated with immunosuppression, and, in some instances, rejection and graft-versus-host disease. Some complications are general; others pertain to the particular organ.

This book is the first to address these complications in a comprehensive manner. It deals with both direct and indirect consequences. As in every surgical procedure, risks and benefits must be considered carefully by the patients and their physicians. This book will aid considerably in arriving at a judicious balance.

William Halsted once said that every surgical operation is an experiment in bacteriology. This book makes clear that every transplant is also an experiment in immunology.

Noel R. Rose

Foreword

Not too long ago it was often stated, and with considerable justification, that organ transplantation was more of a disease than a cure. The immunosuppressive therapy required to control or reverse rejection was the usual villain. Most of the morbidity and mortality were attributable to excessive requirements for steroids in order to prevent rejection. The other maintenance drugs, e.g., azathioprine (or cyclophosphamide), could and often did depress the bone marrow. The long list of complications from such nonspecific immunosuppression ranged from merely annoying to deadly. It was found that every major organ system of the recipient could be affected and in a variety of ways.

In this book, a careful look has been taken at the many adverse ramifications of immunosuppressive therapy in chapters dealing with such diverse topics as the skin, the cardiovascular system, the endocrine system, the liver, the gastrointestinal tract, and the musculoskeletal system. Throughout these chapters, as well as in the Appendix, the ways in which immunosuppression can cause opportunistic infections or malignant tumors have been carefully considered.

In addition, complications more or less specific to different kinds of organ grafts have been covered in chapters dealing with transplantation of the kidney, liver, heart, lung, pancreas, cornea, and bone marrow. Each of these specialty chapters is unique in its own right and reflects the views of some of the most creative members of the transplant community. Virtually all of the chapters give an outstanding survey of the assigned topics. With their look at the dark side of transplantation, the editors and authors have provided an important service to this new medical-surgical specialty.

Thomas E. Starzl

Preface

Transplantation has developed into a well-established discipline in the past decade. Surgical techniques have been expanded to their full application, and added technical support has been utilized to ensure safety of these surgical maneuvers. Advances in the recognition of end-stage disease of kidneys, liver, pancreas, heart, etc., have made possible early selection of appropriate candidates for transplantation. Better ways to diagnose and treat rejection have improved the functional status of transplantable organs. Assuring long-term function of these organs is the ultimate goal of transplantation.

In spite of all previous efforts to maximize posttransplant function, complications still do occur after transplantation. These complications may appear at various stages of the transplant event, that is, during the operative technique in particular, as an expression of the original end-stage disease, or as a consequence of the use of immunosuppressive drugs needed for the management of the allograft response. This book addresses all these complications.

No specific chapter has been assigned to the complications of immunosuppression, in general. Instead, we have dedicated single chapters to the individual problems, such as infectious complications, bone and joint complications, ocular, dermatological, neurological, and psychiatric complications, maternal and fetal complications, endocrine and metabolic complications, and cancer, all secondary in some way to the use of one or more immunosuppressive agents. Individual organs have been discussed separately and, for the sake of completion, an appendix with all complications of immunosuppression has been added.

We hope that this book will serve as the basis to remind the clinician and the student of transplantation of the potential complications that can occur after transplantation and the ways to ameliorate them and, if possible, to attempt to prevent them.

The Department of Surgery of our institution offered an environment conducive to the development of this work. The editorial assistance of Debra A. Gordon is greatly appreciated.

Luis H. Toledo-Pereyra

Contributors

Juhani Ahonen, M.D. Director, Section of Transplantation, Fourth Department of Surgery, Helsinki University Central Hospital, Helsinki, Finland

Leonard C. Alexander, M.D. Chairman, Department of Medicine, Mount Carmel Mercy Hospital, Detroit, Michigan

John C. Baldwin, M.D. Assistant Professor, Department of Cardiovascular Surgery, Stanford University School of Medicine, Stanford, California

Oscar L. Bronsther, M.D.* University of Pittsburgh School of Medicine, Pittsburgh, Pennsylvania

Joseph J. Buckley, M.D. Professor and Head, Department of Anesthesiology, University of Minnesota Health Sciences Center, Minneapolis, Minnesota

Theodore J. Buselmeier, M.D. University of Minnesota, Minneapolis, Minnesota

Frank E. Check, Jr., M.D. Chief, Infectious Diseases, Department of Medicine, Mount Carmel Mercy Hospital, Detroit, Michigan

John W. Cowden, M.D. Associate Professor, Department of Ophthalmology, Kresge Eye Institute, Wayne State University, Detroit, Michigan

---

Present affiliation:
*Assistant Adjunct Professor, Department of Surgery, University of California San Diego Medical Center, San Diego, California.

Carlos O. Esquivel, M.D., Ph.D. Assistant Professor, Department of Surgery, University of Pittsburgh School of Medicine, Pittsburgh, Pennsylvania

Jorge A. Estrin, M.D., Ph.D. Associate Professor, Department of Anesthesiology, University of Minnesota Medical School, Minneapolis, Minnesota

Mark I. Evans, M.D. Director, Division of Reproductive Genetics, Department of Obstetrics and Gynecology, Wayne State University/Hutzel Hospital, Detroit, Michigan

John Gilroy, M.D. Professor and Chairman, Department of Neurology, Wayne State University, Detroit, Michigan

Robert D. Gordon, M.D. Assistant Professor, Department of Surgery, University of Pittsburgh School of Medicine, Pittsburgh, Pennsylvania

Milton M. Green, M.D. Attending Orthopedic Surgeon, Department of Orthopedic Surgery, Mount Carmel Mercy Hospital, and Clinical Professor of Surgery, Wayne State University, Detroit, Michigan

J. Harold Helderman, M.D. Professor of Medicine and Medical Director of Renal Transplant, Division of Nephrology, University of Texas Health Science Center at Dallas, Southwestern Medical School, Dallas, Texas

Hervy H. Hiner, Jr., M.D. Clinical Instructor, Renal Section, Department of Medicine, Baylor College of Medicine, Houston, Texas

Maria Hordinsky, M.D. Assistant Professor, Department of Dermatology, University of Minnesota, Minneapolis, Minnesota

Shunzaburo Iwatsuki, M.D. Associate Professor, Department of Surgery, University of Pittsburgh School of Medicine, Pittsburgh, Pennsylvania

Stuart W. Jamieson, M.D.* Associate Professor, Department of Cardiovascular Surgery, Stanford University School of Medicine, Stanford, California

Jan P. Lerut, M.D.† Transplant Fellow, Department of Surgery, University of Pittsburgh School of Medicine, Pittsburgh, Pennsylvania

---

Present affiliations:
*Professor and Head, Division of Cardiothoracic Surgery, University of Minnesota, Minneapolis, Minnesota.
†Assistant Professor, Department of General Surgery, Catholic University of Leuven Medical School, Leuven, Belgium.

Leonard Makowka, M.D., Ph.D. Assistant Professor, Department of Surgery, University of Pittsburgh School of Medicine, Pittsburgh, Pennsylvania

Robert Mendez, M.D. St. Vincent Medical Center and Clinical Professor of Surgery/Urology, Division of Urology, University of Southern California School of Medicine, Los Angeles, California

Vijay K. Mittal, M.D. Transplant Surgeon, Department of Surgery, Mount Carmel Mercy Hospital, Detroit, Michigan

Sean O'Regan, M.B. Associate Professor, Department of Pediatrics, University of Montreal, Hôpital Ste-Justine, Montreal, Quebec, Canada

Philip E. Oyer, M.D., Ph.D. Associate Professor, Department of Cardiovascular Surgery, Stanford University School of Medicine, Stanford, California

Israel Penn, M.D. Professor, Department of Surgery, University of Cincinnati Medical Center, Cincinnati, Ohio

Oliver W. Press, M.D., Ph.D. Acting Instructor, Division of Oncology, Department of Medicine, Fred Hutchinson Cancer Research Center and University of Washington, Seattle, Washington

Bernard H. Ravitz, M.D. Chief Medical Resident, Department of Medicine, Mount Carmel Mercy Hospital, Detroit, Michigan

Khashayar Sakhaee, M.D. Assistant Professor, Section of Mineral Metabolism, Department of Internal Medicine, University of Texas Health Science Center at Dallas, Southwestern Medical School, Dallas, Texas

Robert T. Schaller, Jr., M.D. Clinical Assistant Professor, Department of Surgery, University of Washington, Seattle, Washington

Norman E. Shumway, M.D., Ph.D. Professor and Chairman, Department of Cardiovascular Surgery, Stanford University School of Medicine, Stanford, California

Robert J. Sokol, M.D. Professor, Chairman, and Chief, Department of Obstetrics and Gynecology, Wayne State University/Hutzel Hospital, Detroit, Michigan

Thomas E. Starzl, M.D., Ph.D. Professor, Department of Surgery, University of Pittsburgh School of Medicine, Pittsburgh, Pennsylvania

Edward B. Stinson, M.D. Thelma and Henry Doelger Professor, Department of Cardiovascular Surgery, Stanford University School of Medicine, Stanford, California

Wadi N. Suki, M.D. Professor, Departments of Medicine and Physiology, Baylor College of Medicine, and Chief, Renal Section, Medical Service, The Methodist Hospital, Houston, Texas

E. Donnall Thomas, M.D. Associate Director, Clinical Research Programs, Fred Hutchinson Cancer Research Center, and Professor, Department of Medicine, University of Washington, Seattle, Washington

Luis H. Toledo-Pereyra, M.D., Ph.D., Ph.D. Chief, Transplantation, and Director, Research, Department of Surgery, Mount Carmel Mercy Hospital, Detroit, Michigan

David H. Van Thiel, M.D. Professor and Chief of Gastroenterology, Department of Medicine, University of Pittsburgh School of Medicine, Pittsburgh, Pennsylvania

Alexander D. Vargas, M.D. Surgeon, St. Vincent Medical Center, and Assistant Clinical Professor of Surgery/Urology, University of Southern California School of Medicine, Los Angeles, California

Lynn Vaughan, M.D. Research Fellow, Departments of Surgery and Dermatology, University of Minnesota, Minneapolis, Minnesota

Robert A. Welch, M.D. Assistant Professor, Division of Maternal-Fetal Medicine, Department of Obstetrics and Gynecology, Wayne State University/Hutzel Hospital, Detroit, Michigan

James I. Whitten, M.D. Chief, Vascular Surgery, Department of Surgery, Mount Carmel Mercy Hospital, Detroit, Michigan

Salem Yazbeck, M.D. Chief, Section of Transplantation, University of Montreal, Hôpital Ste-Justine, Montreal, Quebec, Canada

Contents

Complications of Organ Transplantation

1
Complications of Anesthesia

JORGE A. ESTRIN
University of Minnesota Medical School, Minneapolis, Minnesota

JOSEPH J. BUCKLEY
University of Minnesota Health Sciences Center, Minneapolis, Minnesota

In the last three decades, organ transplantation has emerged as a reliable therapeutic modality for a growing number of patients with end-stage kidney, heart, liver, or pancreas disease [1-4]. The usual indication for transplantation is progressive deterioration of organ function that cannot otherwise be satisfactorily treated. Confronted with this heterogeneous spectrum of gravely ill patients, anesthesiologists have had to develop innovative methods to reduce the prohibitive anesthetic risk in these subjects and to deal with the unique problems created by these new surgical procedures.

Considering the magnitude of the functional derangement that affects patients in end-stage organ failure, one might expect that anesthetic management would be more difficult than in patients less seriously compromised. But firm data on that subject are sparse, and what information exists is largely anecdotal. It is important that careful studies of the entire perioperative period be made if we are to improve the safety and efficiency of this new therapy. Particularly, improved preoperative assessment and preparation and a clearer understanding of the unusual physiological effects of the transplant surgical procedure itself are necessary to assure the best possible chance of success. Finally, the nature and incidence of complications associated with transplant surgery needs systematic study. This chapter will examine our experience in these areas and contrast our methods and results with those of other large centers wherever possible.

I. RENAL TRANSPLANTATION

Anesthetic complications during renal transplantation stem largely from the abnormalities peculiar to the uremic state and from the broad array of multiorgan dysfunction provoked by renal failure [5]. The most frequently reported anesthetic complications during renal transplantation are pulmonary aspiration, cardiac arrhythmias, pulmonary edema, instability of blood pressure, coagulation disorders, and postoperative respiratory distress syndrome [6].

A. Vomiting and Aspiration

Morgan and Lumley [7] were the first to call attention to the danger of regurgitation of gastric contents in renal transplant patients. They urged that a rapid sequence induction technique be employed in all these patients to minimize the risk of aspiration. Although no controlled prospective studies of the incidence of this complication have been made, there is agreement that vomiting and pulmonary aspiration occur more commonly during the induction of or emergence from anesthesia in renal transplant recipients than in normal patients [6]. Several factors explain this tendency: (1) the often urgent nature of the cadaver transplant operation, in which the recipient is hurried to the operating room without adequate restriction of oral intake; (2) the hyperemetic state that uremia and hemodialysis seem to create (hypersecretion, peptic ulcer disease, and gastric atony; all these favor delayed gastric emptying and/or gastroesophageal junction incompetence); and (3) delayed or inadequate termination of the effects of narcotics or muscle relaxants fosters postoperative hypoventilation and hypoxia, conditions that frequently result in aspiration of regurgitated gastric secretions. Regurgitation and aspiration, whether overt or silent, is potentially catastrophic in immunosuppressed, steroid-treated patients, because pulmonary infection and protracted respiratory incompetence are almost inevitable and frequently result in irreversible pulmonary failure and death. This complication can be avoided if the hazard of the full stomach is recognized and if there is systematic application of the rapid sequence technique or awake intubation.

B. Cardiovascular Instability

Patients with end-stage renal failure suffer a significant degree of cardiovascular compromise that significantly limits their survival on chronic dialysis [8,9]. Cardiovascular disease has been estimated to be responsible for 20% late postoperative deaths in patients otherwise successfully transplanted [10]. It is responsible for many of the crises that occur during the perioperative period; hypotension, hypertension, cardiac arrhythmias leading to cardiac arrest, myocardial infarction, and pulmonary edema are examples of the untoward cardiovascular events seen.

Hypertension is a nearly universal complication of renal insufficiency and the uremic state [11]. In fact, the absence of hypertension should cause the anesthesiologist to suspect unidentified antihypertensive therapy, volume depletion due to aggressive dialysis, intake deficit, or salt-wasting renal disease. Blood pressure instability during anesthesia, particularly hypotension during induction and hypertension on awakening, is also commonly observed in these patients. In a retrospective study of 100 anesthetized kidney transplants, Aldrete et al. [12]. found that 55% of patients experienced a fall in blood pressure during induction of anesthesia. In 8% systolic blood pressure was less than 90 torr. Our own experience confirms that finding. In addition, approximately one-third of our recipients required active therapy for postoperative hypertension that was not traceable to pain, CO_2 retention, or other common causes of postsurgical hypertension.

This blood pressure instability is largely related to the defective hemodynamic regulatory mechanisms present in these patients. Two well-defined groups have been identified among uremic hypertensive patients by Vertes et al. [13]. One group comprises the great majority of renal transplant candidates in whom hypertension can be well controlled with dialysis alone (sodium-dependent hypertension). This form of renal hypertension appears to be due to expanded plasma and extracellular fluid volume and increased total exchangeable sodium. In these patients a positive correlation was found between plasma volume and diastolic blood pressure [14-19]. A second, much smaller group of hypertensive uremic patients, whose hypertension is not satisfactorily treatable by dialysis, have elevated renin levels (renin-dependent hypertension) [13]. Pharmacological control of this latter form of hypertension is facilitated by bilateral nephrectomy [20-26].

In general, the more severe the preoperative degree of hypertension the more likely are significant changes in blood pressure during anesthesia, especially if blood pressure is not responsive to dialytic or pharmacological control even after bilateral nephrectomy and if hypertensive encephalopathy or cardiopathy is present. If uremic autonomic neuropathy is present, blood pressure instability, particularly hypotension, can be expected during both dialysis and anesthesia [27,28].

When diabetes mellitus is the basic cause of the renal failure, abnormal intraoperative blood pressure changes can be anticipated, particularly if ischemic heart disease or autonomic diabetic neuropathy are present.

From the foregoing we conclude that renal transplant recipients are at a higher cardiovascular risk because (1) cardiovascular hypertrophy (left ventricular and arteriolar) amplifies the blood pressure responses to acute changes in cardiac loading conditions and adrenergic tone that occur during induction or awakening; (2) autonomic dysfunction associated with baroreceptor reflex resetting and changes in peripheral neurovascular effector organs due to renal disease foster exagerated responses to relatively minor stimulation or depression; and (3) blood volume is a more important determinant of myocardial performance and blood pressure in renal failure patients than in normal subjects due to the frequent abnormal diastolic left ventricular function [29].

The interaction between these predisposing factors and anesthetic or surgical interventions increases the sensitivity of these patients to changes in central adrenergic tone. For example, the sudden decrease in central adrenergic tone that follows anesthetic depression of the vasomotor center produces venular dilatation and reduced preload, which in turn causes a more significant decrease in cardiac output by the dysfunctional, hypertrophic left ventricle. This hemodynamic depression would normally activate sinoaortic baroreceptors and initiate a reflex adrenergic discharge, but in uremic patients the response is blunted by dysfunction of the autonomic pathway [27,28]. Similarly, compensation for anesthetic-induced direct myocardial depression is reduced.

When blood volume is normal or increased, these abnormal hemodynamic responses are usually mild; but when intravascular volume is reduced by repeated dialysis or other substantial fluid loss (e.g., vomiting, diarrhea, sweating), arterial hypotension secondary to anesthesia may be more pronounced. More appropriate control of uremic hypertension, optimization of blood volume, and a slow induction of anesthesia can, in most cases, effectively prevent significant hypotension, but infusion of vasoactive drugs may be necessary if central adrenergic function is seriously impaired.

The incidence and causes of hypertension and tachycardia, which occur during arousal from anesthesia, have not been precisely defined. These disturbances are not related to pain, CO_2 retention, hypoxia, bladder distension, or any of the other well-known causes of postoperative hypertension [30]. The mechanisms involved appear to be (1) an abrupt, "unrestrained" recovery of central adrenergic drive previously depressed by anesthetic drugs; this triggers acute tachycardia and peripheral arteriolar constriction; and (2) an expanded blood volume, which was necessary to maintain hemodynamic stability during anesthesia but in the postoperative period simply heightens cardiac preload and output. This volume overload, the superimposed contracted peripheral vasculature, and the sinus tachycardia result in a hyperdynamic state that requires prompt and aggressive management. That tachycardia rather than bradycardia accompanies the hypertension suggests abnormal sinoaortic mechanoreceptor reflex function.

Preoperative control of hypertension through dialysis and drug therapy can do much to offset postoperative hypertension and tachycardia. This preparation is always possible in patients who receive kidneys from living donors. Blood pressure changes during and after anesthesia are modest in this group. Such preparation is not always possible in cadaver transplant recipients whose operation is often undertaken unexpectedly to accommodate organ preservation limits. It is in this latter group of patients that the most serious blood pressure management problems are seen. Invasive monitoring of the arterial blood pressure and Swan-Ganz catheter assessment of myocardial performance are helpful, even essential, to guide intra- and postoperative blood pressure control. Anesthetic agents are useful in controlling blood pressure intraoperatively but cannot correct the fundamental cause(s) of this type of hypertension (abnormal central adrenergic drive, faulty baroreceptor reflex activity, and volume overload); when the anesthetic is terminated, the hyperdynamic state reappears immediately.

It is our practice to continue or to increase antihypertensive therapy up to and including the day of surgery. This is particularly important with β blockers and clonidine, since sudden withdrawal of these drugs can precipitate a hyperdynamic cardiovascular syndrome. Catastrophic postoperative hypertension and/or myocardial ischemia have been reported after such withdrawal [31,32]. There is no longer any rational basis to withhold antihypertensive agents preoperatively. Rather, it is clearly necessary to continue and perhaps to reinforce any prevalent antihypertensive therapy in order to achieve a more stable intra- and postoperative hemodynamic course.

Several other factors contribute to the potential for cardiovascular complications in renal transplant patients [8,9]. Hyperlipidemia [33], abnormal glucose tolerance, hyperuricemia, hypertension, vascular calcification, and diabetes afflict these subjects and lead to early severe vascular damage. Angina pectoris, claudication, congestive heart failure, recurrent arrhythmias, transient ischemic attacks, and aortic aneurysms are clinical manifestations of this accelerated vascular disease process.

The atherosclerosis prevalent in uremic diabetic patients has special anesthetic implications when considered in relation to the difficulties of blood pressure control discussed above. Uremic diabetic patients are at higher risk of myocardial ischemia than is the general population. Among the younger transplant patient population, hypertension, diabetes, uremia, and the associated accelerated atherogenic processes result in a greater incidence of perioperative myocardial infarction. Two explanations may be offered to explain why coexisting diabetes heightens the risk of myocardial ischemia and infarction. First, cardiologists and anesthesiologists may underestimate the severity of artherosclerosis present in these young patients, who often have severe *asymptomatic* coronary artery disease. Angina pectoris is absent because the coexistent autonomic neuropathy impairs impulse transmission in cardiac afferent pain nerve fibers. Second, control of blood pressure and other factors that affect myocardial oxygen supply-demand balance is especially difficult in this group.

Malignant ventricular arrythmias occur more commonly in diabetic renal failure patients. In fact, a significant incidence of premature ventricular contractions, ventricular tachycardia, and fibrillation have been reported during renal transplantation [12]. Provocative factors, such as hyperkalemia, hypo-

When such abnormal endocrine control mechanisms exist, even a small intravenous dose of potassium may result in severe hyperkalemia.

Hypokalemia may also be encountered in renal transplant candidates because of inadequate diet, excessive use of diuretics, potassium-losing nephropathy, or when renal tubular acidosis is present [42]. Chronic mild hypokalemia is generally well tolerated but can be exacerbated by hyperventilation, rapid correction of metabolic acidosis, infusion of potassium-free fluid, or the administration of insulin, glucose, or catecholamines. When severe hypokalemia develops (less than 2 mEq/L), impaired myocardial contractility, bradycardia, cardiac dysrhythmias, and hypotension usually ensue because of the unresponsiveness of the myocardium and smooth muscle to endogenous catecholamines [43]. Also, the well-known exaggerated response to nondepolarizing muscle relaxant can be expected [44].

Most patients with chronic renal failure have a well-compensated metabolic acidosis [45] that poses no particular problem during transplantation, except occasionally in children suffering renal tubular acidosis [45,46]. Often a serum bicarbonate level of 18 mEq/L and pH of 7.35 represent their uremic steady state of acid-base equilibrium [45]. It is generally unwise to attempt complete correction, which can provoke acute depression of serum potassium and calcium and precipitate serious cardiac arrhythmias, particularly when myocardial ischemia or failure are present.

D. Coagulation Defects

Hemostatic deficits may complicate the management of renal transplant recipients. Platelet plug formation is abnormal secondary to the effects of an extrinsic plasma factor and a decrease in platelet number [47]. Guanidine succinic acid (GSA) found in serum of uremic patients inhibits ADP-mediated platelet factor III release and diminishes platelet aggregation induced by ADP, epinephrine, and collagen. Plasma levels of GSA and platelet dysfunction are effectively corrected by hemodialysis [48,49]. Dialysis can also lower phenol and hydroxyphenol acids present in blood of uremic patients; these acids impair celite-induced platelet factor III activity

Other hemostatic defects not related to uremia may be seen in transplant recipients. For example, a residual heparin effect may follow hemodialysis and chronic antithrombotic therapy instituted to maintain the patency of dialysis shunts or fistulas. Although such coagulopathies are easily recognized and corrected, they occasionally are responsible for troublesome postoperative bleeding and re-exploration of the allograft. Appropriate preoperative hemostatic preparation will effectively forestall such complications.

E. Special Problems in Diabetics

Patients with renal failure due to diabetes are at increased anesthetic risk because of the intercurrent cardiovascular involvement detailed above and the metabolic disturbances that complicate their care.

The catabolic effects of anesthesia and surgery are magnified in diabetic uremic patients not only because of deficient insulin production but also because a sharp rise in other hormones, such as catecholamines, cortisol, somatotropin, and glucagon [51], occurs during and after surgery. These changes stimulate ketogenesis, gluconeogenesis, and glucogenolysis. This reaction resembles accelerated starvation, and its severity is related to the degree of stress imposed [52,53]. A further decrease of an already suppressed insulin release, caused during surgery by excessive catechol release (an α effect), as well as reduced peripheral action of insulin, cause hyperglycemia, accelerated lypolysis, increased free fatty acid blood levels, hepatic ketogenesis, and metabolic acidosis [54,55]. Such hyperglycemia is significant because its osmotic action draws fluid, potassium, and phosphate from the cells and causes intracellular sodium to increase substantially. In the absence of an adequate free water supply, this hyperglycemia can precipitate hyperosmolar nonketotic coma. Uremic and diabetic metabolic acidosis may aggravate hyperkalemia. These serious complications can be avoided by administering an adequate supply of glucose and insulin, by reducing surgical stress response with appropriate anesthesia, and by maintaining proper fluid and electrolyte balance.

The possibility of *hypoglycemia* during surgery in uremic patients should also be recognized. It has been known for some time that the dose of oral hypoglycemic agents must be reduced when renal failure is present because renal excretion of these drugs is decreased [56,57]. Insulin requirements in diabetics also tends to decline during renal failure [56,58] because kidney disposition of plasma insulin (39%) is reduced [59]. Since insulin metabolism may decrease by 50-75% in renal failure [58,59], insulin administration to renal failure patients may cause hypoglycemia [60,61]. Defective transfer of alanine (also present in renal failure) also may cause hypoglycemia [62]. Furthermore, since dialysis improves the metabolic response of uremic patients to insulin, it also can lead to significant hypoglycemia [63]. Normal insulin metabolism is usually restored 2-3 weeks after kidney transplantation [64].

It should be obvious from this review that insulin therapy must be carefully managed in uremic diabetics if serious metabolic disturbances are to be avoided. Frequent blood sugar measurements are essential to identify unpredictably accelerated responses. When dialysis is undertaken, correction of uremic insulin resistance must be anticipated and insulin requirements re-established carefully to avoid hypoglycemia.

low-output syndrome can the anesthesiologist properly anticipate and prepare for the intraoperative difficulties and potential anesthetic complications. For the purpose of this discussion, we will examine the conditions that lead to anesthetic complications, starting with the preparation of the patient for bypass and extending through the entire operation and into the postoperative period.

The prebypass period of the heart transplant operation (from the moment of induction of anesthesia until the patient is placed on total cardiopulmonary bypass) is the most treacherous part of the entire undertaking [79]. During this interval, an individual who is in terminal congestive heart failure must be anesthetized and subjected to sternotomy. Perfusion of vital organs, especially the kidneys, is constantly in jeopardy until extracorporeal can be established. The potential for catastrophic collapse in such highly vulnerable patients and the skills necessary to successfully circumvent the hazards are obvious. Early reports [69, 75-78] of the anesthetic management of heart transplant recipients identified that the commonest causes of systemic arterial hypotension during the prebypass period were myocardial depression or depression of central adrenergic outflow by anesthetic drugs. Other causes were cardiac arrhythmias resulting from gas exchange and electrolyte abnormalities, transient episodes of myocardial ischemia, and surgical manipulation of the heart. Arrhythmias that are usually well tolerated by the normal heart can cause a sudden profound depression of cardiac output in the severely diseased myocardium. The steep ventricular compliance curve upon which these failing hearts operate provides a very narrow range of elevated filling pressures and end-diastolic volumes within which to operate [83]. Thus, errors in blood volume management can precipitate acute cardiac decompensation before cardiopulmonary bypass is established.

Cardiovascular depression is the most common adverse event associated with anesthesia during the prebypass period. The resulting systemic hypotension worsens tissue perfusion and results in acute metabolic acidosis [84]. This acidosis, in turn, further exacerbates the myocardial depression. Renal dysfunction is the second most common problem of the prebypass period. Hypotension and low cardiac output compromise kidney function; glomerular hypoperfusion leads to oliguria and may result in complete renal shutdown. If these disturbances are not rapidly identified and corrected, profound cardiogenic shock ensues. Cardiopulmonary bypass must then be instituted quickly, under difficult conditions, particularly in those patients who have had previous cardiac surgery. The possibility that cardiopulmonary bypass cannot be instituted quickly enough in such circumstances should be seriously considered when planning the cardiac transplant procedure. If acute circulatory failure occurs before cardiopulmonary bypass is available, cerebral edema, renal dysfunction, pulmonary edema, hypoxemia, and severe metabolic acidosis usually follow and will largely negate any benefit of the transplant.

Thus, prevention of acute circulatory failure is the basic anesthetic objective during the prebypass period. This usually requires modification of what might be called "standard" principles of anesthetic management. It is well recognized that low-flow states seen in end-stage congestive heart failure significantly decrease both the dose requirements and the tolerance to anesthetic agents [85]. Proper depth of anesthesia at this time is not only desirable but may be critical in preventing circulatory deterioration. An inappropriately light level of anesthesia may lead to an undesirable adrenergic response and provoke pulmonary and systemic arterial vasoconstriction. Such widespread vasoconstriction increases right and left ventricular impedance to ejection and causes redistribution of blood from the periphery to the central circulation. Such an acute increase in preload, occurring in parallel with the elevated afterload, can result in acute cardiac failure [83]. The adverse effects of increased endogenous catecholamine release in congestive heart failure patients has been recognized recently [86]. Whether the adrenergic responses that follow anesthetic or surgical stimulation can be adequately modulated by doses of anesthetics sufficient only to suppress recall is an important question that has not yet been fully answered. Normally, to achieve depression of central adrenergic tone and to blunt the adrenergic response to surgical stimulation require anesthetic doses significantly greater than those required to provide amnesia and analgesia [87,88]. In patients with advanced cardiomyopathy, the dose of anesthetic that blocks adrenergic responses and depresses consciousness often causes serious myocardial depression so that a truly satisfactory level often cannot be reached without precipitating a circulatory crisis. Lack of any precise pharmacokinetic studies of anesthetics in such patients makes accurate prediction of the clinical responses to anesthetics impossible, and we are left with the necessity to proceed on the basis of experience.

Poor cerebral perfusion likely accounts for the lower anesthetic requirement of patients with advanced cardiac failure; poor myocardial contractility is the cause of their intolerance of anesthesia. This relationship between level of consciousness, myocardial contractility, and adrenergic drive at rest and during surgical stimulation largely determines what effects anesthesia will have upon the heart transplant recipient in the prebypass period. Therefore, induction agents must be given to heart transplant recipients only by careful titration since their effects customarily are delayed because of the patient's prolonged circulation time, and their autonomic and myocardial effects may be magnified. In short, the mode of administration is as important as the choice of anesthetic.

Another deviation from the standard induction technique is required because the heart transplant recipient is usually a potential aspiration risk. Customarily, heart recipients are called from a waiting list, and the logistics of organ donation precludes the usual preoperative fast. They also receive an oral dose of cyclosporine, which must remain in the stomach. Some patients have significant hepatomegaly, ascites, and abdominal distension, which increases intra-abdominal pressure; some are orthopneic and hypoxic and in significant respiratory distress. For these reasons, whenever possible we perform either a rapid sequence induction or an awake endotracheal intubation with the aid of topical anesthesia and a small dose of narcotic. This technique affords early control of pulmonary ventilation and permits the administration of positive end-expiratory pressure, which helps to improve gas exchange and decreases the work of breathing, tissue oxygen demand, and cardiac preload.

We believe it is necessary to begin invasive monitoring *before* the induction of anesthesia. We have frequently discovered these patients to be intensely vasoconstricted, due to a high resting level of adrenergic tone. Myocardial performance often can be substantially improved prior to induction of anesthesia by infusing vasodilators and inotropic agents to effectively manipulate myocardial load, heart rate, and contractility, thereby optimizing myocardial performance and tissue perfusion. The best opportunity to make such precise and beneficial adjustments is in the operating room immediately prior to commencing anesthesia. Furthermore, if subsequent administration of anesthetics adversely affects the preinduction hemodynamic profile, appropriate corrective measures can be applied on a rational and quantitative basis. Tolerance to anesthetics is thus improved, and the prebypass low cardiac output syndrome is forestalled.

Changes in pulmonary gas exchange secondary to congestive heart to failure are well known. Increased venocapillary pressure and interstitial edema reduce the gas exchange surface, cause early small airway closure, and foster alveolar collapse. The resultant decrease in functional residual capacity disturbs O_2 uptake and CO_2 removal. Abnormal regional and global V/Q ratios develop, and dead space is increased. Cardiopulmonary bypass also adversely effects pulmonary function by fostering interstitial lung edema and alveolar collapse. These lung changes due to heart failure and cardiopulmonary bypass not only affect pulmonary gas exchange but also increase pulmonary vascular resistance. The latter may adversely affect the function of the heart homograft [67]. Although pathologic changes in the pulmonary resistance vessels that existed prior to transplantation cannot be changed, every effort should be made to eliminate any intraoperative factors likely to cause pulmonary vasoconstriction. Interstitial pulmonary edema, low lung volume, alveolar collapse, low alveolar oxygen concentration, hypoxia, and metabolic or respiratory acidosis are such factors. By the use of high fractional inspired oxygen concentrations and vasodilator agents and by maintaining an alkaline blood pH and full lung re-expansion before and after cardiopulmonary bypass, it is possible to prevent further worsening of pulmonary vascular resistance. In patients with only mildly elevated pulmonary vascular resistance, mismanagement of its physiological determinants can result in poor performance of the transplanted right heart.

In this regard, it is widely believed that a light level of anesthesia facilitates termination of cardiopulmonary bypass by reducing the depressing effects of anesthetics on the transplanted heart. But "light" anesthesia after bypass may instead have deleterious effects on the heart homograft by fostering high levels of circulating catecholamines, which can cause both pulmonary and systemic vasoconstriction and an undesirable increase in impedance to ventricular ejection. Although there is agreement that the deliberate administration of catecholamines at α-agonist doses is not advisable after bypass [89], the undesirable vasoconstrictive effects of high levels of *endogenous* catecholamines due to inadequate anesthesia have not been as well appreciated.

The transplanted heart should be provided with the best possible conditions for its adequate performance when bypass is terminated. These conditions are met only when the grafted heart works against minimal pulmonary and systemic vascular impedance. This can be achieved by skillful pharmacological manipulation of those physiologic determinants discussed above.

Reversible renal dysfunction (prerenal azotemia) secondary to congestive heart failure is almost always present in heart transplant candidates. Several other processes combine to cause a high incidence of intra- and postoperative renal dysfunction after heart transplantation. Preoperative renal dysfunction, cardiopulmonary bypass, cyclosporine, and pre- and postoperative low cardiac output syndrome may all contribute to this effect. Dilutional hyponatremia and total body potassium depletion as a result of aggressive diuretic therapy are classic extracellular fluid abnormalities in end-stage congestive heart failure. They also can contribute to postoperative renal dysfunction.

Optimizing prebypass blood volume, myocardial performance, and renal perfusion pressure, shortening the cardiopulmonary bypass period, maintaining adequate posttransplant cardiac output and systemic pressure, and careful titration of cyclosporine with frequent measurements of the drug's blood level are at present the best means to prevent further deterioration of renal function. In our series, severe posttransplant renal dysfunction has been a good predictor of postoperative mortality. Maintenance of adequate urine output is an important objective during open cardiac surgery since it is an indicator of adequate tissue perfusion and helps to control fluid balance during bypass. Adequate urine output is best accomplished by optimizing myocardial performance and blood volume and by administering diuretics only after all else has been done to optimize renal blood flow.

Chronic hepatic congestion secondary to congestive heart failure, tricuspid insufficiency, severe systemic venous hypertension, poor nutrition or the administration of coumadin derivatives to combat thromboembolic disease all may cause significant preoperative hemostatic defects. Thrombocytopenia may also be present. Although surgery under these conditions should usually be avoided, the availability of a donor heart becomes an overriding reason to proceed. Significant blood loss may then occur during the prebypass period (particularly in previously operated patients) and require blood transfusion. Even under the best conditions, blood transfusion affects the brittle equilibrium of the failing heart, which has extreme sensitivity to the infusion of citrated blood products. Preoperative correction of this coagulopathy is difficult and risky. Patients in congestive heart failure tolerate poorly the volume expansion required to acutely correct the effects of chronic anticoagulation or hepatic dysfunction. The volume of fresh-frozen plasma required simply aggravates the congestive heart failure. An alternative approach is to delay correction of the coagulopathy until cardiopulmonary bypass is established. Then fresh-frozen plasma can be added to the pump oxygenator prime to assure that adequate concentrations of plasma coagulation factors will be present following cardiopulmonary bypass.

Weaning the transplanted heart recipient from cardiopulmonary bypass involves several important considerations. Factors that determine the ease of this important phase of the operation are (1) the adequacy of preservation of the graft and its reperfusion; (2) the status of the systemic and pulmonary circulations when the weaning process is begun; (3) the physical, chemical, and hematologic characteristics of the blood reperfusing the myocardium; (4) the peculiar characteristics of the denervated heart; (5) the depth of anesthesia; (6) the recovery from hypothermia; and (7) the gas exchange status. The interaction among these factors is complex and to some degree uncontrolled, but the anesthesiologist can influence several of them favorably. Although a detailed examination of this dynamic interaction is outside the limits of this discussion, we have determined that certain anesthetic practices interfere with successful weaning. As mentioned earlier, "light" anesthesia associated with significantly elevated levels of endogenous circulating catecholamines can cause intense pulmonary and systemic vasoconstriction that impairs the immediate performance of the graft. Intense systemic vasoconstriction induced by deep hypothermia during cardiopulmonary bypass alters tissue perfusion patterns and results in metabolic acidosis during rewarming. Metabolic acidosis is an important additional stimulus for catecholamine release and also has a direct negative inotropic effect. Graft performance also may be impaired if electrolyte abnormalities exist, such as low serum calcium. Pulmonary vascular resistance can be adversely affected by incomplete lung re-expansion, inadequate pulmonary ventilation, or the administration of protamine. It should also be remembered that the preservation of the ischemic graft and its reperfusion are critical factors that determine its ultimate function and that time spent reperfusing the graft while on bypass is an essential element that permits the graft to recover adequately before it is called upon to sustain the recipient's circulation. Rebuilding depleted myocardial energy stores, restoring transmembrane ionic gradients, and clearing cellular and interstitial myocardial acidosis are processes that require adequate myocardial reperfusion. Near ideal humoral, thermal, and hemodynamic conditions are necessary for adequate graft recovery from ischemia. Increased diastolic stiffness of an ischemic heart homograft requires higher filling pressures, which in turn adversely affects coronary perfusion pressure, causing further myocardial ischemia. Attempting to obtain better graft performance by increasing filling pressure alone leads to the premature expenditure of barely repleted energy stores and results in additional ischemic insult.

All other conditions being equal, the time spent thoroughly reperfusing the grafted myocardium is an important determinant of outcome. When an insufficiently reperfused graft is caused to eject against elevated systemic and pulmonary vascular resistances, not only will it promptly fail but ultimate full recovery from ischemia is impaired. If an attempt is made to shorten this reperfusion process by infusing inotropes, graft failure may ensue [89].

In our view, excessive systemic and pulmonary vasoconstriction and insufficient recovery from preservation ischemia are two formidable deterrents to resumption of adequate graft function, which, if it is not achieved, results in the low postoperative cardiac output syndrome. Isoproterenol has been recommended as the catecholamine of choice in heart transplantation because it causes vasodilation, both systemic and pulmonary, and at the same time increases heart rate by its action on the homograft's dysfunctional sinus node. However, isoproterenol causes wasteful use of myocardial energy stores. We prefer instead to use volume expansion and vasodilators to optimize myocardial loading and atrial pacing to optimize the heart rate. Extending the reperfusion time as the means to ensure full recovery from ischemia, and using β_1 agonists only if cardiac output is inadequate despite ideal heart rate and loading conditions, seems to us to be the most logical approach to successful weaning.

Most cardiac transplant patients can be extubated within 24 hr, by which time graft function is usually stable. Graft dysfunction, pulmonary edema, renal failure, and sepsis are the most common indications for prolonged tracheal intubation and respiratory support.

Postoperative sepsis is the most prominent cause of mortality among heart transplant recipients. Consequently, strict aseptic technique must be observed during every anesthetic invasive intervention must be observed in these nutritionally deficient, immunosuppressed heart transplant recipients.

III. LIVER TRANSPLANTATION

Liver transplantation has been attempted since 1963. However, it has not been until recently that satisfactory results have been obtained [3]. A better understanding of the pathophysiologic changes of end-stage hepatic failure and their anesthetic and

7. Morgan, M., and Lumley, J.: Anaesthetic considerations in chronic renal failure. Anaesth. Intensive Care 3(3):218-226, 1975.
8. Lowrie, E. G., Lazarus, J. M., Hampers, C. L., and Merrill, J. P.: Cardiovascular disease in dialysis patients. N. Engl. J. Med. 290(13):737-738, 1974.
9. Lindner, A., Charra, B., Sherrard, D. J., and Scribner, B. H.: Accelerated atherosclerosis in prolonged maintenance hemodialysis. N. Engl. J. Med. 290(13):697-701, 1974.
10. Rao, K. V.: Status of renal transplantation: A clinical perspective. Med. Clin. N. Am. 68(2):427-453, 1984.
11. Schoenfeld, P. Y., and Humphreys, M. H.: A general description of the uremic state. In: Brenner, B. M., and Rector, F. C., eds., The Kidney, Philadelphia: W. B. Saunders, 1976, pp. 1423-1447.
12. Aldrete, J. A., Daniel, W., O'Higgins, J. W., Homatas, J., and Starzl, T. E.: Analysis of anesthetic-related morbidity in human recipients of renal homografts. Anesth. Analg. 50(3):321-329, 1971.
13. Vertes, V., Cangiano, J. L., Berman, L. B., and Gould, A.: Hypertension in end-stage renal disease. N. Engl. J. Med. 280(18):978-981, 1969.
14. de Planque, B. A., Mulder, E., and Dorhout Mees, E. J.: The behavior of blood and extracellular volume in hypertensive patients with renal insufficiency. Acta Med. Scand. 186:75-81, 1969.
15. Bianchi, G., Ponticelli, C., Bardi, U., Redaelli, B., Campolo, L., et al.: Role of the kidney in salt and water dependent hypertension of end-stage renal disease. Clin. Sci. 42:47-55, 1972.
16. Lucas, J., and Floyer, M. A.: Body fluid distribution and pressure in experimental hypertension. Clin. Sci. 42:2P, 1972.
17. Dathan, J. R. E., and Goodwin, F. J.: The relationship between body fluid compartment volumes, renin and blood pressure in chronic renal failure. Clin. Sci. 42:2P, 1972.
18. James, J. E. A.: Aortic arch baroreceptor activity in experimental hypertensive rabbits. Clin. Sci. 42:2P, 1972.
19. Dustan, H. P., and Page, I. H.: Some factors in renal and renoprival hypertension. J. Lab. Clin. Med. 64(6):948-959, 1964.
20. Wilkinson, R., Scott, D. F., Uldall, P. R., Kerr, D. N. S., and Swinner, J.: Plasma renin and exchangeable sodium in the hypertension of chronic renal failure. Q. J. Med. 39(155):377-394, 1970.
21. Brown, J. J., Curtis, J. R., Lever, A. F., Robertson, J. I. S., de Wardener, H. E., and Wing, A. J.: Plasma renin concentration and the control of blood pressure in patients on maintenance haemodialysis. Nephron 6:329-349, 1969.
22. Verniory, A., Potvliege, P., Van Geertruyden, J., Vereerstraeten, P., Kinnaert, P., et al.: Renin and control of arterial blood pressure during terminal renal failure treated by haemodialysis and by transplantation. Clin. Sci. 42:685-700, 1972.
23. Stokes, G. S., Mani, M. K., and Steward, J. H.: Relevance of salt, water, and renin to hypertension in chronic renal failure. Br. Med. J. 3:126-129, 1970.

cellular and interstitial myocardial acidosis are processes that require adequate myocardial reperfusion. Near ideal humoral, thermal, and hemodynamic conditions are necessary for adequate graft recovery from ischemia. Increased diastolic stiffness of an ischemic heart homograft requires higher filling pressures, which in turn adversely affects coronary perfusion pressure, causing further myocardial ischemia. Attempting to obtain better graft performance by increasing filling pressure alone leads to the premature expenditure of barely repleted energy stores and results in additional ischemic insult.

All other conditions being equal, the time spent thoroughly reperfusing the grafted myocardium is an important determinant of outcome. When an insufficiently reperfused graft is caused to eject against elevated systemic and pulmonary vascular resistances, not only will it promptly fail but ultimate full recovery from ischemia is impaired. If an attempt is made to shorten this reperfusion process by infusing inotropes, graft failure may ensue [89].

In our view, excessive systemic and pulmonary vasoconstriction and insufficient recovery from preservation ischemia are two formidable deterrents to resumption of adequate graft function, which, if it is not achieved, results in the low postoperative cardiac output syndrome. Isoproterenol has been recommended as the catecholamine of choice in heart transplantation because it causes vasodilation, both systemic and pulmonary, and at the same time increases heart rate by its action on the homograft's dysfunctional sinus node. However, isoproterenol causes wasteful use of myocardial energy stores. We prefer instead to use volume expansion and vasodilators to optimize myocardial loading and atrial pacing to optimize the heart rate. Extending the reperfusion time as the means to ensure full recovery from ischemia, and using β_1 agonists only if cardiac output is inadequate despite ideal heart rate and loading conditions, seems to us to be the most logical approach to successful weaning.

Most cardiac transplant patients can be extubated within 24 hr, by which time graft function is usually stable. Graft dysfunction, pulmonary edema, renal failure, and sepsis are the most common indications for prolonged tracheal intubation and respiratory support.

Postoperative sepsis is the most prominent cause of mortality among heart transplant recipients. Consequently, strict aseptic technique must be observed during every anesthetic invasive intervention must be observed in these nutritionally deficient, immunosuppressed heart transplant recipients.

III. LIVER TRANSPLANTATION

Liver transplantation has been attempted since 1963. However, it has not been until recently that satisfactory results have been obtained [3]. A better understanding of the pathophysiologic changes of end-stage hepatic failure and their anesthetic and surgical implications [90,91], as well as improvements in organ preservation [3], the use of cyclosporine [91-93], and advances in anesthetic management [94-96] blood transfusion [97], and surgical techniques [98] all have contributed to better operative results and long-term survival. At present, the survival rate after 1 year exceeds 80% in adults and 60% in children [3]. Thus, liver transplantation is now considered conventional rather than experimental therapy. When we reviewed our experience in the anesthetic and intraoperative management of liver transplant recipients, 2 years ago, we did not expect that most of the problems identified could be overcome to such an extent within such a short time [94]. The most troublesome of these hazards and the means we use to control them will be discussed.

A. Airway Management

With a few exceptions, transplant patients at the University of Minnesota present as regurgitation and pulmonary aspiration risks. Recognizing the presence of increased intra-abdominal pressure due to hepatomegaly, ascites, and incomplete gastric emptying, we have successfully avoided this complication by systematic use of a rapid sequence induction technique and aggressive preoperative management for relief of the ascites. But the risk is real, since large volumes of gastric content are often recovered by tube drainage after the airway has been secured.

Other complications during hepatic transplantation arise as a sequel to three interacting processes: (1) massive blood loss, which this operation usually causes, and the methods employed to accomplish replacement; (2) the hemodynamic and renal effects provoked by clamping the inferior vena cava; and (3) the metabolic and thermal impact when the liver allograft is reperfused.

B. Massive Intraoperative Hemorrhage

Deficiency of plasma coagulation factors I, II, V, VII, IX, and X [101] secondary to hepatic parenchymal failure and thrombocytopenia due to hypersplenism [102]. can be expected in virtually all candidates for liver transplantation. In patients whose disease has progressed to severe hepatic failure, disseminated intravascular coagulation and secondary thrombolysis further impair coagulation mechanisms [103]. This compound hemostatic abnormality makes the control of bleeding doubly difficult during the removal of the diseased liver, particularly when organ and associated vascular structures (especially collateral venous networks) are encased in heavy scar tissue, as in patients previously subjected to palliative operations (e.g., the Kasai procedure). When liver removal is less tedious (e.g., in carcinoma or chronic hepatitis), blood loss is not likely to be so massive. Severe portal hypertension is often present in these patients as well and is another cause of heavy bleeding, since numerous fragile collateral veins must be divided in the course of the dissection.

In the face of these inherent bleeding hazards (coagulopathy and portal hypertension), even when precise and meticulous surgical technique is employed, massive loss of blood may be unavoidable. In our experience the consequences of extensive blood loss and its replacement are the primary factors responsible for morbidity and mortality in these patients. A spectrum of potential physiologic disturbances has been encountered as a result of the massive blood loss that accompanies liver transplantation.

An interaction occurs among the three factors described (coagulopathy, portal hypertension, and surgical technique) that almost guarantees that substantial blood loss will occur and that massive transfusion of stored bank blood will be required to sustain the patient. Massive transfusion can be expected to aggravate the pre-existing coagulopathy [104,105], fostering even more blood loss and setting up a malignant vicious circle. Blood loss during hepatic transplantation is reported at 500-2000 mL/kg of body weight [106,107]. Not only are large amounts of blood lost, but the *rate* of hemorrhage is very great also, which has direct implications as regards transfusion techniques (venous access, blood warming, methods of infusion, and so on) [105] that are critical in the safe management of these patients. Replacement of a patient's entire blood volume in minutes is not infrequent at certain points during this operation. As a result, all the well-known deleterious consequences of massive transfusion (hypothermia, hyperkalemia, hypocalcemia, coagulopathy, citrate toxicity, metabolic acidosis, and others) become additional pathogenic burdens that these very ill patients must bear in addition to ongoing hypovolemia and impaired tissue perfusion [108]. As hypothermia, metabolic acidosis, and hypocalcemia ensue, a cardiogenic component is added to the hypovolemic shock state, and soon thereafter a progressive lactic acidosis develops as tissue perfusion is impaired [108]. Such circulatory failure and metabolic acidosis stimulate the onset of or aggravate the ongoing consumption coagulopathy, and primary or secondary fibrinolysis complicates the bleeding diathesis.

Within this framework of thermal, hemodynamic, hematologic, and metabolic disturbance, it is perhaps not surprising that life-threatening hypotension, ventricular dysrhythmias, and cardiac arrest sometimes occur [95]. Even if resuscitation is successful in this circumstance, the negative impact of circulatory arrest upon various organ systems (renal, pulmonary, cardiac, and neurological) seriously compromises the transplant effort and reduces the likelihood of long-term patient survival.

Thus, extensive blood loss and the vagaries of massive transfusion are the most significant causes of perioperative morbidity and mortality among patients subjected to hepatic transplantation. Patients with severe liver failure are known to be more susceptible than normal patients to the effects of even moderate blood loss and its replacement [109]. These patients are chronically hypervolemic

[109,110]. Their increased blood volume results from a compensatory mechanism activated to maintain tissue perfusion. Blood loss of lesser magnitude than in normal subjects can provoke early deterioration of tissue perfusion [108]. Moreover, the diseased liver cannot effectively dispose of citrate, which is not metabolized at all during the anhepatic phase. Synthesis of clotting factors is seriously impaired, and the liver cannot effectively participate in acid-base control [111-113]. For these reasons, blood loss and replacement in patients with liver failure should be viewed as very hazardous. The eventual outcome in liver recipients depends to a great extent on how massive is the blood loss and how effective is the transfusion. It should also be kept in mind that the rate at which blood is lost is often a more decisive factor than is the volume lost. Rapid transfusion, although effective in combating hemorrhagic hypovolemia, nonetheless imposes several well-known hazards that must be offset if resuscitation is to be successful. Among those is the potentially serious impact of cold, acidic hyperkalemic stored blood, which is deficient in clotting factors and is loaded with citrate. Patients subjected to such a "toxic" load rapidly become cold, acidotic, hypocalcemic, and hyperkalemic, all of which adds a cardiogenic component to the hypovolemic shock syndrome already in progress. Depressed or absent hepatocellular function impairs normal disposition of the citrate, phosphate, and lactate of stored blood and fosters the development of progressive metabolic acidosis [108].

Additional brisk bleeding may also be encountered when the transplanted liver is revascularized (liver washout period). This is a particularly hazardous situation since further rapid transfusion simply adds to the detrimental metabolic and thermal conditions just cited.

What can be done to cope with these blood loss and replacement problems? There is little the anesthesiologist can do to offset the severe portal hypertension other than to urge the surgeon to perform a meticulous surgical dissection. The anesthesiologist can correct the existing hemostatic defects during the liver dissection by infusing an adequate volume of coagulation factors, platelets, and fibrinogen. A blood transfusion technique that has proved essential in countering the heavy bleeding without imposing the problems cited involves adjusting the chemical and thermal characteristics of stored bank blood to the extent that it can then be infused rapidly without cooling the patient and without worsening the metabolic state [97]. To accomplish this goal, the storage lesion of bank blood must be fully corrected by (1) washing the red cells to remove the excess potassium, (2) warming the blood to body temperature, (3) restoring deficient coagulation factors, and (4) optimizing O_2 carrying capacity. This is accomplished with a modified heater-oxygenator and rapid infusion device we have recently described [97]. Cryoprecipitate and platelets must also be simultaneously infused at a rate adequate to maintain a platelet count of at least 250,000 mL^{-1} and a fibrinogen level of 0.4 g per 100 mL [97].

Frequent monitoring of cardiac output, right atrial pressure, and pulmonary artery wedge pressures is essential to track the adequacy of transfusion under these conditions. These parameters must be maintained at the high postinduction levels to maintain adequate tissue perfusion throughout this massive and continuous exchange transfusion [108]. Finally, calcium must be continuously infused to assure a normal *ionized* serum calcium in the face of impending citrate intoxication [112,114,115].

By applying these management modalities (careful surgical dissection, correction of hemostatic defects, use of a rapid infusion device to deliver whatever blood replacement is required, correction of the storage lesion of bank blood *before* it is infused, use of invasive monitoring to guide blood and fluid replacement and to monitor tissue perfusion, and maintenance of a normal ionized calcium level), better control of blood loss and replacement can be achieved and the dangerous hemodynamic, metabolic, and hemostatic complications of massive hemorrhage can be avoided [97].

C. Management of Ventilation

Pulmonary gas exchange is usually not a significant intraoperative problem. However, positive end-expiratory pressure is necessary to restore and maintain functional residual capacity in the face of increased intra-abdominal pressure and retraction upon the diaphragm. We consider continuous monitoring of pulmonary artery wedge pressure essential in assessing the adequacy of left-heart filling and in avoiding circulatory overload. Pulmonary edema secondary to overtransfusion or myocardial dysfunction is the most frequent cause of intraoperative hypoxemia. Hypoxemia can be particularly severe in patients in whom significant intrapulmonary shunting [116] already exists because of cirrhosis, portal hypertension, or α_1-antitrypsin deficiency. Frequent analysis of arterial and venous O_2 tension, saturation, and content is essential in such circumstances to assure that tissue oxygen requirements are met. Hematocrit must also be maintained at about 30% to provide adequate oxygen carrying capacity while reducing intracapillary sludging.

D. Intravascular Volume Deficits

Because of the extensive dissection required in this operation in the presence of portal venous and lymphatic hypertension, third space and insensitive fluid losses are large. Unless aggressive replacement is undertaken early, serious hypovolemia results. To forestall this insidious complication, we have found it necessary to infuse about 10 mL/kg per hour each of potassium-free balanced salt solution and colloid. The latter is given usually in the form of fresh-frozen plasma, platelet, and cryoprecipitate infusions, which are also required to restore hemostatic reserve. The tendency of this rather massive fluid administration to cause transient hemodilution (hematocrit <30), particularly in children, is offset by inducing a simultaneous brisk diuresis with furosemide. The diuresis also serves to reduce the sodium, potassium, calcium, and citrate overload that can be expected during massive transfusion. The objective of this diuresis is to maintain O_2 carrying capacity and the highest concentration of coagulation factors and to avoid dilution as a cause of coagulopathy.

E. Electrolyte Disturbances

Hypernatremia resulting from the high sodium content of the citrated blood infused and the sodium bicarbonate administered to treat metabolic acidosis, and the associated serum hyperosmolarity it produces, can cause serious postoperative neurological dysfunction (obtundation and seizures). Consequently, it is important to exercise restraint in the use of sodium bicarbonate to correct acid-base imbalance. Rather, the basic cause of metabolic acidosis (poor tissue perfusion) should be corrected by restoring blood volume, cardiac output, and oxygen carrying capacity.

Hyperkalemia has been reported as an almost invariable complication of liver transplantation [95,111]. Since metabolic acidosis (resulting from hemodynamic unstability and poor tissue perfusion) and significant renal dysfunction (secondary to inferior vena cava clamping) often complicate the picture during hepatic transplantation, it is not surprising that hyperkalemia results. Thus, exogenous (blood transfusion) and endogenous (from the transplanted liver) potassium loads are imposed in the presence of impaired K^+ disposal mechanisms (metabolic acidosis, insulin resistance from the anhepatic state, renal dysfunction, and preoperative therapy with aldosterone inhibitors). It is perhaps fortunate that liver recipients usually are chronically depleted of potassium as a result of secondary hyperaldosteronism [117,118] and aggressive diuretic therapy for ascites. Still, the sudden, unpredictable rates at which potassium levels change during rapid blood transfusion and implantation of the new liver impose a significant hazard even in potassium-depleted patients. We prevent this dangerous hyperkalemia by transfusing only normokalemic blood during the operation; thus no exogenous K^+ load is imposed. We also prevent metabolid acidosis and, in fact, strive to induce a mild alkalotic state by hyperventilation to foster the uptake of potassium by tissues. We also stimulate renal excretion of potassium with diuretics. The timely administration of calcium chloride also effectively offsets the cardiotoxic effect of potassium. Although this approach reduces the hazard of intraoperative hyperkalemia, it also results in a marked postoperative hypokalemia that must be corrected by controlled continuous infusion of potassium chloride after revascularization of the liver is completed and during the postoperative period [153].

In normal patients, hepatic citrate disposal mechanisms are sufficient to handle the large amount of citrate administered during a rapid blood transfusion. However, when liver failure is present, citrate "toxicity" is more likely to occur, especially if the rate of transfusion is high [112]. As a result, both total and ionized serum hypocalcemia develop during liver transplantation [96]. A transient but significant decrease in ionized serum calcium occurs so predictably during massive blood transfusion that we administer calcium generously during the operation. We have found that surprisingly large doses of calcium are required to maintain a normal ionized serum calcium; this frequently results in a high level of total serum calcium (15-20 mg per 100 mL). We have not observed any ill effects from this hypercalcemia. But if *ionized* serum calcium is allowed to fall during massive transfusion, serious cardiovascular depression soon appears. Citrate overload also fosters postoperative metabolic alkalosis. This alkalosis is aggravated by the postoperative potassium deficit and often requires aggressive therapy [119].

Although early experience [120] suggested that hypoglycemia may develop before and during the anhepatic phase of the operation, we have not seen this complication. On the contrary, severe *hyperglycemia* has developed on occasion. It results from the administration of glucose in crystalloid infusions and in transfused blood and because of the glucose intolerance and insulin resistance characteristic of the anhepatic phase. The consequence of such hyperglycemia is serum hyperosmolarity, especially if serum sodium is also increased, which can result in postoperative obtundation and coma [121].

F. Interruption of Portal and Inferior Vena Cava Blood Flow and Subsequent Revascularization

Another critical event that fosters intraoperative complications is the interruption of inferior vena cava blood flow [98,101]. Clamping the hepatic artery and portal vein produces very little hemodynamic disturbance, but when the inferior vena cava is interrupted, there is immediate reduction of venous return to the heart. Although the hepatic failure patient often has substantial porta caval and splanchnic collateral flow, it is usually not sufficient to compensate for this very significant decrease in venous return. The result is a sudden, sometimes drastic reduction in cardiac output and secondary intense reflex systemic vasoconstriction, a compensatory mechanism to maintain blood pressure. Unless blood loss has been adequately replaced, the arterial hypotension may be so severe that cardiac arrest ensues. It is thus very important that blood loss has been fully replaced before the inferior vena cava is clamped. Low blood pressure and the intense reflex arterial and renal vasoconstriction it provokes are two factors that reduce renal blood flow and urine output during this phase of the operation. A simultaneous rise in caval pressure below the infrahepatic clamp also impedes renal blood flow and urine output; pressure in the inferior vena cava sometimes reaches 60-80 torr. This caval hypertension, coupled with the low mean aortic pressure and the intense reflex renal vasoconstriction, markedly reduces renal perfusion pressure, produces renal ischemia, and reduces urine formation. Such ischemia, inflicted upon kidneys already compromised by chronic hepatic failure [122], is especially undesirable at a time when a large water, sodium, potassium, calcium, and citrate load must be accommodated. Oliguria is particularly undesirable during reperfusion of the transplanted liver, when potassium is washed into the general circulation (see above). Some workers have overcome these deleterious effects of inferior vena cave clamping by shunting caval blood to the axillary vein [123]. We have chosen to manage the problem by maintaining left-heart filling pressure, cardiac output, and blood pressure at levels equal to or higher than preclamp values. The importance of having Swan-Ganz catheter data during this situation is obvious. If the mean aortic pressure is maintained about 50-70 torr above the mean inferior vena caval pressure, urine output is usually well maintained. If inferior vena cava pressure exceeds 50 torr, we transiently unclamp the inferior vena cava and "bleed off" the pressure to 20 torr or less. By this means we have been able to maintain adequate renal function during inferior vena cava clamping without using a shunt.

Another significant event that may cause complications is the sequential vascular unclamping and reperfusion of the transplanted liver. Revascularization is begun once the portal and suprahepatic caval anastomoses are complete and when the infrahepatic cava suture line is partially completed. By opening the portal vein clamp and keeping both the suprahepatic and infrahepatic caval clamps in place, portal blood flow is re-established through the liver and into the inferior vena cava, where it leaks out through the incomplete infrahepatic caval suture line. This serves to "flush out" the hepatic preservation fluid mixture, which has a dangerously high K^+ content [111]. This technique results in significant additional blood loss. The rapid infusion device plays an important role here, for it permits us to transfuse rapidly (1-3 L/min) and precisely with a blood infusate of normal temperature and composition guided by hemodynamic data [97]. Hypovolemia and the undesirable consequences of massive rapid transfusion are thus effectively avoided.

The next hazardous step in the revascularization sequence is completion of the infrahepatic inferior vena cava anastomosis and gradual unclamping of suprahepatic inferior vena cava while the infrahepatic caval clamp remains in place. This permits cold, acidic, and hyperkalemic blood to pass rapidly from the liver to the heart and systemic circulation [111]. This results in a transient, dangerous elevation of serum potassium and a fall in body temperature. Since we have adopted the plan to maintain a modest deficit of serum potassium, we no longer see the life-threatening hyperkalemia that previously occurred at this juncture. Furthermore, the minor fall in core temperature ($<1°C$) is physiologically insignificant if the patient has previously been maintained normothermic. During this final portion of the revascularization, sodium bicarbonate is infused to compensate for the sudden acid load and calcium chloride is given to maintain a normal potassium-calcium ratio and to prevent cardiac arrythmias. Since air embolization [124] is possible at this point we routinely monitor end-tidal CO_2 and continuously observe pulmonary arterial pressures for several minutes after full revascularization. We know of only one instance in our series when air embolism occurred.

The final step in the revascularization process is the unclamping of the infrahepatic inferior vena cava (IVC) which allows the large mass of blood trapped in the lower limbs and renal bed to return to the central circulation [98]. This blood is also acidic and slightly hyperkalemic. If the recipient's hemodynamic status and acid-base balance has been maintained, no deleterious effects follow IVC unclamping; instead, full restoration of venous return improved cardiac output and systemic tissue perfusion. Sodium bicarbonate administration usually is not necessary at this point; the transient mild metabolic acidosis that results as full caval flow resumes is adequately corrected by normal buffer mechanisms. While the inferior vena cava was clamped, blood volume was expanded to maintain cardiac output and blood pressure; it is therefore not uncommon when the inferior vena cava clamps are removed to observe an increase in cardiac filling pressures, reflecting a hypervolemic state. Cardiac output and filling pressures are measured, and if significant hypervolemia is present, phlebotomy is used to correct the relative overload and to prevent pulmonary congestion and edema.

A disorder of coagulation following reperfusion of the new liver has been observed by us and others [113,124]. Reperfusion of previously ischemic tissue may initiate disseminated intravascular coagulation as activated clotting factors and plasmin are released from the ischemic liver. If this release occurs in a patient already depleted of plasma clotting factors and platelets, a significant coagulopathy may be precipitated, the correction of which will require several exchange transfusions. However, if the patient has an adequate hemostatic reserve before the transplanted liver is reperfused, and if the intrahepatic clotting and lysis process is prevented by heparinizing the preservation fluid, disseminated intravascular coagulation can be avoided. Since we have employed those precautions, the only clotting defect we have observed following reperfusion of the liver is a mild prolongation of the thrombin time due to the presence of residual heparin in the circulation. This is easily corrected by protamine infusion.

As mentioned previously, increased intra-abdominal pressure and difficulties in lung ventilation often arise, especially in children, as the abdomen is closed. This is due to (1) passive congestion of the liver, (2) edematous, distended bowel, and (3) ongoing accumulation of blood in the abdomen because of hemostatic deficit or residual portal hypertension. Adequate nasogastric suction to decompress the gastrointestinal tract, avoidance of nitrous oxide, and skillful management of hemostasis and intravascular volume have effectively eliminated most of the factors that cause the "tight abdomen" and impair chest and lung mechanics.

When liver transplant recipients are managed to maintain adequate tissue perfusion and oxygenation and adequate hemostasis, and when a properly preserved liver is implanted skillfully, few serious postoperative problems are seen. Metabolic alkalosis, hypokalemia, systemic hypertension, mild hypernatremia, and hyperosmolarity are the most commonly observed postoperative consequences of our intraoperative management. Conservation of renal function during the operation and its maintenance in the postoperative period obviously is the key to resolving most of these abnormalities. Adult patients usually have only minimal postoperative pulmonary dysfunction and can be extubated within 24-48 hr. Children may require more prolonged ventilatory assistance, although as more precise intraoperative management has occurred, this need has been significantly reduced. Other postoperative problems, related to compromised hepatic circulation (portal vein or hepatic artery thrombosis), are cholangitis, biliary tract obstruction, and renal dysfunction secondary to cyclosporine [118]. Acute posttransplantation hepatic failure may result from poor donor selection, inadequate liver preservation, poor or failed revascularization of the liver, or transplantation into a poorly sustained recipient; these complications are, for the most part, preventable and are seen less frequently as preparation and support techniques of both donor and recipient improve.

IV. PANCREAS TRANSPLANTATION

Among all the transplant surgical interventions at present pursued, pancreas transplantation presents the fewest problems of intraoperative anesthetic management. In fact, intraoperative anesthetic morbidity and mortality during pancreas transplantation does not appear to be different from that encountered in type I diabetic patients undergoing any other intra-abdominal procedure.

Current opinion states that almost all type I diabetic patients ultimately develop microvascular changes secondary to the derangement of carbohydrate metabolism that characterizes diabetes mellitus. Most of these individuals would benefit from a functional pancreas transplantation, which would normalize their carbohydrate metabolism.

Type I diabetic patients should become transplant candidates at an early stage of their disease, before microvascular changes are fully developed. Such patients do not have significant cardiovascular involvement, so that the risk of anesthesia and surgery are reduced. The anesthetic management of such patients should follow the general principles already established, and the reader is referred to the previous reports on this subject [126-128].

There are no significant special considerations related to the effects of various anesthetics on the transplanted pancreas, and no systematic studies are yet available on this issue. Our experience suggests that the impact of anesthetics on the transplanted pancreas is not different than in the normal intact organ, although in vitro studies have demonstrated the inhibition of insulin secretion by halothane [129,130]. At this time we employ a variety of anesthetic agents and techniques for pancreas transplantation, and it does not appear that any specific problems have been provoked by their use, such as graft dysfunction.

Intraoperative blood sugar management is probably more important than any particular anesthetic method [126,127]. Very "tight" blood sugar control by means of continuous infusion of glucose and insulin is the approach we use. We titrate the infusions to keep the blood sugar between 80 and 120 mg per 100 mL throughout the operation and in the immediate postoperative period [131]. We have seen neither significant hypoglycemia nor hyperglycemia, nor have any hyperosmolar syndromes occurred with this tight control of blood sugar. Pancreas transplantation is thus associated with no significantly greater anesthetic risk or intraoperative problems than those expected during the management of any patient impaired by diabetes mellitus. We have, however, frequently observed the development of hypocalcemia following pancreas transplantation. The uptake of calcium by the ischemic, reperfused graft is the most logical explanation for this event. We have occasionally seen postoperative hypokalemia, which is a known side effect of the continuous insulin-dextrose infusion technique [126,127].

ACKNOWLEDGMENT

The authors acknowledge with gratitude the technical assistance of Nadine Hanson and Taunya Laurion in the preparation of this manuscript.

REFERENCES

1. Monaco, A. P.: Clinical kidney transplantation in 1984. Transplant. Proc. 17(1):5-12, 1985.
2. Jamieson, S. W.: Heart and lung: Recent developments in heart-lung transplantation. Transplant. Proc. 17(1):199-203, 1985.
3. Starzl, R. E., Iwatsuki, S., Shaw, B. W., Jr., and Gordon, R. D.: Liver: Orthotopic liver transplantation in 1984. Transplant. Proc. 17(1):250-258, 1985.
4. Groth, C. G.: Pancreas: Clinical pancreatic transplantation. Transplant. Proc. 17(1):302-306, 1985.
5. Muller, M. C.: Anesthesia for the patient with renal dysfunction. Int. Anesthesiol. Clin. 22:169-187, 1984.
6. Strunin, L., Davies, J. M., and Filshie, J. J.: Anesthesia for renal transplantation. Int. Anesthesiol. Clin. 22:189-202, 1984.

7. Morgan, M., and Lumley, J.: Anaesthetic considerations in chronic renal failure. Anaesth. Intensive Care 3(3):218-226, 1975.
8. Lowrie, E. G., Lazarus, J. M., Hampers, C. L., and Merrill, J. P.: Cardiovascular disease in dialysis patients. N. Engl. J. Med. 290(13):737-738, 1974.
9. Lindner, A., Charra, B., Sherrard, D. J., and Scribner, B. H.: Accelerated atherosclerosis in prolonged maintenance hemodialysis. N. Engl. J. Med. 290(13):697-701, 1974.
10. Rao, K. V.: Status of renal transplantation: A clinical perspective. Med. Clin. N. Am. 68(2):427-453, 1984.
11. Schoenfeld, P. Y., and Humphreys, M. H.: A general description of the uremic state. In: Brenner, B. M., and Rector, F. C., eds., The Kidney, Philadelphia: W. B. Saunders, 1976, pp. 1423-1447.
12. Aldrete, J. A., Daniel, W., O'Higgins, J. W., Homatas, J., and Starzl, T. E.: Analysis of anesthetic-related morbidity in human recipients of renal homografts. Anesth. Analg. 50(3):321-329, 1971.
13. Vertes, V., Cangiano, J. L., Berman, L. B., and Gould, A.: Hypertension in end-stage renal disease. N. Engl. J. Med. 280(18):978-981, 1969.
14. de Planque, B. A., Mulder, E., and Dorhout Mees, E. J.: The behavior of blood and extracellular volume in hypertensive patients with renal insufficiency. Acta Med. Scand. 186:75-81, 1969.
15. Bianchi, G., Ponticelli, C., Bardi, U., Redaelli, B., Campolo, L., et al.: Role of the kidney in salt and water dependent hypertension of end-stage renal disease. Clin. Sci. 42:47-55, 1972.
16. Lucas, J., and Floyer, M. A.: Body fluid distribution and pressure in experimental hypertension. Clin. Sci. 42:2P, 1972.
17. Dathan, J. R. E., and Goodwin, F. J.: The relationship between body fluid compartment volumes, renin and blood pressure in chronic renal failure. Clin. Sci. 42:2P, 1972.
18. James, J. E. A.: Aortic arch baroreceptor activity in experimental hypertensive rabbits. Clin. Sci. 42:2P, 1972.
19. Dustan, H. P., and Page, I. H.: Some factors in renal and renoprival hypertension. J. Lab. Clin. Med. 64(6):948-959, 1964.
20. Wilkinson, R., Scott, D. F., Uldall, P. R., Kerr, D. N. S., and Swinner, J.: Plasma renin and exchangeable sodium in the hypertension of chronic renal failure. Q. J. Med. 39(155):377-394, 1970.
21. Brown, J. J., Curtis, J. R., Lever, A. F., Robertson, J. I. S., de Wardener, H. E., and Wing, A. J.: Plasma renin concentration and the control of blood pressure in patients on maintenance haemodialysis. Nephron 6:329-349, 1969.
22. Verniory, A., Potvliege, P., Van Geertruyden, J., Vereerstraeten, P., Kinnaert, P., et al.: Renin and control of arterial blood pressure during terminal renal failure treated by haemodialysis and by transplantation. Clin. Sci. 42:685-700, 1972.
23. Stokes, G. S., Mani, M. K., and Steward, J. H.: Relevance of salt, water, and renin to hypertension in chronic renal failure. Br. Med. J. 3:126-129, 1970.

24. Chrysanthakopouls, S. G., Kastagir, B. K., Jubis, W., and Kolff, W. J.: Hypertension in patients on maintenance hemodialysis: Evaluation of peripheral renin activity and bilateral nephrectomy. Am. J. Med. Sci. 264(1): 9-21, 1972.
25. Donohue, J. P., Bohnert, W. W., Shires, D. L., and Bradley, K. P.: Bilateral nephrectomy: Its role in management of the malignant hypertension of end-stage renal disease. J. Urol. 106:488-491, 1971.
26. Schiff, M., Jr., Brown, R. S., and Lytton, B.: The role of bilateral nephrectomy in the treatment of hypertension of chronic renal failure. J. Urol. 109: 152-155, 1973.
27. Hennessy, W. J., and Siemsen, A. W.: Autonomic neuropathy in chronic renal failure. Clin. Res. 16:385, 1968.
28. Goldberger, S., Thompson, A., Guhal, A., Kramer, N., and Parrish, A.: Autonomic nervous dysfunction in chronic renal failure. Clin. Res. 19:531, 1971.
29. Prys-Roberts, C., Greene, L. T., Meloche, R., and Foex, P.: Studies of anaesthesia in relation to hypertension. II. Haemodynamic consequences of induction and endotracheal intubation. Br. J. Anaesth. 43:531-546, 1971.
30. Fouad, F. M., Estafanous, F. G., and Tarazi, R. C.: Hemodynamics of post-myocardial revascularization hypertension. Am. J. Cardiol. 41:564-569, 1978.
31. Bruce, D. L., Croley, T. F., and Lee, J. S.: Preoperative clonidine withdrawal syndrome. Anesthesiology 51:90-92, 1979.
32. Maling, T. J. B., and Dollery, C. T.: Changes in blood pressure, heart rate, and plasma noradrenaline concentration after sudden withdrawal of propranolol. Br. Med. J. 366-367, August 1979.
33. Bagdade, J. D.: Uremic lipemia: An unrecognized abnormality in triglyceride production and removal. Arch. Intern. Med. 126:875, 1970.
34. Gibson, D. G.: Haemodynamic factors in the development of acute pulmonary edema in renal failure. Lancet (December) 3:1217-1220, 1966.
35. del Greco, F., Simon, N. M., Roguska, J., and Walker, D.: Hemodynamic studies in chronic uremia. Circulation 40:87-95, 1969.
36. Miller, R. D., Way, W. L., Hamilton, W. K., and Layzer, R. B.: Succinylcholine-induced hyperkalemia in patients with renal failure? Anesthesiology 36(2): 138-141, 1972.
37. Brown, M. J.: Hypokalemia from $beta_2$-receptor stimulation by circulating epinephrine. Am. J. Cardiol. 56:3D-9D, 1985.
38. Gonick, H. C., Kleeman, C. R., Rubini, M. E., and Maxwell, M. H.: Functional impairment in chronic renal disease. III. Studies of potassium excretion. Am. J. Med. Sci. 261(5):281-290, 1971.
39. Hiatt, N., Davidson, M. B., and Bonorris, G.: The effect of potassium chloride infusion on insulin secretion in vivo. Horm. Metab. Res. 4:64-68, 1972.
40. Santeusanio, F., Faloona, R., Knochel, J. P., and Unger, R. H.: Evidence for a role of endogenous insulin and glucagon in the regulation of potassium homeostasis. J. Lab. Clin. Med. 81(6):809-817, 1973.
41. Gerstein, A. R., Kleeman, C. R., Gold, E. M., Franklin, S. S., Maxwell, M. H.,

et al.: Aldosterone deficiency in chronic renal failure. Nephron 5:90-105, 1968.
42. Knochel, J. P., and Seldin, D. W.: The pathophysiology of uremia. In: Brenner, B. M., and Rector, F. E., eds., The Kidney, Philadelphia: W. B. Saunders, 1976, pp. 1448-1485.
43. Knochel, P. J.: Diruetic induced hypokalemia. Am. J. Med. 77(5A):18-27, 1984.
44. Feldman, S. A.: Effect of changes in electrolytes, hydration and pH upon the reactions to muscle relaxants. Br. J. Anaesth. 35:546-551, 1963.
45. Relman, A. S.: Renal acidosis and renal excretion of acid in health and disease. Adv. Intern. Med. 12:295-347, 1964.
46. Walser, M.: The conservative management of the uremic patient. In: Brenner, B. M., and Rector, F. C., eds., The Kidney, Philadelphia: W. B. Saunders, 1976, pp. 1613-1642.
47. Harker, L. A., and Slichter, S. J.: The bleeding time as a screening test for evaluation of platelet function. N. Engl. J. Med. 287(4):155-159, 1972.
48. Horowitz, H. I., Cohen, B. D., Martinez, P., and Papayoanou, M. F.: Defective ADP-induced platelet factor 3 activation in uremia. Blood 30(3): 331-340, 1967.
49. Horowitz, H. I., and Papayoanou, M. F.: Activation of platelet factor 3 by adenosine 5′diphosphate. Thromb. Dieth. Hoenonh. 19:18-28, 1968.
50. Rabiner, S. F., and Hrodek, O.: Platelet factor 3 in normal subjects and patients with renal failure. J. Clin. Invest. 47:901-912, 1968.
51. Russell, R. C. G., Walker, C. J., and Bloom, S. R.: Hyperglucagonaemia in the surgical patient. Br. Med. J. 1:10-12, 1975.
52. Allison, S. P., Tomlin, P. J., and Chamberlain, M. J.: Some effects of anaesthesia and surgery on carbohydrate and fat metabolism. Br. J. Anaesth. 41: 588-593, 1969.
53. Clowes, H. A., O'Donnel, T. F., Blackburn, G. L., and Maki, T. N.: Energy metabolism and proteolysis in traumatized and septic man. Surg. Clin. N. Am. 56(5):1169-1184, 1976.
54. Giddings, A. E. B., O'Connor, K. J., Rowlands, B. J., Mangnall, D., and Clark, R. G.: The relationship of plasma glucagon to the hyperglycaemia and hyperinsulinaemia of surgical operation. Br. J. Surg. 63:612-616, 1976.
55. Schwartz, S. S., Horwitz, D. L., Zehfus, B., Langer, B., Moossa, A. R., et al.: Use of a glucose controlled insulin infusion system (artificial beta cell) to control diabetes during surgery. Diabetologia 16:157-164, 1979.
56. Balodimos, M. C.: Diabetic nephropathy. In: Marbel, A., White, P., Bradley, R. F., and Kroll, L. P., eds., Joslin's Diabetes Mellitus, Philadelphia: Lea & Febiger, 1971, pp. 526-561.
57. Cushman, P., Jr., Dubois, J. J., and Dwyer, E.: Protracted tolbutamide hypoglycemia. Am. J. Med. 35:196-204, 1963.
58. Reaven, G. M., Weisinger, J. R., and Swenson, R. S.: Insulin and glucose metabolism in renal insufficiency. Kidney Int. 6(S1):S63-S69, 1974.
59. Rabkin, R., Simon, N. M., Steiner, S., and Colwell, J. A.: Effect of renal

disease on renal uptake and excretion of insulin in man. N. Engl. J. Med. 282(4):182-187, 1970.
60. O'Brien, J. P., and Sharpe, A. R., Jr.: The influence of renal disease on the insulin I^{131} disappearance curve in man. Metabolism 16(1):76-83, 1976.
61. Zubroid, C. G., Evorsole, S. I., and Dana, G. W.: Amelioration of diabetes and striking rarity of acidosis in patients with Kimmelsteil-Wilson lesions. N. Engl. J. Med. 245(14):518-525, 1951.
62. Garber, A. J., Bier, D. M., Cryer, P. E., and Pagliara, A. S.: Hypoglycemia in compensated chronic renal insufficiency. Diabetes 23(12):982-986, 1974.
63. Alfrey, A. C., Sussman, K. E., and Holmes, J. H.: Changes in glucose and insulin metabolism induced by dialysis in patients with chronic uremia. Metabolism 16(8):733-740, 1967.
64. Fuss, M., Bergans, A., Brauman, H., Toussaint, C., Vereerstraeten, P., et al.: ^{125}I-insulin metabolism in chronic renal failure treated by renal transplantation. Kidney Int. 5:372-377, 1974.
65. Dzurik, R., and Krajci-Lazary, B.: The effect of uremic serum on carbohydrate metabolism in rat diaphragm. Experientia 23:798-799, 1967.
66. Bilbrey, G. L., Faloona, G. R., White, M. G., and Knochel, J. P.: Hyperglucagonemia of renal failure. J. Clin. Invest. 53:841-847, 1974.
67. Rider, A. K., et al.: The status of cardiac transplantation, 1975. Circulation 52:531-539, 1975.
68. Pennock, H. K. M., Retuz, B. A., Bieber, C. P., and Stinson, E. B.: Cardiac transplantation in perspective for the future. J. Thorac. Cardiovasc. Surg. 83:168-177, 1982.
69. Garman, J. K: Anesthesia for cardiac transplantation. Clevel. Clin. Q. 48(1):142-146, 1981.
70. Estrin, J. A., and Buckley, J. J.: Anesthetic management during cardiac transplantation. In: Simmons, R. L., Finch, M. E., Ascher, N. L., and Najarian, J. S., eds., Manual of Vascular Access, Organ Donation, and Transplantation, New York: Springer Verlag, pp. 232-236, 1984.
71. Stinson, E. B., Dong, E., Jr., Iben, A. B., and Shumway, N. E.: Cardiac transplantation in man. III. Surgical aspects. Am. J. Surg. 118:182-187, 1969.
72. Lower, R. R., Stofer, R. C., Hurley, E. J., Dong, E., Fr., Cohn, R. B., and Shumway, N. E.: Successful homotransplantation of the canine heart after anoxic preservation for seven hours. Am. J. Surg. 104:302-306, 1962.
73. Watson, D. C., Reitz, B. A., Baumgartner, W. A., Raney, A. A., et al.: Distant heart procurement for transplantation. Surgery 86(1):56-59, 1979.
74. Oyer, P. H., Stinson, E. B., Jamieson, S. W., Hunt, S., et al.: One year experience with cyclosporin A in clinical heart transplantation. Heart Transplant. 1(4):285-290, 1982.
75. Ozinsky, J.: Cardiac transplantation—the anaesthetist's view: A case report. S. Afr. Med. J. 41:1268, 1967.
76. Keats, A. S., Strong, M. J., Girgis, K. Z., and Goldstein, A., Jr.: Observa-

tions during anesthesia for cardiac homotransplantation in ten patients. Anesthesiology 30:192, 1969.
77. Plaiement, B., Wielhorski, W. A., Grondin, P., Lepage, G., and Drrda, I.: Anesthetic management in nine heart transplantations. Laval Med. 41:186, 1970.
78. Fernando, N. A., Keena, R. L., and Boyan, C. P.: Anesthetic experience with cardiac transplantation. J. Thorac. Cardiovasc. Surg. 75:531, 1978.
79. Cohn, J. N.: Treatment of heart failure in perspective: An overview. In: Cohn, J. H., ed., Drug treatment of heart failure, New York: Yorke Medical Books, 1983, pp. 1-12.
80. NcKee, P. A., Castelli, W. P., McNamara, P. M., and Kannel, W. B.: The natural history of congestive heart failure: The Framingham study. N. Engl. J. Med. 245(26):1441-1446, 1971.
81. Cohn, J. N.: Vasodilator therapy for heart failure: The influence of impedance on left ventricular performance. Circulation 48:5-8, 1973.
82. Liang, C. S., Sherman, L. G., Doherty, J. U., Wellington, K., Lee, V. W. and Hood, W. B., Jr.: Sustained improvement of cardiac function in patients with congestive heart failure after short-term infusion of dobutamine. Circulation 69(1):113-119, 1984.
83. Parmley, W. W.: Pathophysiology of congestive heart failure. Am. J. Cardiol. 56:7A-11A, 1985.
84. Fulop, M., Horowitz, M., Aberman, A., and Jaffe, E. R.: Lactic acidosis in pulmonary edema due to left ventricular failure. Ann. Intern. Med. 79:180-186, 1973.
85. Kemmotsu, O., Hashimoto, Y., and Shimosata, S.: The effects of fluroxene and enflurane on contractile performance of isolated papillary muscles from failing hearts. Anesthesiology 40(3):252-260, 1974.
86. Francis, G. S., Goldsmith, S. R., and Cohn, J. N.: Relationship of exercise capacity to left ventricular performance and basal plasma norepinephrine levels in patients with congestive heart failure. Am. Heart J. 104:725-731, 1982.
87. Murphy, M. R., and Hug, C. C., Jr.: The anesthetic potency of fentanyl in terms of its reduction of enflurane MAC. Anesthesiology 57:485:488, 1982.
88. Sprigge, J. S., Wynands, J. E., Whalley, D. G., Bevan, D. R., Townsend, G. E., et al.: Fentanyl infusion anesthesia for aortocoronary bypass surgery: Plasma levels and hemodynamic response. Anesth. Analg. 61:972-978, 1982.
89. Lazar, H. L., Buckberg, G. D., Foglia, R. P., Manganaro, A. J., and Maloney, J. V., Jr.: Detrimental effects of premature use of inotropic drugs to discontinue cardiopulmonary bypass. J. Thorac. Cardiovasc. Surg. 82:18-25, 1981.
90. Farman, J. F.: Anaesthesia in the presence of liver disease and for heaptic transplantation. Br. J. Anaesth. 44:946-952, 1972.
91. Starzl, T. E., Klintmalm, G. B., Porter, K. A., Iwatsuki, S., and Schroter, G. P. J.: Liver transplantation with use of cyclosporin A and prednisone. N. Engl. J. Med. 305(5):266-269, 1981.
92. Calne, R., and Williams, R.: Orthotopic liver transplantation. Curr. Prob. Surg. 16:3-44, 1979.

93. Editorial, Transplantation overview: Livergrafting. Transplantation 35(2): 109-111, 1983
94. Estrin, J. A., and Buckley, J. J.: Anesthetic management during liver transplantation. In: Simmons, R. L., Finch, M. E., Ascher, N. L., and Najarian, J. S., eds., Manual of Vascular Access, Organ Donation, and Transplantation, New York: Springer-Verlag, 1984, pp. 285-291.
95. Farman, J. V., Lines, J. G., Williams, R. S., Evans, D. B., Samuel, J. R., et al.: Liver transplantation in man: Anaesthetic and biochemical management. Anaesthesia 29:17-32, 1974.
96. Borland, L. M., Roule, M., and Cook, D. R.: Anesthesia for pediatric orthotopic liver transplantation. Anesth. Analg. 64:117-124, 1985.
97. Estrin, J. A., Belani, K. G., Karnarvas, A. G., Peterson, B. J., Leonard, A. S., and Buckley, J. J.: A new approach to massive blood transfusion during pediatric liver resection. (In press)
98. Ascher, N. L., Simmons, R. L., and Najarian, J. S.: Host hepatectomy and liver transplantation. In: Simmons, R. L., Finch, M. E., Ascher, N. L., and Najarian, J. S., eds., Manual of Vascular Access, Organ Donation, and Transplantation, New York: Springer-Verlag, pp. 255-284, 1984.
99. Najarian, J. S., and Ascher, N. L.: Liver transplantation. N. Engl. J. Med. 311(18):1179-1181, 1984.
100. NIH panel calls liver transplants "therapeutic"; urges wider use. In: Medical World News, Chicago: Abbott Pharmaceuticals, Inc., July 25, 1983.
101. Rapaport, S. I., Ames, S. B., Mikkelsen, S., and Goodman, J. R.: Plasma clotting factors in chronic hepatocellular disease. N. Engl. J. Med. 263(6). 278-371, 1960.
102. Toghill, P. J., Green, S., and Ferguson, R.: Platelet dynamics in chronic liver disease with special reference to the role of the spleen. J. Clin. Pathol. 30:367-371, 1977.
103. Rake, M. O., Flute, P. T., Pannel, G., and Williams, R.: Intravascular coagulation in acute hepatic necrosis. Lancet 1:533-537, 1970.
104. Miller, R. D., Robbins, T. O., Tong, M. J., and Barton, S. L.: Coagulation defects associated with massive blood transfusions. Ann. Surg. 174(5):794-801, 1971.
105. Collins, J. A.: Problems associated with the massive transfusion of stored blood. Surgery 75(2):274-295, 1974.
106. Butler, P., Israel, L., Jenkins, D. E., Nusbacher, J., and Starzl, T.: Blood transfusion during liver transplantation. Transfusion 23:433, 1983.
107. Goldsmith, M. F.: Liver transplants: Big business in blood. JAMA 250(21): 2904-2903, 1983.
108. Fath, J. J., Estrin, J., Konstantinides, F. N., Najarian, J. S., and Cerra, F. B.: The effects of hyperdynamic flow on lactate metabolism during hepatic transplantation: A requirement for aerobic metabolism in endstage cirrhosis. Crit. Care Med. 13(4):268, 1985.
109. Better, O. S., and Schrier, R. W.: Disturbed volume homeostasis in patients with cirrhosis of the liver. Kidney Int. 23:303-311, 1983.

110. Eisenberg, S.: Blood volume in patients with Laennec's cirrhosis of the liver as determined by radioactive chromium-tagged red cells. Am. J. Med. 20:189-195, 1956.
111. Carmichael, F. J., Lindop, M. J., and Farman, J. V.: Anesthesia for hepatic transplantation: Cardiovascular and metabolic alterations and their management. Anesth. Analg. 64:108-116, 1985.
112. Gray, T. A., Sealy, M., Smith, S. C. H., Tomlin, P., and McMaster, P.: Is calcium important for hemodynamic stability during liver transplantation? Transplant. Proc. 17(1):290-292, 1985.
113. Kang, Y. G., Martin, D. J., Marquez, J., Lewis, J. H., Bontempo, F. A., Sahw, B. W., Jr., Starzl, T. E., and Winter, P. M.: Intraoperative changes in blood coagulation and thromboelastographic monitoring in liver transplantation. Anesth. Analg. 64:888-896, 1985.
114. Drop, L. J., and Laver, M. B.: Low plasma ionized calcium and response to calcium therapy in critically ill man. Anesthesiology 43(3):300-306, 1975.
115. Howland, W. S., Ryan, G. M., Bettingole, R. E., and Fortner, J. G.: Coagulation abnormalities associated with liver transplantation. Surgery 68(4): 591-596, 1970.
116. Bashour, F. A., Miller, W. F., and Chapman, C. B.: Pulmonary venoarterial shunting in hepatic cirrhosis. Am. Heart J. 62:350-358, 1961.
117. Laragh, J. H.: Hormones and the pathogenesis of congestive heart failure: Vasopressin, aldosterone, and angiotensin. II. Further evidence of renal-adrenal interaction from studies in hypertension and in cirrhosis. Circulation 25:1015-1023, 1962.
118. Laragh, J. H., Cann, P. J., and Ames, R. P.: Interaction between aldosterone secretion, sodium and potassium balance, and angiotensin activity in man: Studies in hypertension and cirrhosis. Can. Med. Assoc. J. 90:248-256, 1964.
119. Kassirer, J. P., Berkman, P. M., Lawrenz, D. R., and Schwartz, W. B.: The critical role of chloride in the correction of hypokalemic alkalosis in man. Am. J. Med. 38:172-188, 1965.
120. Aldrete, J. A., LeVine, D. S., and Gingrich, T. F.: Experience in anesthesia for liver transplantation. Anesth. Analg. 48(5):802-815, 1969.
121. Machade, M. C. C., Monteiro Da Cunha, J. E., Margarido, N. F., Bacchella, T., Goncalves, L., and Raia, A. A.: Hypersomolar coma associated with clinical transplantation. Int. Surg. 61(6 and 7):368-369, 1976.
122. Shear, L. S., Hall, P. W., and Gabuzda, G. J.: Renal failure in patients with cirrhosis of the liver. Am. J. Med. 39:199-209, 1965.
123. Toledo-Pereyra, L. H., and MacKenzie, G. H.: Orthotopic liver transplantation with the assistance of an external shunt and a nonpulsatile perfusion pump. Transplantation 35(1):102-104, 1983.
124. Mazzoni, G., Koep, L., and Starzl, T.: Air embolus in liver transplantation. Transplant. Proc. 11(1):267-268, 1979.
125. Klintmalm, G. B. G., Iwatsuki, S., and Starzl, T. E.: Nephrotoxicity of cyclosporin A in liver transplant patients. Lancet 2:28, 1981.

126. Houghton, A., Hicky, J. B., Ross, S. A., and Dupre, J.: Glucose tolerance during anaesthesia and surgery. Comparison of general and extradural anaesthesia. Br. J. Anaesth. 50:494-499, 1978.
127. Taitelman, U., Reece, E. A., and Bessman, A. N.: Insulin in the management of the diabetic surgical patient: Continuous intravenous infusion versus subcutaneous administration. JAMA 237(7):658-660, 1977.
128. Walts, L. F., Miller, J., Davidson, M. B., and Brown, J.: Perioperative management of diabetes mellitus. Anesthesiology 55:104-109, 1981.
129. Gingerich, W. P. H., and Paradise, R. R.: Inhibition by halothane of glucose-stimulated insulin secretion in isolated pieces of rat pancreas. Anesthesiology 40(5):449-452, 1974.
130. Ewart, R. B. L., Rusy, B. F., and Bradford, M. W.: Effects of enflurane on release of insulin by pancreatic islets in vitro. Anesth. Analg. 60:878-884, 1981.
131. Thomas, D. J. B., Platt, H. S., and Alberti, K. G. M.: Insulin-sependent diabetes during the perioperative period: An assessment of continuous glucose-insulin-potassium infusion, and traditional treatment. Anaesthesia 39:629-637, 1984.

2

Kidney Transplantation: Vascular Complications and Perirenal Fluid Collections

JAMES I. WHITTEN and LUIS H. TOLEDO-PEREYRA
Mount Carmel Mercy Hospital, Detroit, Michigan

In our personal experience with over 379 renal transplants, vascular complications and incidents of perirenal fluid collections have been uncommon (Tables 1 and 2). Vascular complications in this chapter are divided into early and late, based on their occurrence after transplantation. Early complications include hemorrhage from the wound, the transplanted kidney, or the arterial or venous anastomosis, such as thrombosis of the renal artery or spontaneous rupture of the kidney. Late complications include the development of anastomotic or mycotic aneurysms of the renal artery and renal artery stenosis (Table 3). Perirenal fluid collections, such as lymphoceles and seromas, are also included in this chapter. Urinomas are discussed in the chapter on urologic complications.

I. EARLY VASCULAR COMPLICATIONS

A. Hemorrhage

1. Intraoperative Nonanastomotic Hemorrhage

Intraoperative nonanastomotic hemorrhage may occur from untied or torn hilar vessels in the donor kidney. The bleeding will be evident when the clamps are removed after vascular anastomosis. Bleeding should be controlled by clamping and tying or suture.

Table 1 Vascular Complications in Renal Transplant Recipients at Mount Carmel Mercy Hospital, 1972-1985

Renal artery stenosis	4/379	(1.0%)
Anastomotic aneurysm	1/379	(0.02%)
Renal artery thrombosis[a]	1/379	(0.02%)
Renal vein thrombosis	1/379	(0.02%)
Spontaneous rupture	1/379	(0.02%)

[a]Same patient with anastomotic aneurysm and thrombosis.

Table 2 Perirenal Fluid Collections in Renal Transplant Recipients at Mount Carmel Mercy Hospital, 1972-1985

Hematoma	5/379	(1.3%)
Seroma	4/379	(1.0%)
Lymphocele	7/379	(1.8%)

Table 3 Vascular Complications After Renal Transplantation

Early vascular complications
Hemorrhage
Intraoperative nonanastomotic
Vascular anastomosis
Wound
Spontaneous rupture
Thrombosis
Renal artery thrombosis
Renal vein thrombosis
Late vascular complications
Massive hemorrhage
Renal artery stenosis
Aneurysm
Anastomotic aneurysm
Mycotic aneurysm

2. Vascular Anastomosis

Bleeding from the arterial or venous anastomosis can be a serious complication after renal transplantation that may occur either intraoperatively or postoperatively [1-4]. During surgery, bleeding should be obvious once the clamps are removed after completion of the vascular anastomosis. Usually this bleeding can be controlled by simple packing around the anastomosis with dry gauze sponges. If this is not successful, then Gelfoam pledgets soaked with topical thrombin will usually suffice. If bleeding is brisk from the anastomosis, then additional sutures will be required to obtain hemostasis. In any event, if meticulous attention to hemostasis and the vascular anastomosis is undertaken, then postoperative bleeding should be rare.

3. Wound

Wound hemorrhage posttransplantation can develop especially if the patient has been recently dialyzed. The incidence is reduced if regional heparinization is used. Platelet abnormalities may still contribute to bleeding; however, if meticulous care in securing hemostasis is observed, postoperative bleeding should generally not be a problem.

B. Spontaneous Rupture

This complication is extremely rare after renal transplantation, occurring in approximately 0.8-9.6% of kidney transplants [5-7]. Most ruptures occur within the first 2 weeks after surgery. They are diagnosed by pain, swelling over the graft, oliguria, and vascular collapse. Hematuria may also be present. Spontaneous rupture is almost always preceded by the classic signs of allograft rejection. There are several possible causes of renal allograft rupture. They include renal biopsy, ischemic damage at the time of harvest or implantation, urinary obstruction, emboli secondary to perfusion, and trauma. Cortical ischemia, edema, and acute rejection are present in most cases. Rupture usually occurs on the convex surface along the longitudinal axis of the kidney. Multiple stellate graft ruptures are also occasionally seen in association with graft rejection. All renal allograft ruptures occur in conjunction with acute rejection, major occlusion of renal vessels, or hyperacute or accelerated rejection.

Some transplant programs perform routine capsulotomies at the time of transplantation; however, this technique remains controversial as a measure to prevent spontaneous rupture [8]. The best prophylaxis is probably early diagnosis and aggressive treatment of acute rejection episodes. If detection and intervention is too late, the most common treatment is transplant nephrectomy. However, repair may be made in selected cases. When a ruptured graft is left in place, rerupture may occur. Overall mortality for renal rupture has been reported at 10%

[8,9]. In our transplant experience of over 379 cases, spontaneous rerupture has occurred in only 1 case. This was in a patient who had a posttransplant biopsy. The biopsy was done on the longitudinal convex border of the kidney and the rupture occurred at this same place. The kidney could not be saved.

C. Thrombosis

1. Renal Artery Thrombosis

In our experience, thrombosis of the renal artery is a relatively rare complication. Goldman et al. reported only 6 cases in 525 transplants [2]. Thrombosis may occur as a result of a failure to recognize and tack down an intimal flap. It occurs most often with end-to-side anastomosis to the external iliac artery. If end-to-end anastomosis to the internal iliac artery is done and there is a large disparity in size between recipient and donor artery, the gathering of the anastomosis may predispose to both stenosis and thrombosis. The incidence of thrombosis is also more common in multiple anastomosis in kidneys with multiple renal arteries [1]. Internal damage secondary to perfusion or rough handling with retrieval may also predispose to thrombosis. Delayed thrombosis is usually secondary to rejection but may be also secondary to stenosis.

Renal artery thrombosis should be suspected if there is a sudden cessation of urine output in a functioning kidney. Immediate exploration and thrombectomy should be carried out if salvage of the transplanted kidney is to be done. Delay for arteriography will probably result in irreversible damage. In our experience, however, a marked decrease in urine output not infrequently occurs. First the Foley is irrigated to make sure it is not plugged with a clot. The central venous pressure (CVP) is determined, and if it is low, a fluid challenge is done. If the CVP is high, then a Lasix challenge is given. If there is no resulting increase in urine output, then usually an arteriogram is done to rule out thrombosis or renal artery stenosis. Since in our experience renal artery thrombosis is so rare, we do not immediately explore the kidney. In most instances the cause of decreased output is acute renal failure, and eventually function returns. In some, accelerated rejection is the cause and it is hard to reverse these cases.

2. Renal Vein Thrombosis

This complication has been reported in the literature in 1-4% of transplants [3, 10]. Again, this complication is rare in our experience. Thrombosis is thought to occur as a result of intimal injury during organ retrieval or transplantation, from kinking of the anastomosis or iliac vein, as an extension of thrombosis from the iliac-venous system, from pressure on the iliac from a lymphocele, urinoma, hematoma, or silent left iliac vein compression syndrome, or occasionally from severe rejection [1]. Renal vein thrombosis should be suspected if there is oliguria or anuria, reduction of renal function, graft swelling, or massive proteinuria or hematuria. Ipsilateral leg swelling may also develop from deep vein thrombosis. The confirmatory test for renal vein thrombosis is venography. However, angiography will be suggestive of its presence. If the thrombosis is incomplete, then heparin should be instituted and/or thrombectomy should be done. If the thrombosis is complete, then nephrectomy will be necessary. Heparinization should be done in either event since the patient is at risk for pulmonary embolism.

II. LATE COMPLICATIONS

A. Massive Hemorrhage

Massive hemorrhage can occur because of infection from perinephric abscess or mycotic aneurysms from hematoma infection and, rarely, from infected urinary leakage. It may present with intense graft site pain or back pain radiating to the flank and to the rectum, a drop in hematocrit, or vascular collapse. Obviously, expeditious exploration to control the hemorrhage is necessary to avoid the patient mortality associated with this complication, which can be as high as 50% [1-4].

B. Renal Artery Stenosis

This complication has been reported in the literature in 0.6-13.5% of patients receiving renal transplants [11]. These figures, however, may underestimate the actual occurrence of renal artery stenosis, since this complication is only investigated in patients with postoperative hypertension. The presence of bruit over the iliac vessel should also arouse suspicion of renal artery stenosis. Diminished renal function may also be present. If hypertension cannot be controlled with drug therapy, further investigation as to its etiology is usually conducted, especially if renal function is compromised. Renal biopsy is useful to rule out rejection. Subintimal fibrosis, which may be demonstrated by biopsy, is also specific for renal artery stenosis. Selective renal vein renin determinations may also be helpful. Arteriograms, however, are necessary to demonstrate the type and degree of stenosis present. If the stenosis is greater than 50%, it is considered hemodynamically significant.

The various types of renal artery stenosis may be classified by their location and etiology. Posttransplant stenosis is evidenced as (1) a short stenotic segment localized to the area of anastomosis, (2) a lesion in the donor artery, or (3) stenosis secondary to renal allograft rejection [1].

Renal artery stenosis localized to the area of the anastomosis is most commonly encountered and is more frequently seen after end-to-end vascular procedures. One of the causes of renal artery stenosis is thought to be technical

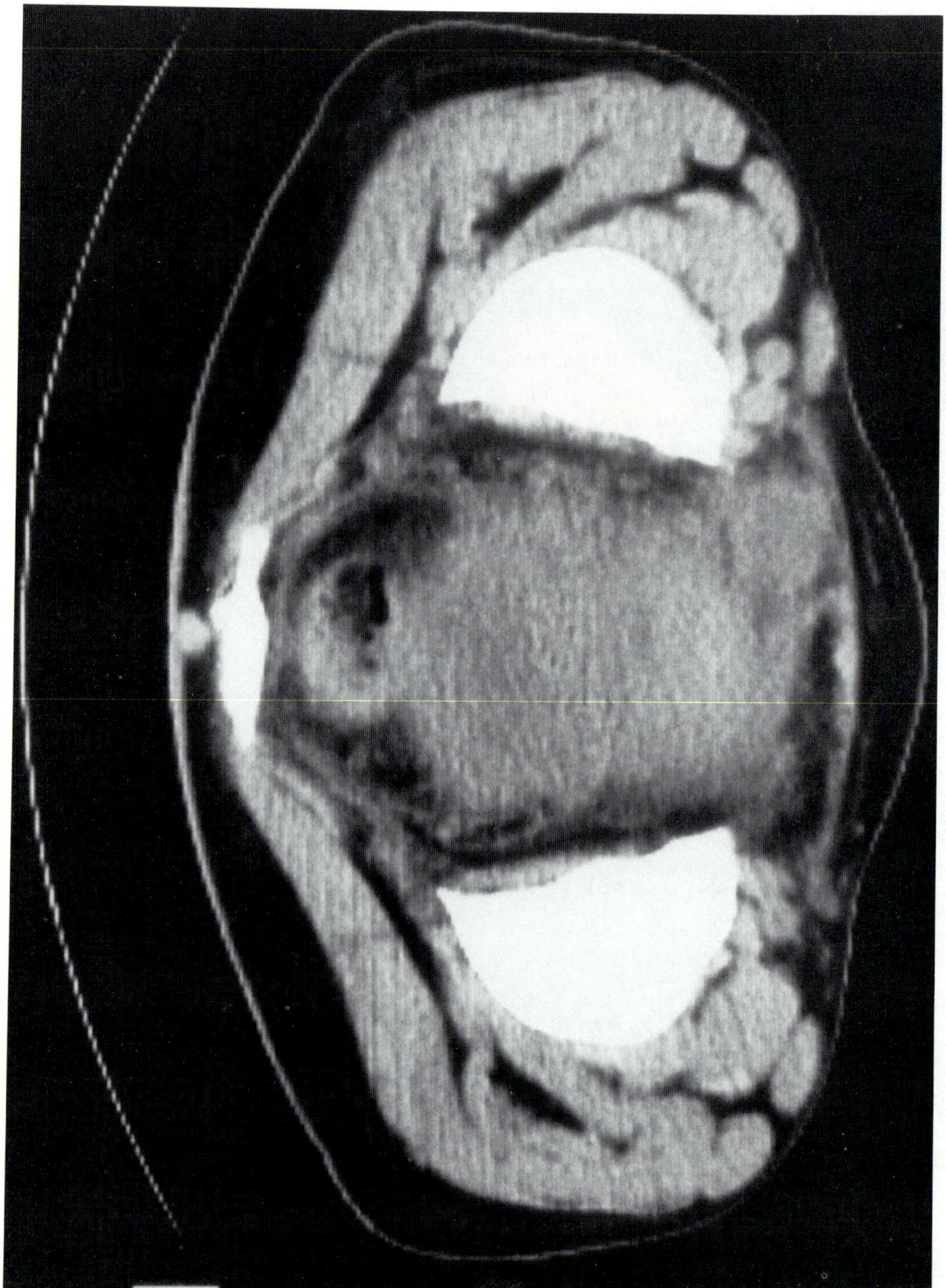

Figure 2 CT scan shows large pelvic collection due to perinephric hematoma

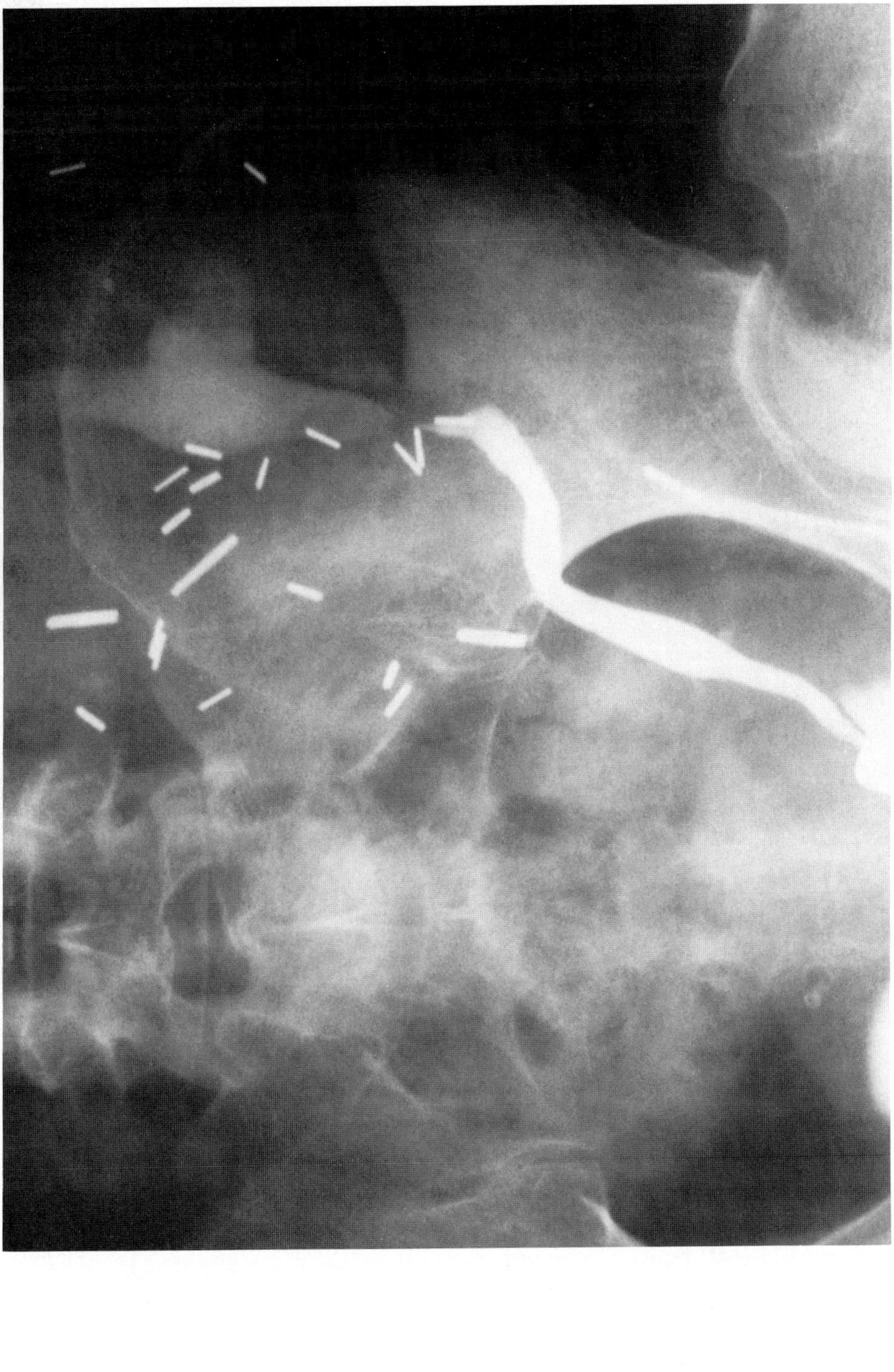

Figure 3 Retrograde pyelogram shows obstruction at the UPJ.

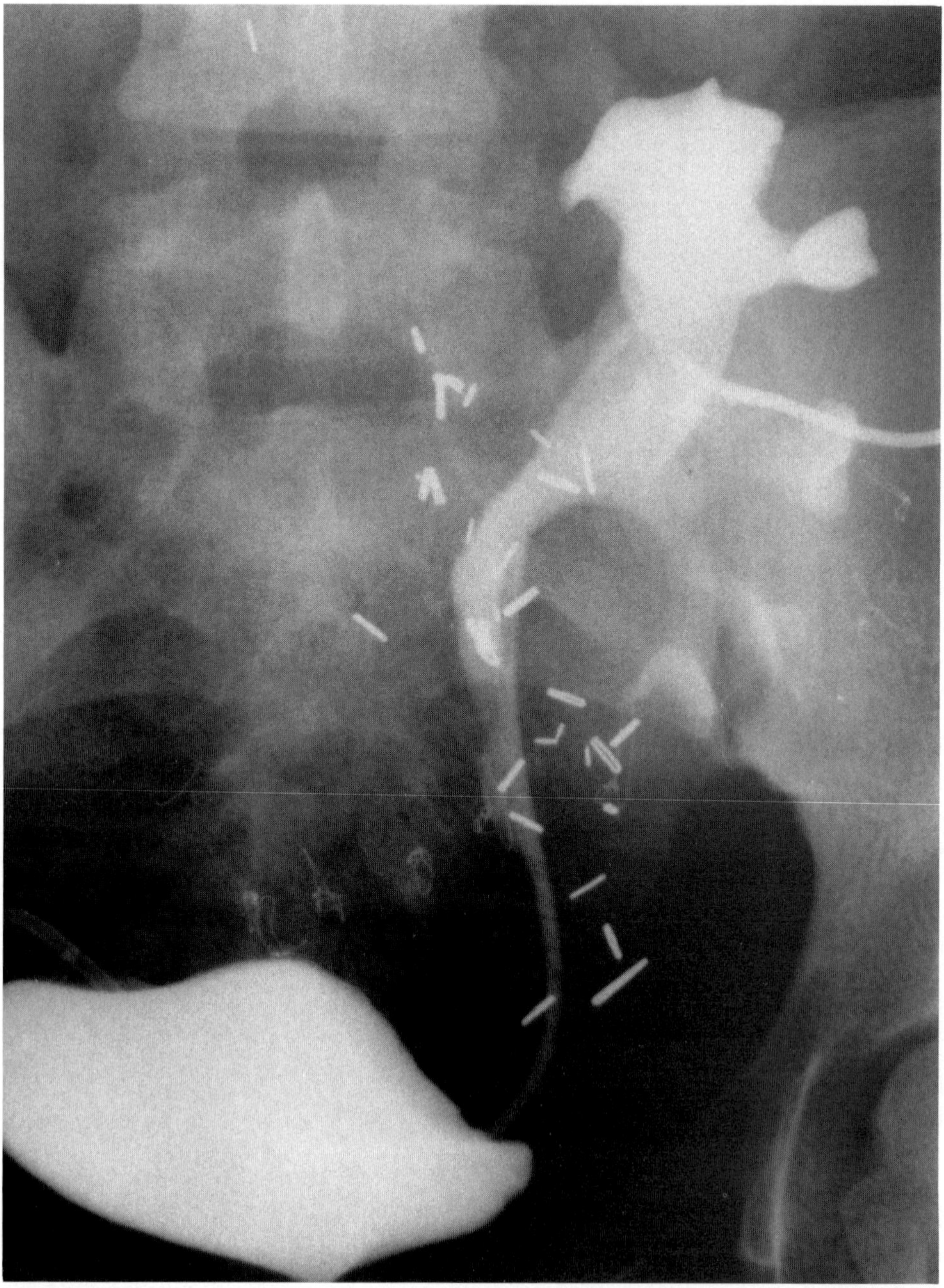

Figure 4 Distal ureteral obstruction treated by antegrade placement of the ureteral stent.

IV. URETERAL FISTULAS

The development of a ureteral fistula after renal transplantation is the most serious of all complications since it involves a high morbidity and mortality rate. Prevention of this complication is based upon the recognition of factors involved in the etiology of this problem. It appears that vascular insufficiency is the most important factor in the development of the ureteral fistula [20,24,49,59]. This vascular compromise is usually inflicted at the time of the donor nephrectomy by partial devascularization and may be aggravated by rejection, leading to ureteral ischemia and subsequent necrosis. Isolated ureteral rejection probably does not occur [56], but in the presence of renal rejection, the ureter can also be involved [3,20,49,56] and may add to the burden of compromised vascular insufficiency.

An incidence of 0.5-10% of ureteral necrosis have been reported in the literature [54,57,59]. We found in 172 consecutive transplants performed in 1984 an incidence of 1.6%. Some authors report a higher incidence of ureteral necrosis in living related transplants, due to the hilar dissection usually performed in these cases at the time of donor nephrectomy [4,34,56], but others find that the incidence is about the same [57]. Also, it has been found with a higher incidence in kidneys with multiple vessels [56], but others disagree (52-54]. Most probably, when the fistula develops in kidneys with multiple vessels it is due to the inadvertent division of a lower polar vessel. Although a ureteral fistula has also been found by some to have a higher incidence in the diabetic patient [51], our own experience and that from other large centers do not confirm this observation [57,59].

A. Diagnosis

Clinical signs and symptoms are seen early and usually are present before the fifth week after transplantation. Very rarely, symptoms and signs are manifested late and have been reported up to 6 months posttransplantation [34]. Late occurrence of a ureteral fistula most probably comes about because of borderline ureteral vascular insufficiency aggravated by progressive graft rejection. The patient usually presents with pain and swelling over the graft area, fever, progressive creatinine elevation, oliguria, cutaneous urinary drainage, or sepsis. Signs and symptoms of a ureteral fistula may mimic acute rejection or a vascular problem. Therefore, prompt and accurate evaluation is imperative for appropriate treatment. We prefer noninvasive diagnostic procedures, such as an initial ultrasound study; this will usually reveal the presence of periureteral collection and/or hydronephrosis. A renal scan may well show the isotope extravasating out of the ureter. When the serum creatinine is below 2 mg per 100 mL, an intravenous pyelogram can be diagnostic. Unfortunately, this is infrequently the case. A cystogram is necessary in most cases to rule out a vesical fistula. A CT or MRI scan

can be extremely helpful when other more simple procedures are nondiagnostic (Fig. 5). Without doubt, a retrograde pyelogram [17] or antegrade pyelogram [28] are usually very accurate to diagnose the site and extent of the ureteral fistula (Fig. 6). Our success with retrograde studies has generally been poor.

B. Treatment

We advocate early definitive operative treatment, as do others [56], because of the mortality and morbidity accompanying these cases. There are, however, selected cases of high-risk individuals or anatomic considerations in which a conservative approach can be taken [8,12,29]. We and others [4,17,28,34,57,59] have used percutaneous endourologic techniques, via placement of a nephrostomy tube alone as a temporary measure or in combination with the passage of an antegrade stent [8,61], with some success.

When a surgical procedure is needed, surgical reconstruction depends on the extent and location of the ureteral slough, the conditions of the ureter, and the presence of a native ureter. If the ureteral necrosis occurs only at the distal end of the ureter, reimplantation of the viable ureter may be performed. Secondary pyeloureteral (P-U) or uteroureteral (U-U) anastomosis is usually the procedure of choice in these cases, when the native ureter is present [49,54]. When a P-U or U-U is performed, many transplant surgeons believe that an ipsilateral nephrectomy should be performed to avoid complication of the native ipsilateral kidney [49] or the procedure should be performed end to side [3,25]; however, most recently this approach has been challenged [7,54], since most native kidneys to which ureters have been ligated remain asymptomatic, or if a complication should occur, a nephrectomy can be performed in a second stage. In our center, we have elected to leave the native kidney in situ and have observed no complications. The use of stents and a nephrectomy tube is controversial [45, 49,56], but some authors strongly advocate their use [17].

When the native ureter is absent, many alternatives are available to solve the problem: a vesicoureteral anastomosis through a psoas hitch can be performed with good results, and the bladder can be mobilized efficiently to reach the renal pelvis [49]. If the opposite native ureter is present, a contralateral ureteroureterostomy can be performed. A Boary flap is an alternative that can be utilized when a psoas hitch is not feasible [63]. A calycovesicostomy is also a procedure that can be performed in selected cases [13]. Finally, on occasion, when the life of the recipient is threatened by clinical instability and/or sepsis, a nephrectomy is a judicious modality to solve the problem.

C. Outcome

Although the prognosis of the recipient with a ureteral fistula appears to have improved in recent years, it is still the cause of significant morbidity and mortality [34,57]. Graft survival can be expected to be around 63% [54,57].

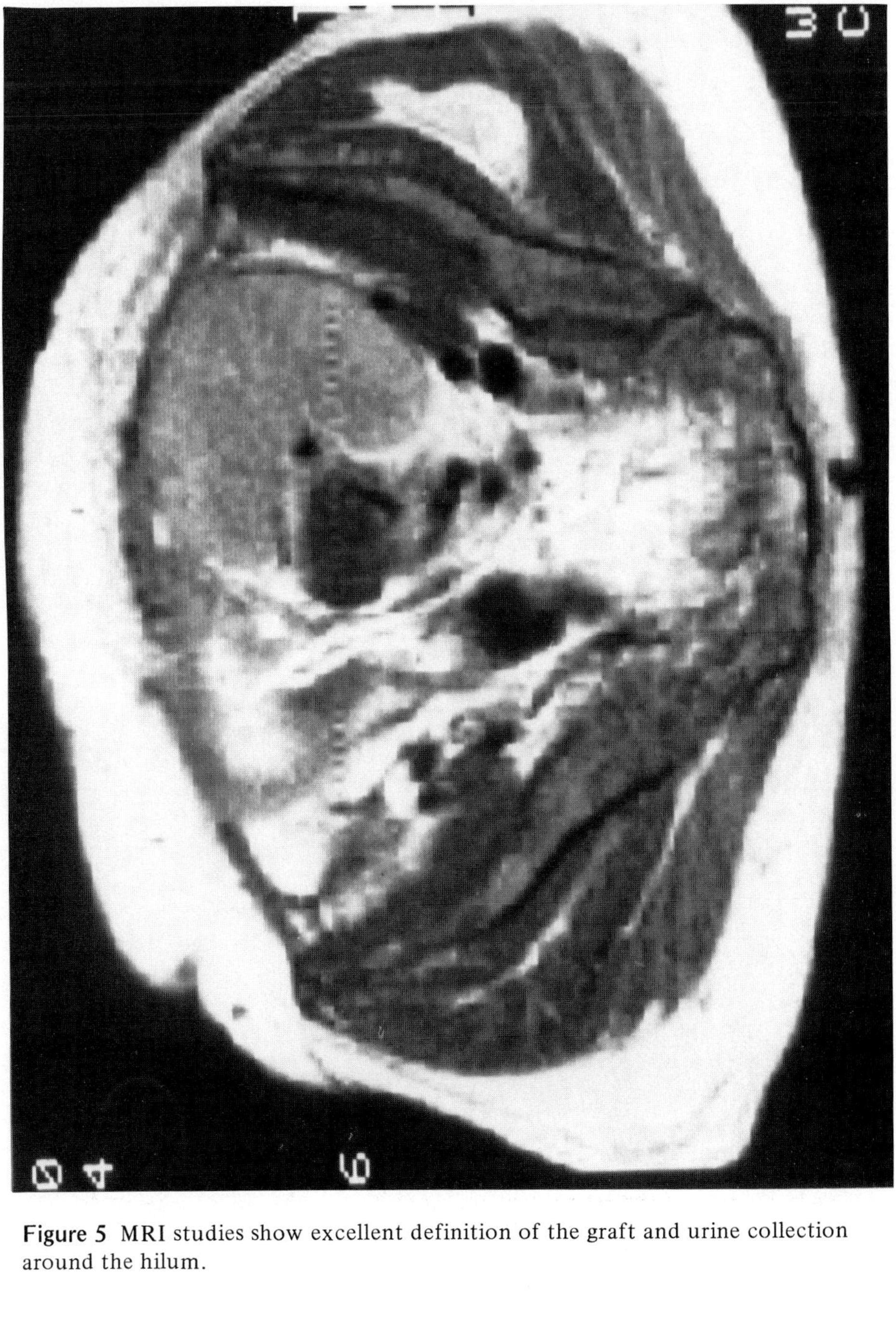

Figure 5 MRI studies show excellent definition of the graft and urine collection around the hilum.

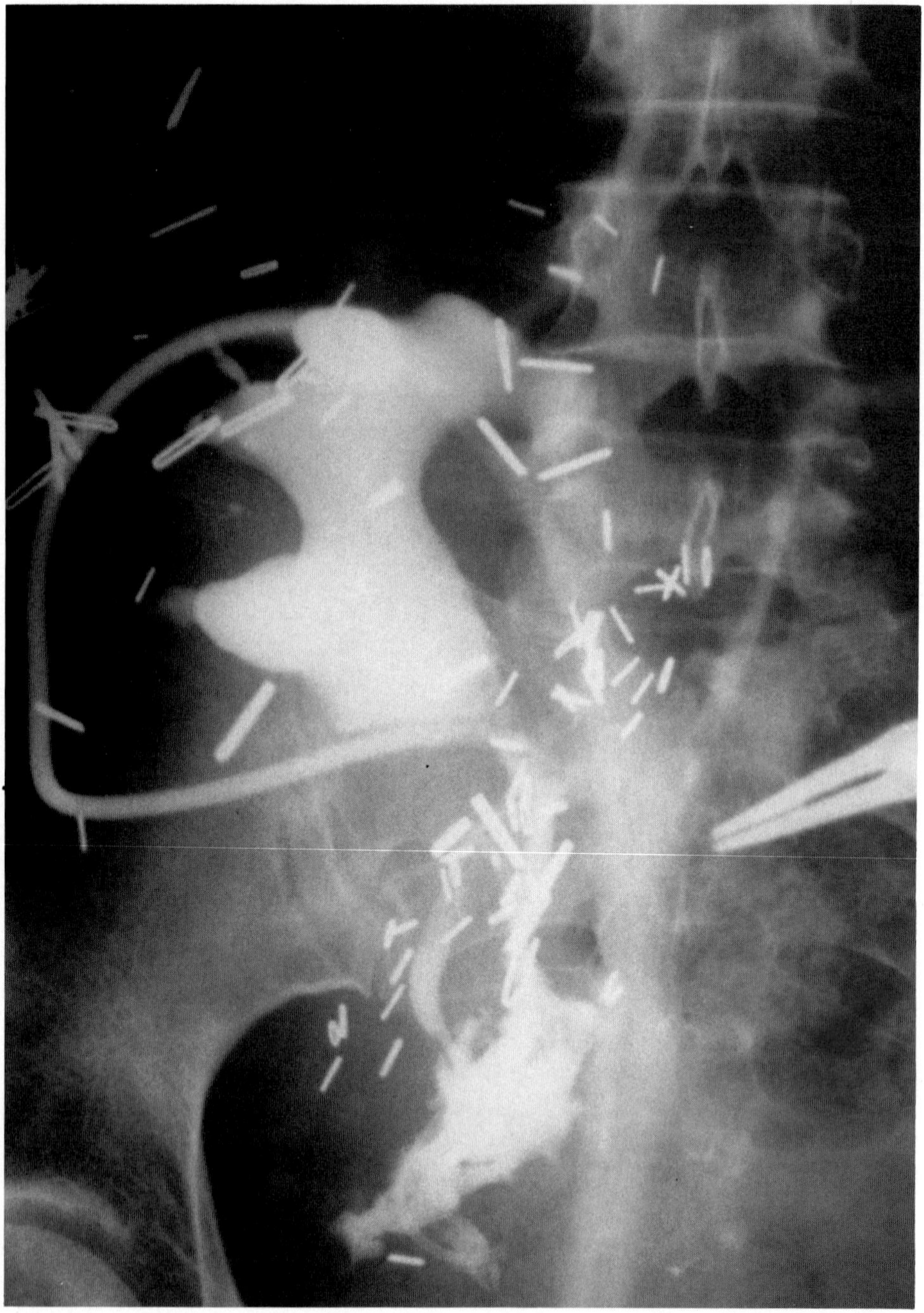

Figure 6 Urinary fistula diagnosed by antegrade pyelogram.

V. VESICAL FISTULAS

A vesical fistula may develop at the site of the anterior cystotomy closure or at the ureteral hiatus. Most often, the fistula arises from the anterior cystotomy suture line. To prevent this complication, a three-layer watertight closure has been recommended by many authors. We utilize a three-layer running closure of Vicryl. The first layer of mucosa is closed with 4-0 Vicryl and the other two layers with 2-0 Viscral. In bladders that have been previously operated, the cystostomy should be performed away from previous scars since at that site the vascular supply of the bladder may be compromised. A cystostomy tube is almost never required, and a short period of catheter drainage from 2 to 5 days is generally utilized.

The incidence of vesical fistula varies from 0.6 to 4.4% [34,54,57,58]. We found only 1 vesical fistula in 172 consecutive transplants performed in 1984, an incidence of 0.5%. Some reports reveal a higher incidence in the diabetic patient [51,58], and a longer catheter drainage period is the common method of choice. However, other authors do not confirm this observation [57,65]. An increased incidence of bladder fistula has been described following retransplantation [48], due to the formation of vesical scars.

A. Diagnosis

The signs and symptoms of a vesical fistula are usually manifested in the first 2 weeks posttransplantation [57]. If there is a drain, extravasation of the urine may be seen early. If there is no drain or the drain site has already healed, the urinary output is diminished, the serum creatinine may be elevated, and a mass is palpable above the pubis. There may be fever or pain in the suprapubic area or around the allograft. The diagnosis is usually suspected by an ultrasound study, which will demonstrate a perivesical fluid collection. Radioisotope studies may show urinary extravasation but will not confirm the source of the fistula. The most accurate diagnostic test is the cystogram. In selective cases, the use of methylene blue is extremely helpful.

B. Treatment

Our treatment of choice has been continuing vesical catheter drainage, and at times a sump drainage apparatus is used. This almost always resolves the problem within 2-4 weeks. Other centers also advocate a conservative approach, particularly when the fistula is relatively small [44,49,54]. Immediate repair has been the treatment of choice in some transplant centers [34,46,65].

VI. CALYCEAL FISTULAS

Calyceal fistulas are related to segmental renal ischemia as a result of ligation of an accessory renal artery [16]. Multiple arterial vessels occur in 20-25% of cases; therefore, a meticulous dissection should be performed by the surgeon performing the donor nephrectomy so that the arterial supply to each kidney is assessed and reported accurately. In living related donors, a preoperative arteriogram is mandatory. If an accessory artery is transected at the time of harvesting, bench surgery should be performed prior to transplantation to reconnect the divided vessel [34].

According to the literature, the incidence of calyceal fistula varies from 1.3 to 2.2% of cases [34,54]. High morbidity and mortality have been reported with this complication [16].

A. Diagnosis

It is usually difficult to recognize the diagnosis in these cases. A high index of suspicion is needed and should be kept in mind if some problem occurred during the donor nephrectomy, especially if an accessory vessel was ligated. At the time of transplantation an area of ischemia may indicate arterial interruption to a renal segment. Clinically, urinary extravasation may be present through the wound. More often, a mass, fever, and/or sepsis will manifest. The diagnosis may be defined by an excretory urogram, but at the time, only a retrograde study will be diagnostic. A CT scan and/or angiography may be helpful in selective cases.

B. Treatment

Calcyceal fistulas have been treated by nephrostomy drainage [64] or segmental resection with closure with or without the aid of omentum [2,15,55].

VII. RENAL RUPTURE

Spontaneous graft rupture is a serious complication usually presenting with dramatic symptomatology at the graft site and signs of acute blood loss. Usually the rupture occurs within the first 3 weeks posttransplantation but can present as late as 170 days [32,33,49]. The most common etiology is acute rejection; however, other factors contributing to this problem have been described, such as ischemic damage (acute tubular necrosis, ATN), renal biopsy, emboli secondary to perfusion, trauma, urinary obstruction, and lymphatic occlusion of the graft [33,39,42,49,50].

In some series the incidence has been reported as high as 4% [42,50]. However, most authors believe it to be of rare occurrence. It is seen twice as often in

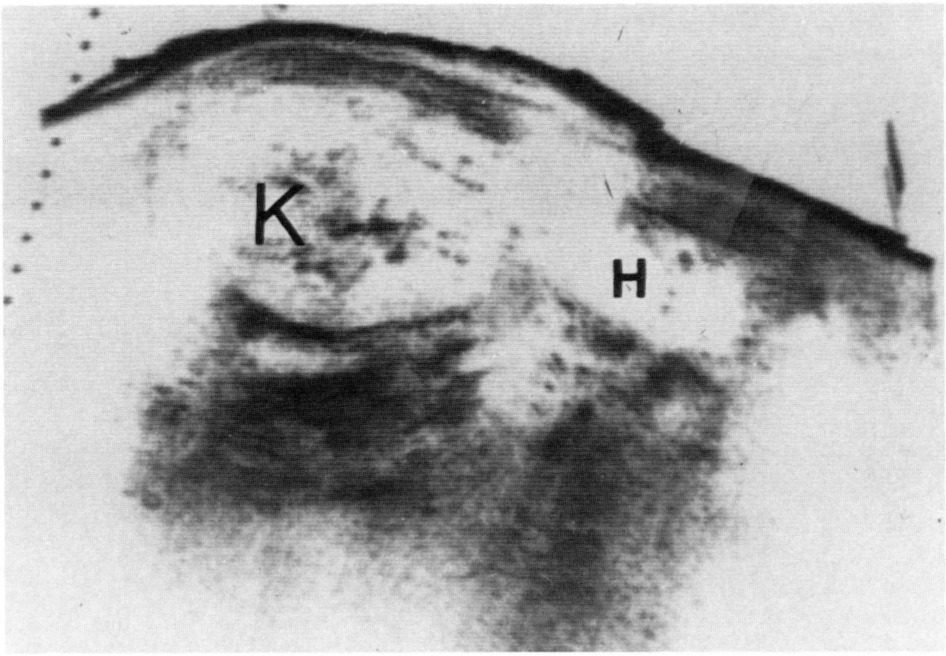

Figure 7 Ultrasound study shows a perirenal collection in a case of spontaneous renal rupture.

cadaveric transplants. The rupture usually occurs on the convex border of the kidney along its long axis.

A. Diagnosis

Clinical presentation is acute, and usually there is pain and swelling over the graft site, oliguria, and/or hematuria. As a result of blood loss, hypovolemia or shock may be present. When the diagnosis is suspected, it can be confirmed by ultrasonography or CT scan (Fig. 7). IVP or retrograde pyelography or more rarely angiography may be of help to verify the diagnosis.

B. Treatment

Surgical exploration of the graft should be performed after the diagnosis is suspected. Review of the literature reveals a high incidence of graft removal in up to 74% of cases. A nephrectomy is performed in most cases because of patient instability or severe damage to the graft. In selective cases, repair of the kidney may be attempted after drainage of the perinephric hematoma is accomplished. Simple suturing or the use of a peritoneal patch has been attempted [33,49]. However, 28.5% of these cases will rerupture once again [33]; therefore, if the graft is repaired, careful observation of the recipient for the next few weeks is mandatory. Routine capsulotomy [27] is not recommended by most transplant surgeons since serious complications can arise from this technique [33,50].

C. Outcome

The mortality after allograft rupture has been described as high as 9% with a graft loss of approximately 74% [33].

VIII. SCROTAL COMPLICATIONS

Since long-term survival can be expected in the graft majority of patients following renal transplantation, the prevention of scrotal complications has become an important goal in the management of these patients. In the past, division of the spermatic cord to gain better exposure or to prevent ureteral obstruction [23] was usually accomplished by the transplant surgeon. However, this practice may lead to several complications, such as hydrocele, testicular atrophy, testicular necrosis, or recurrent pain. Apart from the morbidity associated with these problems, the patient may stand the risk of infertility. Review of the literature indicates that 74.4% of testicles develop a complication after cord ligation [47]. Therefore, it is important to preserve the cord at the time of transplantation. This can be accomplished simply by methodically separating and dissecting the cord from the neighboring structures, which usually does not jeopardize the surgical procedure. The ureter should pass below the cord toward the bladder [5]. Epididymitis as a result of infection related to urethral catheter is rarely seen. A short-term catheter drainage may prevent this complication. A hydrocele is the most common complication that occurs after division of the spermatic cord and has been reported in 67% of cases [47]. The cause is probably related to lymphatic interruption. Testicular atrophy has been reported in 13.8% of cases following cord ligation due to interruption of the arterial supply. Testicular atrophy of the contralateral side can occur, probably as a result of uremia [14]. Genital edema may present as a result of vascular blockage, perinephric collections, or lymphatic interruption at the level of the iliac region. We have seen a case of scrotal edema and a case of labial edema as a result of extensive dissection of the iliac vessel with interruption of the lymph drainage of the genitalia. In many cases, the scrotal complication is asymptomatic, but in some the condition may become progressive. A symptomatic hydrocele should be treated by hydrocelectomy, and simple puncture should be avoided to avoid infection.

Epididymitis is treated with broad-spectrum antibiotics; however, in severe cases an orchiectomy should be performed to avoid sepsis. In testicular atrophy an orchiectomy is only indicated when symptomatic.

REFERENCES

1. Anderson, E. E., Glenn, J. F., Siegler, H. F., and Stickler, D. L.: Ureteral implantation in renal transplantation. Surg. Gynecol. Obstet. 134:494, 1972.
2. Anderson, E. E., Glenn, J. F., Siegler, H. F., and Stickler, D. L.: Urologic complications in renal transplantation. J. Urol. 107:187, 1972.
3. Anderson, M. J., and Middleton, R. G.: Secondary pyeloureterostomy with intact ureter. J. Urol. 128:247, 1982.
4. Barry, J. M., Lawson, R. K., Strong, B., and Hodges, C. V.: Urologic complications in 173 kidney transplants. J. Urol. 112:567, 1974.
5. Barry, J. M.: Spermatic cord preservation in kidney transplantation. J. Urol. 127:1076, 1982.
6. Barry, J. M.: Unstented extravesical ureteroneocystostomy in kidney transplantation. J. Urol. 128:918, 1983.
7. Baquero, A., Ginsberg, P. C., Kaschak, D., Rya, R., Schneeberg, A., Solish, L., and Bannett, A. D.: Experience with pyeloureterostomy associated with simple ligation of native ureter without ipsilateral nephrectomy in renal transplantation. J. Urol. 133:386, 1985.
8. Berger, R. E., Ansell, J. S., Tremann, J. A., Hetz, J. H., Rattazzi, L. C., and Marchiolo, T. L.: The use of self-retained ureteral stents in the management of urologic complications in renal transplant recipients. J. Urol. 124:781, 1980.
9. Burleson, R. L., and Marbarger, P. D.: Prevention of lymphocele formation following renal allotransplantation. J. Urol. 127:18, 1982.
10. Colfry, A. J., Jr., Schlegel, J. U., Lindsey, E. S., and McDonald, J. C.: Urological complication of renal transplantation. J. Urol. 112:564, 1974.
11. Corriere, J. N., Perloff, L. J., Barker, C. F., Henderson, L. W., Schoenberg, H. W., and Murphy, J. J.: The ureteropyelostomy in human renal transplantation. J. Urol. 110:24, 1973.
12. Desai, S. G., McRoberts, J. W., Hellebuch, A. A., and Luke, R. G.: Conservative non-operative management of ureteral fistulas following renal allografts. J. Urol. 112:572, 1974.
13. Ehrlich, R. M., Whitmore, K., and Fine, R. N.: Calycovesicostomy for total ureteral obstruction after renal transplantation. J. Urol. 129:818, 1983.
14. Freeman, R. M., Lawson, R. L., and Feary, M. O.: Gynecomastia: An endocrinologic complication of hemodialysis. Ann. Intern. Med. 69:67, 1968.
15. Fox, M., and Tottenham, R. C.: Urinary fistula from segmental infarction in a transplanted kidney: Recovery following surgical repair. Br. J. Urol. 44: 336, 1972.

16. Goldman, M. H., Burleson, R. L., Tilney, N. L., Vineyard, G. C., and Wilson, R. E.: Calyceal-cutaneous fistulae in renal transplant patients. Ann. Surg. 184:679, 1976.
17. Goldstein, I., Cho, S. I., and Olsson, C. A.: Nephrostomy drainage for renal transplant complications. J. Urol. 126:159, 1981.
18. Greenberg, S. H., Wein, A. G., Perloff, L. J., and Barker, C. F.: Uretero-pyelostomy and ureteroneocystostomy in renal transplantation postoperative urologic complications. J. Urol. 118:17, 1977.
19. Helling, T. S., Thomas, C. Y., Jr.,.Moore, J. D., and Koontz, P. J.: The surgical approach to obstructive problems of the transplant ureter. Transplant. Proc. 14:751, 1982.
20. Hriko, G. M., Birtch, A. G., Bennett, A. H., and Wilson, R. E.: Factors responsible for urinary fistula in the renal transplant recipient. Ann. Surg. 178: 609, 1973.
21. Jordan, M. L., Novick, A. C., Geisinger, M., Stowe, A., et al.: Imaging of the transplanted kidney with nuclear magnetic resonance. Transplant. Proc. 17: 32, 1985.
22. Kartheuser, A. H., Lefevre, Y. J., Squifflet, J. P., et al.: Anterior extravesical ureteroneocystostomy: The procedure of choice in kidney transplantation. Transplant. Proc. 17:176, 1985.
23. Karmi, S. A., Dagher, F. J., Ramos, E., and Young, J. D., Jr. Spermatic cord: Cause of ureteral obstruction in renal allotransplant recipients. Urology 11: 380, 1978.
24. Khauli, R. B., Novick, A. C., Choi, H. K., Stowe, N. T., and Straffon, R. A.: Preservation of the ureteral blood supply in rat renal transplantation. Microsurgery 4:225, 1983.
25. Kinnaert, P., Hall, M., Janssen, F., Vereerstraeten, P., Toussaint, C., and Geertruyden, J. V.: Ureteral stenosis after kidney transplantation: True incidence and long term follow up after surgical correction. J. Urol. 133: 17, 1985.
26. Koehler, P. R., Kanemoto, H. H., and Maxwell, J. C.: Ultrasonic "B" scanning in the diagnosis of complications in renal transplant patients. Radiology 119:661, 1976.
27. Lee, H. M., Madge, G. E., Mendez-Picon, G., and Chateerjee, S. N.: Surgical complications in renal transplant recipients. Surg. Clin. North Am. 58:285, 1978.
28. Lieberman, R. P., Crummy, A. B., Glass, N. R., and Belzer, N. O.: Fine needle antegrade pyelography in the renal transplant. J. Urol. 126:155, 1981.
29. Lieberman, R. P., Glass, N. R., Crummy, A. B., Sollinger, H. W., and Belzer, F. O.: Non-operative percutaneous management of urinary fistulas and strictures in renal transplantation. Surg. Gynecol. Obstet. 155:667, 1982.
30. Lieberman, S. F., Keller, F. S., Barry, J. M., and Rosch, J.: Percutaneous antegrade transluminal ureteroplasty for renal allograft ureteral stenosis. J. Urol. 128:122, 1982.
31. List, A. R., Blohme, J., Brynger, H., and Nilson, A. E.: Balloon dilatations

for ureteral strictures in graft kidneys. A viable alternative to further surgery. Transplantation 35:105, 1983.
32. Lord, R. S., Belzer, F. O., and Kountz, S. L.: Delayed spontaneous rupture of the allografted kidney. Arch. Surg. 100:667, 1970.
33. Lord, R. S., Effaney, D. F., Hayes, J. M., and Tracy, G. D.: Renal allograft rupture; cause, clinical features and management. Ann. Surg. 177:268, 1973.
34. Loughlin, K. R., Tilney, N. L., and Richie, J. P.: Urologic complications in 718 renal transplant patients. Surgery 95:297, 1984.
35. Mathew, T. H., Kincaid-Smith, P., and Vicraman, P.: Risks of vesicoureteric reflux in the transplanted kidney. N. Engl. J. Med. 297:414, 1977.
36. Marchiolo, T. L., and Tremann, J. A.: Technique for treating stricture at a ureteroneocystostomy. Surgery 73:634, 1973.
37. Marx, W. L., Halazs, N. A., McLaughlin, A. P., and Gittes, R. F.: Urological complications in renal transplantation. J. Urol. 112:561, 1974.
38. Malek, G. H., Uehling, D. T., Daouk, A. A., and Kisken, W. A.: Urological complications of renal transplantation. J. Urol. 109:449, 1970.
39. Martin, D. C., Goodwin, W. E., Kauman, J. J., Mims, M. M., Goldman, R., Rubini, M., and Gonick, H.: Kidney transplants: 92 cases. Results, lessons learned, future prospects. J. Urol. 100:227, 1968.
40. McDonald, J. C., Rohr, M. S., and Frentz, G. D.: External ureteroneocystostomy and ureteroureterostomy in renal transplantation. Ann. Surg. 190: 663, 1979.
41. Morley, P., Barnett, E., and Bell, P.: Ultrasound in the diagnosis of fluid collections following renal transplantation. Clin. Radiol. 26:199, 1975.
42. Murray, J. E., Wilson, R. E., Tilney, N. L., Cooper, W. C., et al.: Five years experience in renal transplantation with immunosuppressive drugs. Ann. Surg. 168:416, 1968.
43. Novick, A. C., Irish, C., Steinmuller, D., Buonocore, E., and Cohen, C.: The role of computerized tomography in renal transplant patients. J. Urol. 125:15, 1981.
44. O'Donnohue, E. P. N., Chisholm, G. D., and Shackman, R.: Urinary fistulae after renal transplantation. Br. J. Urol. 45:28, 1973.
45. Olsson, C. A., Manick, J. A., Schmitt, G. W., Idelson, B. A., Williams, L. E., Lemann, J., Jr., Harrington, J. T., and Nabseth, D. C.: Nephrostomy in renal transplantation. Am. J. Surg. 121:467, 1971.
46. Palmer, J. M., and Chatterjee, S. N.: Urologic complications in renal transplantation. Surg. Clin. North Am. 58:305, 1978.
47. Penn, I., Mackie, G., Halgrimson, C. G., and Starzl, R. E.: Testicular complications following renal transplantation. Ann. Surg. 176:697, 1972.
48. Pfeffermann, R., Vidne, B., Leapuran, S., et al.: Urologic complications in renal primary and retransplantation. Am. J. Surg. 131:242, 1976.
49. Smith, R. B., and Ehrlich, R. M.: The surgical complications of renal transplantation. Urol. Clin. North Am. 3:621, 1976.
50. Salaman, J. R., Calne, R. Y., Pena, J., Sells, R. A., White, H. J. O., and Yoffa,

D.: Surgical aspects of clinical renal transplantation. Br. J. Surg., 56:413, 1969.
51. Simmons, R. L., Kjelstrand, C. M., Kyriakides, D. K., et al.: Surgical aspects of transplantation in diabetic patients. Kidney Int. 6(19):129, 1974.
52. Simmons, R. L., Tallent, M. B., Kjellstrand, C. M., and Najarian, J. S.: Kidney transplantation from living donors with bilateral double renal arteries. Surgery 69:201, 1969.
53. Spanos, P. K., Simmons, R. L., Kjellstrand, C. M., Buselmeier, T. J., and Najarian, J. S.: Kidney transplantation from living related donors with multiple vessels: A problem revisited. Am. J. Surg. 125:554, 1973.
54. Schiff, M., Jr., McGuire, E. J., Weis, R. M., and Lytton, B.: Management of urinary fistulas after renal transplantation. J. Urol. 115:251, 1976.
55. Schiff, M., Jr., McGuire, E. J., and Webster, J.: Successful management of calyceal fistulas following renal transplantation. Arch. Surg. 110:1129, 1975.
56. Starzl, R. E., Groth, C. G., Putnam, C. W., Penn, I., et al.: Urological complications in 216 human recipients of renal transplants. Ann. Surg. 172:1, 1970.
57. Sagalowsky, A. I., Ransler, C. W., Peters, P. C., et al.: Urologic complications in 505 renal transplants with early catheter removal. J. Urol. 129:929, 1983.
58. Salvatierra, O., Jr., Kountz, S. L., and Belzer, F. O.: Prevention of ureteral fistula after renal transplantation. J. Urol. 112:445, 1974.
59. Salvatierra, O., Jr., Olcott, C., IV, Amend, W. J., Cochrum, C. K., and Feduska, N. J.: Urological complications of renal transplantation can be prevented or controlled. J. Urol. 117:421, 1977.
60. Schweitzer, R. T., Cho, S. I., Kountz, S. L., and Belzer, F. O.: Lymphoceles following renal transplantation. Arch. Surg. 104:43, 1972.
61. Streem, S. B.: Endourologic management of renal transplant complications. Cleve. Clin. Q. 51:349, 1984.
62. The 17th Report of the Human Renal Transplant Registry. ACS/NIH Organ transplant registry third scientific report. JAMA 226:1197, 1973.
63. Toguri, A. G., Emtage, J. B., and Jarzylo, S. V.: Management of total ureteral loss after kidney transplantation. Can. J. Surg. 26:198, 1983.
64. Williams, G., Birtch, A. G., Wilson, R. E., Harrison, J. H., and Murray, J. E.: Urological complications of renal transplantation. Br. J. Urol. 42:21, 1970.
65. Waltzer, W. C., Zincke, H., and Myers, R. P.: Urinary tract reconstruction in renal transplantation. Urology 16:233, 1980.
66. Zincke, H., et al.: Late ureteral obstruction mimicking rejection after transplantation. Urology 9:504, 1977.

4

Kidney Transplantation: Wound Complications

JUHANI AHONEN
Helsinki University Central Hospital, Helsinki, Finland

Early reports on renal transplantation [1,2] indicated high rates of wound complications. However, considerable improvement even in this respect has taken place during the last years. In this chapter the basic principles of wound healing, the effects of uremia and immunosuppressive therapy, and the most common healing complications are reviewed.

I. BASIC PRINCIPLES IN WOUND HEALING

The aim of the wound-healing process is to re-establish the integrity and tensile strength of the tissue involved. The healing process is usually described as successive phases: inflammation, proliferation, and maturation (Fig. 1).

The inflammatory phase in wound healing starts immediately after wounding and lasts in the human for 3-4 days [3]. The initial event is blood coagulation, followed by dilation of blood vessels in the tissue surrounding the wound. This leads to edema and cellular infiltration. The first cells to invade the wound area are polymorphonuclear leukocytes (PML). They do not have a role in the healing process; their function is to protect the tissue against invading microorganisms [4]. Later monocytes appear; they mature into macrophages. They phagocytose dead cells and tissue debris, but most importantly by secreting soluble substances [3,4] activate resting primitive mesenchymal cells to become fibroblasts. A similar function has been ascribed to the thrombocytes in the initial blood clot [5]. During the inflammatory phase there is practically no increase in the tensile strength [6]. In the fibrin scaffold formed

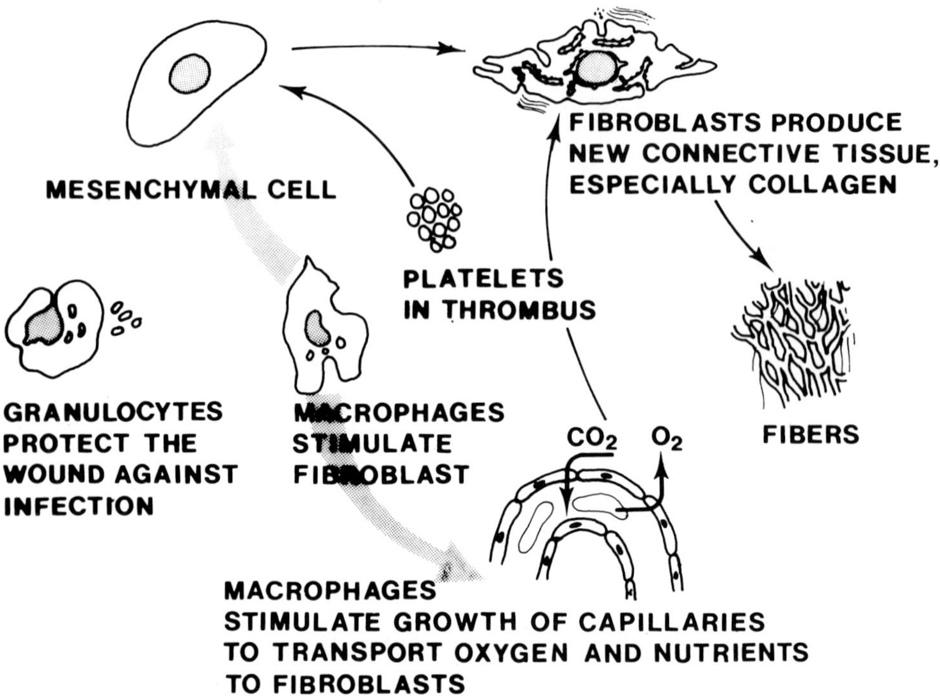

Figure 1 Successive phases in the healing process.

in the wound clot, fibrin seems to be associated with plasma-derived fibronectin [7]. This scaffold is important for fibroblast adherence [8].

The proliferation phase follows the inflammatory phase; now the tensile strength increases substantially [6], so that toward the end of this phase, which usually lasts for 10 days, stitches can safely be removed from a sutured wound. Characteristic of this phase is proliferation of fibroblasts, which immediately start to produce collagen and other extracellular substances. Another important feature is the growth and development of new capillaries to supply the actively synthesizing cells with oxygen. The newly formed capillaries are very sensitive; even small reductions in circulating blood volume cause closure of these, with reduced tissue pO_2 as a result [9]. Another feature to be remembered is the absolute necessity of vitamin C for the synthesis of collagen [10].

During the maturation phase, which lasts for several months, the tensile strength of the wound increases most. The strength of a scar is due to collagen produced by fibroblasts. During the maturation phase there is a constant synthesis and breakdown of collagen [11]. The net amount of collagen is not increased, but the fibers are organized into stronger bundles [12], which are orientated according to the stress forces. If there is a disturbed balance between synthesis and breakdown of collagen, the result is a hypertrophic scar or a keloid.

II. COMPLICATIONS IN WOUND HEALING

The initial inflammatory phase in wound healing is of utmost importance, almost all the complications derive from disturbances during this period. This is especially so in the case of the most important complication: wound infection. The factors in wound infection can be described as follows:

$$\text{Rate of infection} = \frac{\text{Number of bacteria} \times \text{virulence}}{\text{Local resistance}}$$

It is usually estimated that a minimum of 10^6 bacteria are needed for infection to occur [13].

The most important determinant in wound infection is, however, the local resistance against infections. All operations are contaminated to a certain degree when conventional sterile techniques are used; infection can occur only if the resistance is compromised.

As earlier mentioned, leukocytes (PMN) invade the wound area in a few hours; they are most important cells in resistance against infection. They are attracted to the area by complement factors released in connection with the injury. Their efficacy is related to the local oxygen tension; they enter even hypoxic wounds, but their microbial killing capacity is reduced by low tissue oxygen tension, in particular if the invading organisms are *Staphylococcus aureus, Escherichia coli,* or *Klebsiella* [13]. Leukocytes have a definitive capacity to ingest and digest foreign material, devitalized tissue, or bacteria. If they have to remove much dead tissue or foreign material, their phagocytic capacity may be overwhelmed, thus leaving bacteria free to multiply and invade. This means that surgical technical factors are most important in preventing wound infections, especially in clean and clean contaminated operations.

A. Clinically Relevant Factors in Wound Infections

The first and the most relevant factor in preventing wound infections in operations like kidney transplantation (clean contaminated, if the urinary bladder is entered) is the surgical technique. Bad technique lets into the wound lots of dead or dying tissue and foreign material (sutures (Table 1).

Other factors of importance that have been identified are as follows:

Table 1 Factors in Wound Infection

Determinants of wound infection:
Magnitude of bacterial contamination
Local host defense against infection
Virulence of the bacteria
Local host defenses reduced by:
Dead and dying tissue in the wound: avoid by sharp dissection; careful use of diathermy; avoidance of many ligatures
Foreign bodies in the wound: avoid by use of least irritating suture materials; avoid unnecessary sutures and ligatures
Local circulatory disturbances: avoid tight sutures; no subcutaneous ligatures; careful hemostasis

Hypovolemia and *Vasoconstrictors* induce hypoxia into the wound; if this occurs within a few hours after wounding, leukocyte function in the wound is compromised.

Obesity: the massive subcutaneous tissue in these patients must often be sutured to avoid dead spaces; this increases the risk of infection [14].

Diabetes mellitus: it is not fully known whether the worsened local resistance is due to microvascular changes in diabetes or to the postulated defective phagocytic function of the leukocytes [13].

Defective preoperative nutrition has been shown to lead to decreased PMN chemotaxis, decreased number of circulating lymphocytes, and reduced T-helper-T-killer suppressor ratio and blastogenesis when lymphocytes are stimulated in vitro by phytohemagglutinin (PHA) and a decreased mixed lymphocyte culture response. This anergic state predisposes to infections.

Preoperative shave, if performed a few hours before operations, leads to microscopic skin lesions where bacteria colonize.

B. Effect of Uremia on Wound Healing

Experimental studies have confirmed the widespread clinical impression that woung healing is disturbed in uremia. Kursh et al. [15] showed that when rats were made uremic by 70% nephrectomy skin wound tensile strength development was delayed and collagen accumulation into subcutaneously implanted sponges was reduced. Further experiments by the same group indicated, however, that if the uremic animals were pair fed with controls the rate of wound healing was similar and delayed in both groups. This means that it is not the uremic state itself, but the consequent defective nutrition, that is responsible for healing disturbances.

This corroborates well with other results on the role of nutrition in wound healing [16]. Only very severe anemia can negatively affect the rate of wound healing. Heughan et al. [17] showed that healing proceeded at a normal rate at a hematocrit value of 20%. Blood volume is of critical importance in maintaining adequate oxygen supply to the wound granulation tissue via the newly formed capillaries [9]. The bleeding disorders associated with uremia can lead to postoperative hematomas and thus delay healing. The coagulation defect is due to one or several dialyzable compounds that affect thrombocyte function [18] and can be corrected by dialysis.

C. Effect of Immunosuppressive Treatment on Wound Healing

Glucocorticosteroids delay the rate of wound healing by modifying the initial inflammatory phase [19]. The number of lymphocytes, monocytes, and macrophages is diminished during the inflammatory phase in experimental granulation tissue under methylprednisolone treatment [20]; this results in a reduced number of fibroblasts and a decreased amount of collagen later. However, within 3 weeks the differences disappear [21]. This means that glucocorticosteroids delay the rate of wound healing but do not permanently suppress it. The number of polymorphonuclear leukocytes is not affected, but the development of new capillaries is. The increased susceptibility to infection of glucocorticoid-treated healing tissue could thus be explained by the diminished supply of oxygen, which leads to impaired micro-organism killing capacity of the leukocytes.

Cyclosporine does not impair the formation of experimental granulation tissue [22], which corroborates well with clinical observations that cyclosporine treatment is not associated with healing disturbances.

Azathioprine and its combination with other drugs has not been studied in this respect (Table 2).

Table 2 Effects of Immunosuppressive Drugs on Wound Healing

Glucocorticosteroids delay healing by interfering with the monocyte-macrophage function; inhibiting the growth of new capillaries in the wound, leading to disturbed granulocyte and fibroblast function
Azathioprine suppresses cell proliferation, but has a weak effect on a healing wound
Cyclosporine does not have any direct negative effects on wound healing but may enhance it by activating macrophages

III. WOUND INFECTIONS IN RENAL TRANSPLANT RECIPIENTS

A. Primary Transplant Wound

Renal transplantation is classified as a clean, contaminated operation when the bladder is opened and urine is not infected and as a contaminated operation if urine is infected. The renal transplant recipient runs a high risk of infection, because of the uremic, malnourished state and immunosuppressive therapy; this is especially true if the primary transplant wound is reopened (reoperations or transplant nephrectomy) because the patient is at that time often on established immunosuppression. Wound infection is always a serious complication; in the renal transplant recipient it can be catastrophic, leading to a slowly healing open wound and, in the worst case, to infection of the arterial anastomosis and massive bleeding or to life-threatening sepsis.

In clean contaminated wounds, infection rates from 5 to 15% are commonly reported. Early reports of renal transplant wounds gave figures from 14 to 34%. Belzer et al. [23] reported an infection rate under 1% in primary wounds. We had an infection rate exceeding 10% in the 1970s; then more attention was given to this problem. At present the wound infection rate is around 3% (120-140 renal transplantations per year). In about 90% of cases *S. aureus* has been isolated from the infected wound; in the United States the most common causative agents are gram-negative bacteria.

Since wound infections have serious consequences in renal transplantation, proper measures, based on the understanding the basic biologic principles of wound healing, should be undertaken to prevent them. Attention must be directed to the patient's nutritional status, blood pressure must be brought under control, and clotting disorders should be corrected. This usually requires starting dialysis treatment before transplantation. Since obesity is a risk factor we do not accept overweight patients on our waiting list.

The cornerstone in prevention of wound infections is adequate surgical technique. Sharp dissection to minimize unnecessary tissue damage should be used. Complete control of hemostasis is necessary. The use of diathermy is a somewhat controversial issue. It causes certain damage to the surrounding tissue, but so is the case when forceps crushes the tissue and a ligature strangulates. As a rule of thumb, it can be said that a vessel with a diameter up to 2 mm can be controlled by diathermy; larger vessels should be ligated. It is definitely better to isolate the vessel and clamp and ligate it, than to cut and then clamp, since about five times more tissue is strangulated into the ligature in the latter case.

Because transplant recipients are immunosuppressed during the operation, it is generally agreed that prophylactic antibiotics should be used. The value of local antibiotics has been repeatedly proven [24]. Belzer et al. [25] uses bacitracin-neomycin solution; polymyxin could be added if *Pseudomonas* is the problem. Local antibiotics must always be combined with systemic antibiotics because antibiotics must be present in the surrounding tissue to combat bacterial invasion from the wound itself. Principles in the selection and use of systemic antibiotics are as follows:

Safe agent with low systemic and no nephrotoxicity
Activity against expected pathogens
Administer immediately preoperatively
Short course of one to three doses postoperatively.

The choice of suture materials for closing the wound is also of importance today, when a wide variety are available. Sutures made of natural fibers potentiate infection more than synthetic materials; this is well correlated with tissue reaction to them. Of absorbable multifilament sutures, polyglycolic and polyglactic acid elicit the least inflammatory response in tissue and are thus recommended for ligatures and suturing muscles and fascia. Polydioxanone is a monofilament synthetic absorbable suture, which in our hands has been shown to be well suited for constructing the anastomosis between ureter and bladder. Of the nonabsorbable materials nylon and polypropylene are the least reactive; the former is recommended for skin closure, the latter for vascular anastomosis. Interrupted sutures are recommended for skin closure; with a localized abscess in the wound, the whole length need not be opened. If glucocorticosteroids are used, sutures must be left in place for up to 2 weeks to avoid dehiscence. Stitch abscesses can develop when stitches are in place for so long. Stitches can be removed after a week and replaced by tapes. Tape closure can also be used primarily; this is known [26] to decrease the risk of infection, but they are tedious and difficult to use for primary closure of the wound. For wound dressing simple porous tape is adequate, although recent experimental evidence speaks for the use of occlusive dressings [27].

The use of drains merits a careful weighing of potential benefits and harmful effects. Sterile collections of blood are not major irritants to tissues, but hematomas enhance bacterial virulence [28]. Drains, as foreign material in wounds, impair resistance to infection. They also can act as a conduit for bacteria to invade. We do not routinely use any drains or splints in renal transplantation but rely on careful hemostasis, and we never accept a kidney in which blood vessels of the ureter seem to be compromised. If the reason for drainage arises, we use suction drainage for 12-24 hr.

B. Transplant Nephrectomy and Reoperations for Complications

Very high infection rates, 17-50%, have been reported in transplant nephrectomies [23,29]. The patients subjected to this operation are uremic, often mal-

[30] have described femoral neuropathy in adults who have undergone renal transplantation. We have similarly seen such femoral neuropathy in two patients. The neuropathy resolved. Although Vaziri et al. attributed this complication possibly to uremia or nerve compression, in our experience the neuropathy occurred after a prolonged cessation of arterial perfusion and thus may have been ischemic in origin.

E. Ocular Complications

Posterior subcapsular cataracts may occur in children with renal transplants. The incidence reported is extremely variable, 3.4-60% [28,31-34]. Though usually mild on occasion, cataract extraction may be required to obtain sufficient vision to facilitate school work [28,34]. The dose of steroids required during the first year appears to be a major determinant of cataract incidence and severity [31]. Other ophthalmologic abnormalities frequently seen in children postrenal transplantation include hypertensive retinopathy, associated with the high incidence of hypertension in this population group.

F. Hypertension

An extremely high incidence of hypertension is seen in children after renal transplantation [20,22,29,35-38]. Hypertension may be associated with the more technically difficult aspects of engraftment, resulting in areas of ischemia within the graft. Also, it has been suggested that the use of adult kidneys in small children may result in renal ischemia and thus contribute to the development of hypertension. The incidence of hypertension, up to 100%, commonly resolves with time and decreasing steroid dosage [39]. It is seen more commonly in patients who have undergone frequent rejection episodes, which may contribute to renal ischemia, and also those who have therefore required high-dose steroid therapy. Early hypertension can be secondary to fluid and sodium retention, acute tubular necrosis, acute rejection, or high-dose steroid therapy.

Hypertension can also be secondary to chronic rejection or renal artery stenosis. Renal artery stenosis is not uncommon and is a potentially correctable cause of hypertension [35,37]. Tunnel stenosis of the donor artery, possibly due to high perfusion pressure, has been reported with the use of kidneys from very young donors [4]. However, hypertension may occur in children posttransplantation who have no discernible cause of hypertension, that is, in the absence of arterial stenosis, rejection, or recurrent disease [40]. Hypertension may complicate the course of transplantation even in infants [41,42]. The phenomenon of hypertension in pediatric renal transplantation was investigated to determine whether the utilization of adult kidenys in children was a causative factor. Studies on transplantation of adult dog kidneys to puppies did not verify this thesis [43]. Hypertension is a common, as in adults, accompaniment of acute rejection and has resulted in convulsions [16] and death due to hypertensive encephalopathy [42]. Therefore, aggressive therapy is required when treating severe hypertension in pediatric patients. Viral myocarditis has occurred posttransplantation in two children [16].

G. Metabolic Complications

Endocrinologic abnormalities are uncommon in pediatric patients after renal transplantation. The majority of endocrinologic abnormalities are observed in patients with cystinosis. Because of progressive fibrosis and evolution of the thyroid gland in cystinotic patients, thyroid replacement therapy is commonly required [44,45]. Similarly in these patients, transient diabetes probably due to a similar phenomenon occurring in the pancreas, has been reported [16,45], although diabetes has also occurred in noncystinotic recipients [22]. Lipid abnormalities are also common in pediatric patients and reflect those seen in adult patients, that is, mainly type II or type IV hyperlipoproteinemia [46-50].

H. Liver Abnormalities

Hepatic complications of renal transplantation are mainly restricted to those involving infection acquired pre- or posttransplantation [51]. Recent indications that chronic hepatitis of A, B, or non-A, non-B origin may have deleterious consequences to patient survival posttransplantation raises the possibility that a similar phenomenon, although not yet reported, may be occurring in children [51]. Previous reports on the transplantation of pediatric patients with abnormalities of hepatic function are limited but have not to date indicated a deleterious outcome [52]. Fennell et al. [52] reported that, in 7 of 12 children who had elevated transaminase levels, enzyme levels returned to normal posttransplantation. Malekzadeh et al. noted an association between elevated enzyme levels and azathioprine therapy [53]. Hepatitis posttransplantation with a positive Australia antigen test [16,54] has also been described. Of eight patients, three had elevated transaminase levels associated with cytomegalovirus seroconversion [55].

I. Infection

Children are subject to all the same infectious complications seen in adults, and these are a major cause of death [29]. Thus cytomegalovirus infection [29,55], urinary tract infections [56,57], and others, so commonly seen in adults, are also seen in children. Rarer infections, such as that with mycobacterium, *Aspergillus fumigatus,* and *Histoplasma capsulatum,* have also been reported [6,29,58]. Varicella infection poses special problems in immunosuppressed children [44, 59]. It is necessary to stop azathioprine therapy while maintaining minimal steroid therapy in these children. The severe form of varicella infection may be complicated by prolonged fever, liver involvement, and thrombocytopenia and may be fatal. Recurrent varicella may occur. Zoster immune globulin should be administered to children at risk with renal transplantation who are exposed to varicella. As in adults, complicated cytomegalovirus versus infection has been noted in children [29,55]. Patients who have had splenectomy are at risk for pneumococcal sepsis [60] and thus require prophylactic antibiotherapy [61]. *Pneumocystis* has been a cause of death in pediatric patients [6,29]. The use of prophylactic sulfonamide therapy is effective in preventing infection with this organism [61]. Infections with *Nocardia asteroides* have [6,62] been reported. Fungal infections, systemic and involving the urinary tract, have occurred in children with transplants [57,63]. Urinary tract infection appears to be extremely common after transplantation in children who had end-stage renal disease of urologic origin [56]. Wound infection also appears common in this group. The use of prophylactic antibiotic therapy [64], although controversial [65], particularly in this group seems advisable.

J. Musculoskeletal Complications

The final height achieved by children who reach adulthood who receive renal transplants is approximately 3 standard deviations less than the mean [66]. Growth is usually better after successful engraftment than in patients on dialysis [16,67], but in general growth is still quite inadequate [68,69]. A major proportion of the height deficit is attributable to poor growth associated with chronic renal failure prior to dialysis or during chronic dialysis therapy [70]. Growth retardation may be substantial if renal failure is present in infancy [71].

Growth appears to be inversely related to skeletal maturation. Children with a bone age of less than 12 years at the time of transplant grow better than more mature children [70,72]. Inglefinger et al. [73] reported that 8 children aged less than 7 years at the time of transplant showed catch-up growth, whereas only 1 of 16 aged 7-11 years and none of 76 older than 11 years had accelerated growth. It is suggested that the apparently better growth in the children with a bone age of less than 12 years may be related in part to a greater degree of growth retardation in younger children. Posttransplantation growth is influenced by steroid dosage, adequacy of transplant function, and growth potential, the latter factor calculated from bone age, stature, and chronological age.

Low-dose prednisone (less than 0.2-0.3 mg/kg per day) is accompanied by better growth rates than is high-dose therapy. Alternate-day steroid therapy appears to be more conducive to normal growth rates, according to some studies [74-76]. However, others have shown no difference. Although such therapy has been suggested to be associated with an increased incidence of rejection, this has not been a problem in children [77].

Persistent phosphaturia with or without secondary hyperparathyroidism has been considered a contributory factor to growth retardation [23]. However, no relationship was noted between plasma phosphate levels and growth in a recent study on prepubertal children [78].

Aseptic necrosis of bone, especially in weight-bearing regions, is a frequent complication of renal transplantation and has been described in children [57,79]. Although usually involving the femoral head or condyle, it has also involved the tibial plateaus and tali [6,29,62]. Steroid-induced osteopenia, ischemia of bone due to fat embolism or vascular changes, persistent secondary hyperparathyroidism, and hypophosphatemia have been suggested as pathogenic factors [80].

Spontaneous fractures involving the femur and the ulna and vertebral compression fractures have also been observed in children posttransplantation [6,29, 57,62,81]. Slipped capital femoral epiphyses and femoral neck atrophy may also may also occur [6,62]. These fractures may be due to osteopenia induced by uremic bone disease following transplantation. Immunosuppressive therapy may also be a contributory or aggravating factor. Steroid-induced myopathy may complicate the recovery of children posttransplantation [16].

K. Malignant Tumors

Although the development of malignant tumors is a recognized complication of adult transplantation, a few, reported in pediatric patients, had reticulum cell sarcoma, lymphosarcoma, and dysgerminoma [82]. Patients as young as 5 years of age have had tumors [83]. Squamous cell carcinoma [2,84], hepatoblastoma [42], and lymphosarcoma [20] have also been reported. However, it has been suggested that the potentially longer life span of the pediatric patients theoretically increases the potential for development of malignancy [3].

L. Dermatologic Complications

Acne due to steroid therapy can be very distressful for the young transplanted patient. Dermatologic complications, such as warts, have also been observed in children [85]. One report describes an antibody-mediated bullous skin eruption caused by chronic allograft rejection [86]. The eruption resolved after graft removal.

M. Recurrence of Original Disease

Recurrence of the original renal disease that resulted in renal failure has been described in pediatric patients. Henoch-Schonlein purpura nephritis had been observed to recur in the transplant kidney and result in graft loss [82,87]. A recent report suggests that membranoproliferative glomerulonephritis type II, previously thought to follow a relatively benign course posttransplantation, may in fact result in a high incidence of graft loss [93]. The recurrence of membranoproliferative glomerulonephritis type I has been reported in transplants in 7 of 23 pediatric patients [94-99]. IgA nephropathy (Berger's disease) has also recurred in transplanted pediatric patients [100]. Focal segmental sclerosis can also recur in transplant kidneys [102]. The recurrence of membranous nephropathy, systemic lupus, and polyarteritis nodosa in adults, although not in children, has been reported.

Hemolytic uremic syndrome also has been reported to recur in the renal transplants of pediatric patients [103,104].

Although transplantation for primary oxalosis frequently results in graft loss, a successful long-term course can be achieved by the use of pyridoxine, neutral phosphate, noncalciuric diuretics, and a high fluid intake to minimize calcium oxalate deposition in the graft [105].

Cystinosis does not recur in the transplanted kidney although cystine accumulation may occur in mesangial cells of native origin [44].

N. Psychosocial Problems

Younger children appear to recover from the stress of operation better than teenagers. The latter group commonly suffer from a lack of self-esteem. Noncompliance is not uncommon among pediatric renal transplants [107]. In particular, girls may regard their appearance posttransplantation as repugnant, and this causes such problems in social relationships that they may not consider having a transplant worth the resulting psychic stress. They may then stop immunosuppressive therapy—the cause of their cushingoid appearance. They may also avoid clinic visits. Two patients have commited suicide posttransplantation [2]. Difficulties may also be encountered in returning the child to school, the child's reluctance stemming from short stature, scars, and cushingoid appearance [108, 109].

II. SURGICAL COMPLICATIONS

With increasing experience with kidney transplantation in children, its indications have been broadened and complications have become more apparent and are reported more frequently. The majority of surgical complications reported in adults are now observed and reported in children. Urologic complications are most frequent, followed by vascular complications.

A. Urologic Complications

Urologic complications are frequent and serious in children because of the increased incidence of obstructive uropathy as the cause of end-stage renal disease in this group. The incidence of this complication is estimated at around 30%

[110] and is comparable to that reported in adults, but in more recent reports this figure is decreasing [2,20].

Urinary leaks constitute the vast majority of urologic complications [2,22,57, 110]. Obstructive uropathy in the recipient and young age of the donor, as well as the cadaveric origin of the kidney, are contributing factors to the occurrence of ureteral and bladder leaks [22,111]. The leaks may come from the bladder, the ureter, and the calices and result from technical problems leading to ureteral tip necrosis, total ureteral necrosis, dislodgement of the ureteral anastomosis from the bladder, and reflux or obstructive uropathy. Surgical repair must be attempted as soon as possible, but the diagnosis may be delayed for a long period. Although the repair is more frequently successful than in adults, urinary leaks are still associated with an important mortality and morbidity rate [20], and removal of the transplant may be preferable to a tenuous urinary repair. Some authors have reported success with a nonsurgical approach [57,112].

Obstructive ureteral complications have been reported in children [20] and result usually from improper ureteral reimplanatation or from ischemia of the ureter leading to stricture or external compression. Transplanted kidneys are usually followed by ultrasonography; if cortical atrophy is noted to be progressing or the renal function is deteriorating, surgical repair is indicated. This complication responds to ureteral reimplantation or endoscopic dilatation. Ureteropelvic obstruction may be present in the donor and can become evident after transplantation. It sometimes requires surgical repair.

Ureteral necrosis and obstruction at the level of the pelvic brim has been reported by Lawson et al. [28], due to compression by a large adult kidney placed intraperitoneally in a small child. The ureter was posterior to the kidney and compressed against the pelvic brim when the abdomen was closed tightly.

Vesicoureteral reflux, in either the transplanted or the autogenous ureter, is a serious complication and needs surgical correction if there is a progressive dilatation of the urinary tract or intractable urinary infection. Calculi developed in 5% of Warshaw's patients [20] and were removed surgically. Urinary incontinence was present in one patient of the same series and did not respond to surgical treatment.

A special case must be made of the utilization of defunctionalized bladder for ureteral reimplantation. Salvatierra et al. have emphasized that ureteral integrity depends on adequate blood supply derived from the perihilar fatty tissue [113]. Therefore the frequency of ureteral leaks would not be expected to be higher in patients with abnormal lower urinary tract. The present tendency is to use the patient's own bladder even if it had been defunctionnalized, repeatedly infected, or subjected to numerous operations [20,114-116]. The indications for urinary diversion are limited to patients with neurogenic bladder, previous cystectomy, anomalies of the cloaca type, and documented daytime urinary incontinence. More recently, Gonzalez et al. [117] have emphasized the

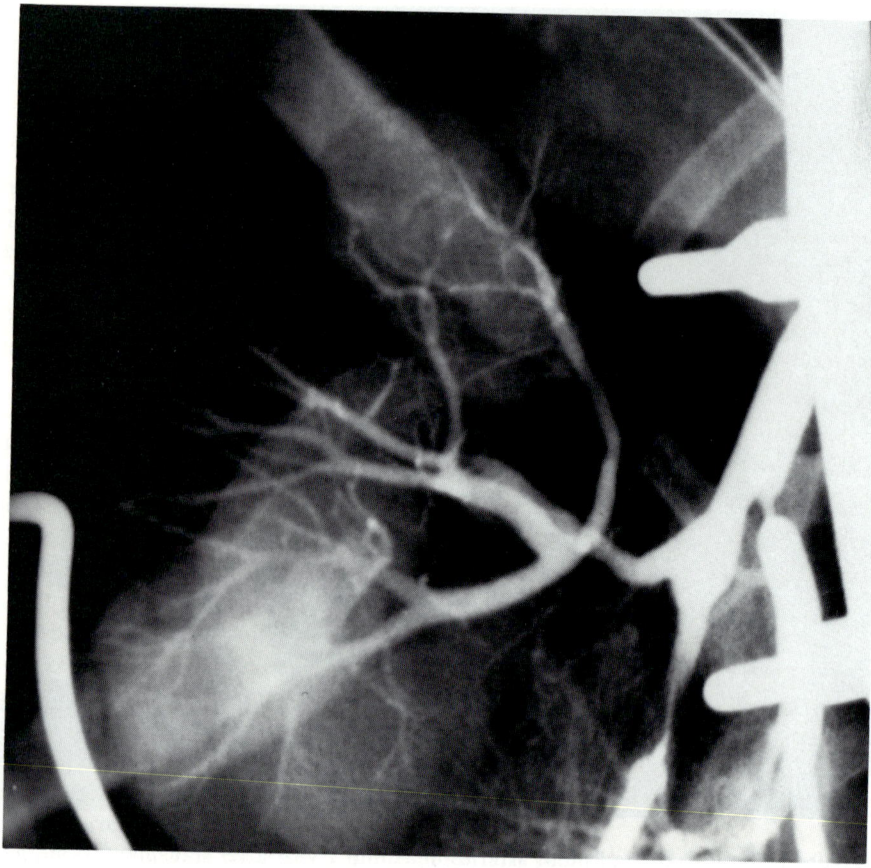

Figure 2 After transluminal angioplasty, blood pressure normalized, blood urea nitrogen fell to 18 mg/dl, and plasma creatinine to 0.9 mg/dl.

to adhesions because of previous intra-abdominal operations or because of the necessary transperitoneal approach in small children.

Pancreatitis is reported in children and may be lethal [4]. Large doses of steroids and hyperparathyroidism are clear predisposing factors to this complication. In most cases, pancreatitis in the transplant patient is mild and responds well to medical treatment. The doses of prednisone should be decreased in these patients.

REFERENCES

1. Miller, L. C., Lum, C. T., Bock, G. H., Simmons, R. L., Najarian, J. S., and Mauer, S. M.: Transplantation of the adult kidney into the very small child. Am. J. Surg. 145:243, 1983.
2. Najarian, J. S., Mauer, S. M., and Howard, R. J.: Kidney transplantation. In: Ravitch, M. M., Welsh, K. J., Benson, C. D., Aberdeen, E., and Randolph, J. G., eds., Pediatric Surgery, Vol. 2, Chap. 116, pp. 1293, Chicago: Year Book Medical Publishers, 1979.
3. Arbus, G. S., Hardy, B. E., Balfe, J. W., Churchill, B. M., Steele, B. T., Baumal, R., and Curtis, R. N.: Cadaveric renal transplants in children under 6 years of age. Kidney Int. 24:S111, 1983.
4. Trompeter, R. S., Haycock, G. B., Bewick, M., and Chantler, C.: Renal transplantation in very young children. Lancet 1:373, 1983.
5. Herrin, J. T.: Pediatric renal transplantation. Kidney Int. 18:519, 1980.
6. Lilly, J. R., Giles, G., Hurwitz, R., Schroter, G., Takagi, H., Gray, S., Penn, I., Halgrimson, C. G., and Starzl, T. E.: Renal homotransplantation in pediatric patients. Pediatrics 47:548, 1971.
7. Better, O. S.: Tubular dysfunction following kidney transplantation. Nephron 25:209:1980.
8. Vaziri, N. D., Nellans, R. E., Brueggemann, R. M., Barton, C. H., and Martin, D. C.: Renal tubular dysfunction in transplanted kidneys. South. Med. J. 72:530, 1979.
9. Wilson, D. R., and Siddiqui, A. A.: Renal tubular acidosis after kidney transplantation. Ann. Intern. Med. 79:352, 1973.
10. Battle, D. C., Mozes, M. F., Manaligod, J., Arruda, J. A. L., and Kurtzman, N. A.: The pathogenesis of hyperchloremic metabolic acidosis associated with kidney transplantation. Am. J. Med. 70:786, 1981.
11. Mookerjee, B., Gault, M. H., and Dossetor, J. B.: Hyperchloremic acidosis in early diagnosis of renal allograft rejection. Ann. Intern. Med. 71:47, 1969.
12. Wilson, D. R., and Siddiqui, A. A.: Renal tubular acidosis after kideny transplantation. Natural history and significance. Ann. Intern. Med. 79: 352, 1973.
13. Better, O. S., Chaimowitz, C., Navey, Y., et al.: Syndrome of incomplete renal tubular acidosis after cadaver kidney transplantation. Ann. Intern. Med. 71:39, 1968.
14. Briggs, W. A., Kommami, N., Wilson, R. E., and Merrill, J. P.: Kidney transplantation in Fanconi syndrome. N. Engl. J. Med. 286:25, 1972.
15. Friedman, A., and Chesney, R.: Fanconi's syndrome in renal transplantation. Am. J. Nephrol. 1:45, 1981.
16. Chantler, C., Carter, J. E., Bewick, M., Counahan, R., Cameron, J. S., Ogg, C. S., Williams, D. G., and Winder, E.: 10 years experience with regular hemodialysis and renal transplantation. Arch. Dis. Child. 55:434, 1980.

17. Hutcheon, R. A., Kaplan, B. S., and Drummond, K. N.: Distal renal tubular acidosis in children with chronic hydronephrosis. J. Pediatr. 89:372, 1976.
18. Parfitt, A. M.: Hypercalcemic hyperparathyroidism following renal transplantation: Differential diagnosis, management, and implications for cell population control in the parathyroid gland. Min. Electrolyte Metab. 8:92, 1982.
19. Diethelm, A. G., Edwards, R. P., and Whelchel, J. D.: The natural history and surgical treatment of hypercalcemia before and after renal transplantation. Surg. Gynecol. Obstet. 154:481, 1982.
20. Warshaw, B. L., Edelbrock, H. H., Ettenger, R. B., Malekzadeh, M. H., Pennisi, A. J., Uittenbogaart, C. H., and Fine, R. N.: Renal transplantation in children with obstructive uropathy. J. Urol. 123:737, 1980.
21. Moorhead, J. F., Ahmed, K. Y., Varghese, Z., Wills, M. R., Baillod, R. A., and Tatler, G. L. V.: Hypophosphataemic osteomalacia after cadaveric renal transplantation. Lancet 1:694, 1974.
22. Fine, R. N., Korsch, B. M., Stiles, Q., Riddell, H., Edelbrock, H. H., Brennan, L. P., Grushkin, C. M., and Lieberman, E.: Renal homotransplantation in children. J. Pediatr. 76:347, 1970.
23. Ingelfinger, J. R.: Factors affecting growth following renal transplantation in childhood. Dial. Transplant. 11:1075, 1982.
24. Frei, D., Guttmann, R. D., and Gorman, P.: A matched-pair control study of postrenal transplant polycythemia. Am. J. Kidney Dis. 11:36, 1982.
25. Ianhez, L. E., DaFanseca, J. A., Chocair, P. R., Maspes, V., and Sabbaga, E.: Polycythemia after kidney transplantation. Urol. Int. 32:382, 1977.
26. Schramek, A., Adller, O., Hashimonai, M., Better, O. S., and Tuma, S.: Hypertensive crisis, erythrocytosis, and uraemia due to renal-artery stenosis of kidney transplants. Lancet 1:70:1975.
27. Dagher, F. J., Ramos, E., Ersler, A. J., Alongi, S. V., Karmi, S. A., and Caro, J.: Are the native kidneys responsible for erythrocytosis in renal allorecipients. Transplantation 28:496, 1979.
28. Lawson, R. K., Talwalkar, Y. B., Musgrave, J. E., Campbell, R. A., and Hodges, C. V.: Renal transplantation in pediatric patients. J. Urol. 113:225, 1975.
29. Najarian, J. S., Simmons, R. L., Tallem, M. B., Kjellstrand, C. M., Buselmeier, T. J., Vernier, R. L., and Michael, A. F.: Renal transplantation in infants and children. Ann. Surg. 174:583, 1971.
30. Vaziri, N. D., Barton, C. H., Ravikumar, G. R., Martin, D. C., Ness, R., and Saiki, J.: Femoral neuropathy: A complication of renal transplantation. Nephron 28:30, 1981.
31. Fine, R. N., Offner, G., Wilson, W. A., Mickey, M. R., Pennisi, A. J., and Malekzadeh, M. H.: Posterior subcapsular cataracts in renal transplantation. Ann. Surg. 182:585, 1975.
32. Belzer, F. O., Schweitzer, R. T., and Holliday, M.: Renal homotransplantation in children. Am. J. Surg. 124:270, 1972.
33. Cerrili, J., Evans, W. E., and Satoz, F. F.: Renal transplantation in infants and children. Transplant. Proc. 4:633, 1972.

34. Lawson, R. K., Campbell, R. A., and Hodges, C. V.: Renal transplantation in infants and small children. Transplant. Proc. 3:358, 1970.
35. Ingelfinger, J. R., Lazarus, J. M., Levey, R. H., Lowrie, E. G., Topar, M., and Grupe, W. E.: Hypertension in pediatric renal transplant patients. Pediatr. Res. 9:376, 1976.
36. Laplante, M. P., Kaufman, J. J., and Goldman, R.: Kidney transplantation in children. Pediatrics 46:665, 1970.
37. Malekzadeh, M. H., Brennan, L. P., Payne, V. C., and Fine, R. N.: Hypertension after renal transplantation in children. J. Pediatr. 86:370, 1975.
38. Fine, R. N., Edelbrock, H. H., Brennan, L. P., Grushkin, C. M., Korsch, B. M., Riddell, H., Stiles, Q., and Lieberman, E.: Cadaveric renal transplantation in children. Lancet 1:1087, 1971.
39. Jacquot, C.. Idatte, J. M., Bednorsian, J., Weiss, Y., Safor, M., and Bariety, J.: Long term blood pressure changes in renal homotransplantation. Arch. Intern. Med. 138:233, 1978.
40. Ingelfinger, J. R., Grupe, W. E., and Levey, R.: Post-transplant hypertension in the absence of rejection or recurrent disease. Clin. Nephrol. 15:236, 1981.
41. Rizzochi, G., Malekzadeb, M. H., Pennissi, A. J., Ettenger, R. B., Uittengogaart, C. H., and Fine, R. N.: Renal transplantation in children less than 5 years of age. Arch. Dis. Child. 55:532, 1980.
42. Moel, D. I., and Butt, K. M. H.: Renal transplantation in children less than 2 years of age. J. Pediatr. 99:535, 1981.
43. Inglefinger, J. R., and Caldicott, W. J. H.: Cardiovascular function in pups receiving allografts from adult dogs. Pediatr. Res. 15:935, 1981.
44. Langlois, R. P., O'Regan, S., Pelletier, M., and Robitaille, P.: Kidney transplantation in uremic children with cystinosis. Nephron 28:273, 1981.
45. Broyer, M., Donckerwolcke, R. A., Brunner, F. P.. Brynger, H., Jacobs, C., Kramer, P., Selwood, N. H., Wing, A. J., and Blake, P. H.: Combined report on regular dialysis and transplantation of children in Europe, 1980. Proc. Eur. Dial. Transplant. Assoc. 18:60, 1981.
46. Broyer, M., Tete, M.-J., Laudat, M.-H., and Goldstein, S.: Plasma lipids in kidney transplanted children and adolescents: Influence of pubertal development, dietary intake and steroid therapy. Eur. J. Clin. Invest. 11:397, 1981.
47. Pennisi, A. J., Heuser, E. T., Mickey, M. R., Lipsey, A., Malekzadeh, M. H., and Fine, R. N.: Hyperlipidemia in pediatric hemodialysis and renal transplant patients. Am. J. Dis. Child. 130:957, 1976.
48. Saldanha, L. F., Hurst, K. S., Amend, J. C., Lazarus, J. M., Lowrie, E. G., Ingelfinger, J., Grupe, W., and Levey, R.: Hyperlipidemia after renal transplantation in children. Am. J. Dis. Child. 130:951, 1976.
49. Ibels, L. S., Alfrey, A. C., and Weil, R.: Hyperlipidemia in adult, pediatric and diabetic renal transplant recipients. Am. J. Med. 64:634, 1978.
50. El-Bishti, M., Counahan, R., Jarrett, R. J., Stimmler, L., Wass, V., and Chantler, C.: Hyperlipidaemia in children on regular haemodialysis. Arch. Dis. Child. 52:932, 1977.
51. Parfrey, P. S., Forbes, R. D. C., Hutchinson, T. A., Beaudoin, J. G., Dauphi-

nee, W. D., Hollomby, D. J., and Guttman, R. D.: The clinical and pathological course of hepatitis B liver disease in renal transplant recipients. Transplantation 37:461, 1984.
52. Fennell, R. S., III, Andres, J. M., Plaff-William, W., and Richard, G. A.: Liver dysfunction in children and after renal transplantation. Pediatrics 67: 855, 1981.
53. Malekzadeh, M. H., Grushkin, C. M., Wright, H. T., Jr., and Fine, R. N.: Hepatic dysfunction after renal transplantation in children. J. Pediatr. 81: 279, 1972.
54. Henriksson, C., Jorgen Andersen, H., Gustafsson, A., and Gelin, L.-E.: Renal transplantation in children. Acta Paediatr. Scand. 64:833, 1975.
55. Fine, R. N., Grushkin, C. M., Malekzadeh, M., and Wright, H. T., Jr.: Cytomegalovirus syndrome following renal transplantation. Arch. Surg. 105:564, 1972.
56. Krieger, J. N., Stubenbord, W. T., and Darracott Vaughan, E., Jr.: Transplantation in children with end stage renal disease of urologic origin. J. Urol. 124:508, 1980.
57. Fennell, R. S., III, Garin, E. H., Pfaff, W., Brient, B., Iravani, A., Walker, R. D., and Richard, G. A.: Renal transplantation in children and adolescents. Clin. Pediatr. 18:518, 1979.
58. Lichtenstein, I. H., and MacGregor, R. R.: Mycobacterial infections in renal transplant recipients: Report of five cases and review of the literature. Infect. Dis. 5:216, 1983.
59. Feldhoff, C. M., Balfour, H. H., Jr., Simmons, R. L., Najarian, J. S., and Mauer, S. M.: Varicella in children with renal transplants. J. Pediatr. 98:25, 1981.
60. Hodson, E. M., Najarian, J. S. Kjellstrand, C. M., Simmons, R. L., and Mauer, S. M.: Renal transplantation in children ages 1 to 5 years. Pediatrics 61:458, 1978.
61. Mauer, S. M., and Howard. R. J.: Renal transplantation in children. In: Edelman, C. M., ed., Pediatric Kidney Disease, vol. 1, Chap. 36, Boston: Little, Brown, 1978, p. 518.
62. Fine, R. N., and Grushkin, C. M.: Hemodialysis and renal transplantation in children. Clin. Nephrol. 1:243, 1973.
63. Rifkind, D., Marchioro, T. L., Schneck, S. A., and Hill, R. B., Jr.: Systemic fungal infections complicating renal transplantation and immunosuppressive therapy. Am. J. Med. 43:28, 1973.
64. Peters, C., Peterson, P., Marabella, P., Simmons, R. L., and Najarian, J. S.: Continuous sulfa prophylaxis for urinary tract infection in renal transplant recipients. Am. J. Surg. 146:589, 1983.
65. Griffin, P. J. A., and Salaman, J. R.: Urinary tract infections after renal transplantation: Do they matter? Br. Med. J. 1:710, 1979.
66. Chantler, C., Broyer, M., Donckerwolcke R. A., Brynger, H., Brunner, F. P., Jacobs, C., Kramer, P., Selwood, N. H., and Wing, A. J.: Growth and rehabilitation of long-term survivors of treatment for end-stage renal failure in childhood. Proc. Eur. Dial. Transplant. Assoc. 18:329, 1981.

67. Donkerwolcke, R. A., Chantler, C., Broyer, M., Brunner, F. P., Brynger, H., Jacobs, C., Kramer, P., Selwood, N. H., and Wing, A. J.: Combined report or regular dialysis and transplantation of children in Europe, 1979. Proc. Eur. Dial. Transplant. Assoc. 17:87, 1980.
68. Fine, R. N., Malekzadeh, M. H., Pennisi, A. J., Ettenger, R. B., Uittenbogaart, C. H., Negrete, V. F., and Korsch, B. M.: Long-term results of renal transplantation in children. Pediatrics 61:641, 1978.
69. Travis, L. B., Chesney, R., McEnery, P., Moel, D., Pennisi, A., Potter, D., Talwalkar, Y. B., and Wolff, E.: Growth and glucocorticoids in children with kidney disease. Kidney Int. 14:365, 1978.
70. Jones, R. W. A., Bishti, M., and Chantler, C.: The promotion of anabolism in children with chronic renal failure. In: Wharton, B. A., ed., Nutrition in Children. Proceedings of the Pediatric Conference of the Royal College of Physicians 1979, Topics in Pediatrics, vol. 2, Tunbridge Wells: Pitman Medical, 1980, pp. 90-109.
71. Jones, R. W. A., Rigden, S. P., Barrett, T. M., and Chantler, C.: The effects of chronic renal failure in infancy on growth, nutritional status, and body composition. Pediatr. Res. 16:784, 1982.
72. Grushkin, C. M., and Fine, R. N.: Growth in children following renal transplantation. Am. J. Dis. Child. 125:514, 1973.
73. Ingelfinger, J. R., Grupe, W. E., Harmon, W. E., Feinback, S. K., and Levey, R. H.: Growth acceleration following renal transplantation in children less than 7 years of age. Pediatrics 68:255, 1981.
74. Potter, D. E., Holliday, M. A., Wilson, C. J., Salvatierra, O., Jr., and Belzar, F. O.: Alternate day steroids in children after renal transplantation. Transplant. Proc. 7:79, 1975.
75. McEnery, P. T., Gonzalez, L. L., Martin, L. W., and West, C. D.: Growth and development of children with renal transplants. Use of alternate day steroid therapy. J. Pediatr. 813:806, 1973.
76. Hoda, Q., Hasinoff, D. J., and Arbus, G. S.: Growth following renal transplantation in children and adolescents. Clin. Nephrol. 3:6, 1975.
77. Brietenfield, R. V., Hebert, L. A., Lemann, J., Jr., Piering, W. F., Kauffman, H. M., Sampson, D., Kalbfleisch, J., and Beres, J. A.: Stability of renal transplant function with alternate-day corticosteroid therapy. JAMA 244:151, 1980.
78. Bosque, M., Munian, A., Bewick, M., Haycock, G., and Chantler, C.: Growth after renal transplants. Arch. Dis. Child. 58:110, 1983.
79. Nielsen, H. E., Melsen, F., and Christensen, M. S.: Aseptic necrosis of bone following renal transplantation. Acta Med. Scand. 202: 1977.
80. Squifflet, J. P., Pirson, Y., Van Cangh, P., Otte, J. B., Van Ypersele de Strihou, C., and Alexandre, G. P. J.: Renal transplantation in children. Transplantation 32:278, 1981.
81. Nielsen, H. E., Melsen, F., and Christensen, M. S.: Spontaneous fractures following renal transplantation. Min. Electrolyte Metab. 2:323, 1979.
82. Antone, S.: Clinical aspects of kidney transplantation in children. In: Rubin,

M. I., and Barrett, R. M., eds., Pediatric Nephrology, Chap. 4, Baltimore: Williams & Wilkins, 1975, pp. 877.
83. Penn, I.: Malignant lymphomas in organ transplant recipients. Transplant. Proc. 13:736, 1981.
84. Caterson, R. J., Furber, J., Murray, J., McCarthy, W., Mahony, J. F., and Sheil, A. G. R.: Carcinoma of the vulva in two young renal allograft recipients. Transplant. Proc. 16:559, 1984.
85. Ingelfinger, J. R., Grupe, W. E., Topar, M., and Levey, R. H.: Warts in a pediatric renal transplant population. Dermatologica 155:7, 1977.
86. Feehally, J., Reilly, D. T., Walls, J., and Wood, R. F. M.: An antibody-mediated bullous skin eruption caused by chronic renal allograft rejection. Transplantation 34:295, 1982.
87. Baliah, T., Kim, K. H., Anthone, S., Anthone, R., Montes, M., and Andres, G. A.: Recurrence of Henoch-Schonlein purpura glomerulonephritis in transplanted kidneys. Transplantation 18:343, 1974.
88. Cameron, J. S.: Glomerulonephritis in renal transplants. Transplantation 34:237, 1982.
89. Levy, M., Ami Moussa, R., Habib, R., Gagnadoux, M. F., and Broyer, M.: Anaphylactoid purpura nephritis and transplantation (abstract). Kidney Int. 22:326, 1982.
90. Sakai, T., Tanaka, T., and Kasai, N.: Recurrence of Henoch-Schonlein purpura glomerulonephritis in transplanted kidney (abstract). International Congress of Nephrology, Florence, 1975.
91. Weiss, J. H., Bhathena, D. B., Curtis, J. J., Lucas, B. A., and Luke, R. G.: A possible relationship between Henoch-Schonlein syndrome and IgA nephropathy (Berger's disease). An illustrative case. Nephron 22:582, 1978.
92. Bar-On, H., and Rosenmann, E.: Schonlein-Henoch syndrome in adults. A clinical and histological study of renal involvement. Isr. J. Med. Sci. 8:1702, 1972.
93. Eddy, A., Sibley, R., Mauer, S. M., and Kim, Y.: Renal allograft failure due to recurrent dense intramembranous deposit disease. Clin. Nephrol. 21:305, 1984.
94. Broyer, M., Gagnadoux, M. F., Beurton, D., Pascal, B., and Louville, J.: Transplantation in children: Technical aspects, drug therapy and problems related to primary renal disease. Proc. Eur. Dial. Transplant. Assoc. 18:313, 1981.
95. Curtis, J. J., Wyatt, R. J., Bhathena, D., Lucas, B. A., Holland, N. H., and Luke, R. G.: Renal transplantation for patients with type I and type II membranoproliferative glomerulonephritis. Serial complement and nephritic factor measurements and the problem of recurrence of disease. Am. J. Med. 66:216, 1979.
96. Levy, M., and Arsan, A.: Récidive de la maladie originale sur le rein transplanté. Semin. Nephrol. Pediatr. (Paris), March 6-7, 1978.
97. McLean, R. H., Geiger, H., Burke, B., Simmons, R., Najarian, J., Vernier, R. L., and Michael, A. F.: Recurrence of membranoproliferative glomerulo-

nephritis following kidney transplantation. Serum complement component studies. Am. J. Med. 60:60, 1976.
98. Zimmerman, S. W., Hyman, L. R., Uehling, D. T., and Burkholder, P. M.: Recurrent membranoproliferative glomerulonephritis with glomerular properdin deposition in allografts. Ann. Intern. Med. 80:169, 1974.
99. Brinere, J.: Glomerular lesions in renal allografts. Adv. Intern. Med. 49: 1, 1982.
100. Berger, J., Yaneva, H., Nabarra, B., and Barbanel, C.: Recurrence of mesangial deposition of IgA after renal transplantation. Kidney Int. 7:232, 1975.
101. Mathew, T. H., Mathews, D. C., Hobbs, J. B., and Kincaid-Smith, P.: Glomerular lesions after renal transplantation. Am. J. Med. 59:177, 1975.
102. Ettenger, R. B., Heuser, E. T., Malekzadeh, M. H., Pennisi, A. J., Uittenbogaart, C. H., and Fine, R. N.: Focal glomerulosclerosis in renal allografts. Association with the nephrotic syndrome and chronic rejection. Am. J. Dis. Child. 131:1347, 1977.
103. Cerelli, G. J., Nelsen, C., and Dorfmann, L.: Renal homotransplantation in infants and children with the hemolytic-uremic syndrome. Surgery 71:66, 1972.
104. Folmann, R., Arbus, G. S., Churchill, B., Gaum, L., and Huber, J.: Recurrence of the hemolytic uremic syndrome in a 3½-year-old child, 4 months after second renal transplantation. Clin. Nephrol. 10:121, 1978.
105. Scheinman, J. I., Najarian, J. S., and Mauer, S. M.: Successful strategies for renal transplantation in primary oxalosis. Kidney Int. 25:804, 1984.
106. DeShazo, C. V., Simmons, R. L., Bernstein, D. M., DeShazo, M. M., Willment, J., Kjellstrand, C. M., and Najarian, J. S.: Results of renal transplantation in 100 children. Surgery 76:461, 1974.
107. Korsch, B. M., Fine, R. N., and Negrete, V. F.: Noncompliance in children with renal transplants. Pediatrics 61:872, 1978.
108. Bernstein, D. M.: After transplantation the child's emotional reactions. Am. J. Psychiatry 172:109, 1971.
109. Malekzadeh, M. H., Pennesi, A. J., Uittenbogaart, C. H., Korsch, B. M., Fine, R. N., and Main, M. E.: Current issues in pediatric renal transplantation. Pediatr. Clin. North Am. 23:857, 1976.
110. Edelbrock, H. H., Riddel, H., Mickelson, J. C., Grushkin, C. M., Leberman, E., and Fine, R. N.: Urologic aspects of renal transplantation in children. J. Urol. 106:934, 1971.
111. Fine, R. N., Brennan, L. P., Edelbrock, H. H., Riddell, H., Stiles, Q., and Lieberman, E.: Use of pediatric cadaver kidneys of homotransplantation in children. JAMA 210:477, 1969.
112. Desai, S. G., McRoberts, J. W., Hellebusch, A. A., and Luke, R. G.: Conservative non-operative management of ureteral fistulas following renal allografts. J. Urol. 112:572, 1974.
113. Salvatierra, O., Jr., Kountz, S. L., and Belzer, F. O.: Prevention of ureteral fistula after renal transplantation. J. Urol. 1122:445, 1974.

114. Firlit, C.: Use of defunctionalized bladders in pediatric renal transplantation. J. Urol. 116:634, 1976.
115. Cerilli, J., Anderson, G. W., Evans, W. E., and Smith, J. P.: Renal transplantation in patients with urinary tract abnormalities. Surgery 79:248, 1976.
116. Tunner, W. S., Whitsell, J. C., II, Rubin, A. L., Stenzel, K. H., Davis, D. S., Riggio, R. R., Schwartz, G. H., and Marshall, V. F.: Renal transplantation in children with corrected abnormalities of lower urinary tract. J. Urol. 106:133, 1971.
117. Gonzalez, R., Lapointe, S., Sheldon, C. A., and Mauer, M. S.: Undiversion in children with renal failure. J. Pediatr. Surg. 19:632, 1984.
118. Beckerhoff, R., Uhllschmid, G., and Vetter, W.: Plasma renin and aldosterone after renal transplantation. Kidney Int. 5:39, 1974.
119. Grossman, R. A., Dafoe, D. C., Shoenfeld, R. B., Ring, E. J., Maclean, G. K., Oleaga, J. A., Freiman, D. B., Najia, Perloff, L. J., and Barker, C. F.: Percutaneous transluminal angioplasty treatment of renal transplant artery stenosis. Transplantation 6:339, 1982.
120. Sniderman, K. W., Sprayregen, S., and Sos, T. A.: Percutaneous transluminal dilatation in renal transplant artery stenosis. Transplantation 30:440, 1980.
121. Rao, K. V., Smith, E. J., Alexander, J. W., Fidler, J. P., Pemmaruju, S. R., and Pollack, V. E.: Thromboembolic disease in renal allograft recipients. Arch. Surg. 111:1086, 1976.
122. Yazbeck, S., and O'Regan, S.: Microsurgery for Brescia-Cimino fistula construction in pediatric patients. Nephron 38:109, 1984.
123. Burleson, R. L., and Marbarger, P. D.: Prevention of lymphocele formation following renal allotransplantation. J. Urol. 127:18, 1982.
124. Poisson, J., Le Guillou, M., Scetbon, V., Leroux-Robert, C. E., and Küss, R.: Rupture spontanée du rein allotransplanté. J. Urol. Nephrol. 7-8:575, 1973.
125. Henriksson, C., Andersen, H. J., Gustafsson, A., and Gelin, L. E.: Renal transplantation in children. Acta Paediatr. Scand. 64:833, 1975.

6

Kidney Transplantation: Infectious Complications

FRANK E. CHECK, JR., BERNARD H. RAVITZ, and
LEONARD C. ALEXANDER
Mount Carmel Mercy Hospital, Detroit, Michigan

A recent prospective study identified infection requiring hospitalization in approximately one-third of renal allograft recipients over a 4-year period [1]. Of these episodes, 50% were associated with a viral etiology, 30% bacterial, 16% polymicrobial, and 3% fungal [1]. Multiple factors, including geographic location, determine the specific type of infecting agents, and each transplant program tends to have variability among the types of infections reported [2]. Alterations of host defense mechanisms secondary to immunosuppressive therapy appear to play the major role in the development of such infections. This chapter is not a complete review of the literature but rather a selective view of renal transplant (RT)-associated infections with emphasis on clinical relevance.

Rifkind et al. in a 1967 editorial implicated high-dose steroid therapy in the pathogenesis of RT infections and suggested that utilization of antilymphocyte globulin (ALG) might ameliorate this problem [3]. Randomly, retrospectively selected records from 40 RT patients from our institution from 1973 to 1981 revealed a statistically significant lesser number of bacterial isolates (including wound, urine, sputum, and blood) and less mortality at 30 and 60 days post-transplant in the steroid-ALG-treated group versus the higher dose steroid-treated group without ALG therapy. A decline in infectious related deaths in patients treated with ALG in a controlled fashion has been described [4]. Eickhoff and associates demonstrated a relationship between "high-dose" prednisone therapy and hyperglycemia with lethal infectious complications [5]. Lymphocytopenia and monocytopenia are reproducible phenomena following steroid therapy and result in a neutrophilic leukocytosis [6]. Thus the white blood cell (WBC) and differential count may not be helpful in assessing the possibility of infection. In most current immunosuppressive regimens humoral responses are preserved [7] and T-cell lymphocytic functions are depressed [8]. Thus, one can expect some magnitude of antibody responsiveness in this group of patients despite cellular derangements. The cyclic fungal polypeptide cyclosporine alters helper and effector T cells and NK (natural killer) cells [9]. More recently, cyclosporine treatment was associated with a decreased incidence of cytomegalovirus disease [1].

The role of the polymorphonuclear leukocyte is very important since an absolute decrease in this cell line [10] and chemotactic defects [11] are probably important in the pathogenesis of infections. Golshan et al. demonstrated that depressed granulocytic adherence early postoperatively and at the time of rejection crises was the major defect in granulocytic function in RT patients [12]. Chemotactic activity improved progressively posttransplantation despite immunosuppression and was supranormal during rejection crises [12]. Phagocytosis was enhanced early postoperatively and during rejection crises [12]. Bactericidal activity, interestingly, was unaffected in RT recipients of live related donors but depressed in recipients of cadaveric kidneys [12]. Appreciating the inherent difficulties in performing these studies, the decrease of granulocyte adherence must be considered a risk factor of infection especially at peak times of steroid administration. The presence of multifactorial alterations of host defense mechanisms make simplistic explanations of the increased risk of infection in RT recipients untenable.

I. VIRAL INFECTIONS

Peterson et al. reviewed 194 episodes of fever in 433 RT recipients, and 55% of these episodes were related to viral agents, especially cytomegalovirus (CMV) [13]. Concomitant infections with both CMV and either Epstein-Barr virus (EBV) or varicella zoster virus (VZV) has also been noted [1]. VZV and herpes simplex virus also are frequently responsible for clinical disease in this type of patient.

A. Cytomegalovirus

In the series of Peterson et al., 87% of CMV disease developed within the first 3 months of transplantation [1]. The source of CMV may include latent virus in the hematopoietic system or other organs of the RT recipient, exogenous blood [14], and possibly latent virus in the transplanted kidney [15]. Cocultivation techniques by Naraqi et al., however, were unable to detect latent CMV in renal tissue allografts [16]. Whether serological status has a bearing on the severity of disease is not completely clear, although some believe seronegative recipients have more symptomatic disease [17]. Simmons et al. previously commented on two clinical syndromes associated with CMV infection: (1) fever, leukopenia, and renal dysfunction were associated with normal in vitro lymphocyte function, the development of antibody to the virus, typically findings of cellular rejection at kidney biopsy, the absence of any plasma factor suppressive for immune function, and spontaneous recovery from this illness; and (2) a second, smaller group of patients with fever, leukopenia, renal dysfunction, absence of CMV antibody response (diagnosis made by viral isolation), presence of a plasma suppressive factor, depressed lymphocyte function, progressive disease with bacterial, protozoal, and/or fungal superinfection, extensive gastrointestinal hemorrhage, and death as the usual outcome [18]. Fiala et al. have described stabbing arthralgias of knees, hips, ankles, sacroiliac joints, and wrists associated with active CMV infection [19]. Luby et al. have implicated CMV with hepatic function abnormalities after renal transplant. These abnormalities have occasionally persisted in some patients beyond 120 days [20]. CMV is most commonly isolated from the urine, frequently from oropharyngeal secretions and less commonly from the blood [21]. Pass et al. demonstrated CMV shedding in 76% of recipients of cadaver kidneys 16 days posttransplant, but in only 33% of recipients of living, related donor kidneys [21]. They have also demonstrated increased risk of morbidity due to CMV in RT patients who receive both a poorly matched graft and antithymocyte globulin [22]. Richardson et al. reported that CMV may result in acute renal allograft dysfunction related to a diffuse glomerulopathy distinct from the usual histopathologic pattern of rejection [23]. If clinically significant CMV infection is present, strong consideration should be given to decreasing or discontinuing immunosuppression [24], and secondary bacterial and/or protozoal invaders should be sought and promptly treated [17]. Currently there is no uniformly effective antiviral agent against CMV, although studies continue with a guanosine analog similar to acyclovir [25]. Ideally, prevention of CMV disease should be the goal. A live attentuated vaccine, Towne-125, can induce a CMV-specific immune response, but this vaccine was unable to prevent reinfection with different strains of CMV [26]. Research in this area continues. The selection of seronegative donor kidneys for seronegative recipients is another strategy but may not always be practicable [17].

B. Varicella Zoster Virus

Peterson et al. described 11 of 103 RT recipients with VZV infection, and this was the second most common viral infection [1]. In this group of 11 patients, visceral dissemination (meningoencephalitis) occurred in only 1 patient [1]. Luby et al. documented the occurrence of clinically unsuspected zoster without an eruption in unexplained unilateral pain syndromes and the occurrence of asymptomatic rises in titers of CF antibody to VZV [27]. Luby et al. also noted that the course of most patients with VZV infection was benign [27]. Despite the limited reported occurrence of dissemination, the utilization of antiviral therapy with intravenous acyclovir in this setting appears to be increasing.

C. Herpes Simplex Virus

Pass et al. identified herpes simplex virus (HSV) from 70% of RT recipients, and this was isolated most often from the oropharynx [21]. Shedding of HSV reached a peak within the first month posttransplantation when immunosuppression was most intense [21]. In a prospective study by Armstrong et al., rises in HSV antibody titer occurred in 38% of RT recipients and was second only to CMV [28]. Naraqi et al. concluded that HSV infections primarily occurred via the endogenous reactivation of latent HSV [29]. Pass et al. noted a relationship between the level of HSV antibody and a history of herpetic lesions in prospective RT recipients and the development of HSV lesions and viral shedding posttransplantation [30]. Fatal dissemination [30], chronic mucocutaneous ulceration [30], keratoconjunctivitis [30], meningoencephalitis [30], hepatitis [31]; and other problems have been described with HSV infection in RT patients. Pass et al. noted mucocutaneous lesions in 20 of 32 (63%) seropositive patients [30]. These lesions in our population have been primarily orofacial and often have demonstrated a hemorrhagic crust. These lesions may persist for weeks, and viral shedding continues [30], necessitating the need for contact isolation. In our patient population with HSV type I orofacial lesions, therapy with intravenous acyclovir has usually resulted in prompt resolution. Wade et al. demonstrated oral acyclovir to be safe and effective in the prevention of HSV reactivation after marrow transplantation [32]. Further studies need to be performed to determine if oral acyclovir would be appropriate in RT recipients at high risk for HSV reactivation.

D. Epstein-Barr Virus

Reactivation of Epstein-Barr virus (EBV) also occurs posttransplant, and Armstrong et al. have demonstrated serological rises in 32% of patients after renal transplant [28]. In a study by Cheeseman et al., 21 of 41 RT recipients had EBV isolated from at least one throat washing, and the frequency of EBV excretion increased gradually to 50% in the fifth month and beyond after transplantation [33]. Interestingly, in this group virus excretion and antibody elevations appeared to be independent of each other [33]. Rising anti-R EBV antibody titers were associated with leukopenia and fever and in single cases with atypical lymphocytosis and in another with fleeting pulmonary infiltrates and persistent cough [33]. EBV has also been implicated in the pathogenesis of lymphoproliferative diseases occurring in immunosuppressed recipients of organ transplants [34]. Hanto et al. have described a RT recipient who developed an EBV-associated polyclonal B-cell lymphoproliferative disease that underwent regression on two occasions with intravenous acyclovir treatment [34].

E. Hepatitis B Virus

Hepatitis B infection is seen in the RT recipient, but in our experience this has been a rare event. Pirson et al. demonstrated that HBs antigenemia in RT recipients results in significantly increased hepatic disease and decreased patient survival in the late posttransplant period [35]. The transplanted kidney may be the source of the hepatitis B virus [36], and pretransplant screening should be performed. Hepatitis B vaccine may be beneficial in the seronegative candidate considered for renal transplantation.

II. BACTERIAL INFECTIONS

Bacterial pathogens are still an important cause of infection in the RT patient, and in a recent survey by Peterson et al. approximately one-third of the infections were related to bacteria [1]. Primary sites of infection include the genitourinary (GU) tract, pulmonary system, surgical wound, and central nervous system. When bacteremia occurs, it usually arises from the GU tract [2]. In our experience, surgical wound or deep soft tissue infections in patients with diabetes mellitus are associated with the greatest morbidity and mortality. In the report by Peterson et al., 10 of 24 patients with bacteremic infections had polymicrobial infections and 70% of these infections were fatal [1].

III. FUNGAL INFECTIONS

Fungal infections have been uncommon in our experience. Primary sites of involvement include pulmonary, central nervous system, soft tissue, and GU tract. Skin biopsy may be helpful in disseminated fungal infections. Geographic history may be important in suggesting the reactivation of such agents as *Coccidioides* and *Histoplasma.*

IV. INFECTIONS IDENTIFIED BY ORGAN SYSTEM

The chronology and types of infection posttransplantation have been described by Rubin et al. [37] (summarized in Fig. 1). The trauma of GU catheterization and transplant surgery in the presence of immunosuppression auger early posttransplant infections at these sites. The etiologic agents that are responsible for infection at these sites are frequently an epidemiological reflection of the microbes existing in the hospital environment visited by these patients [37].

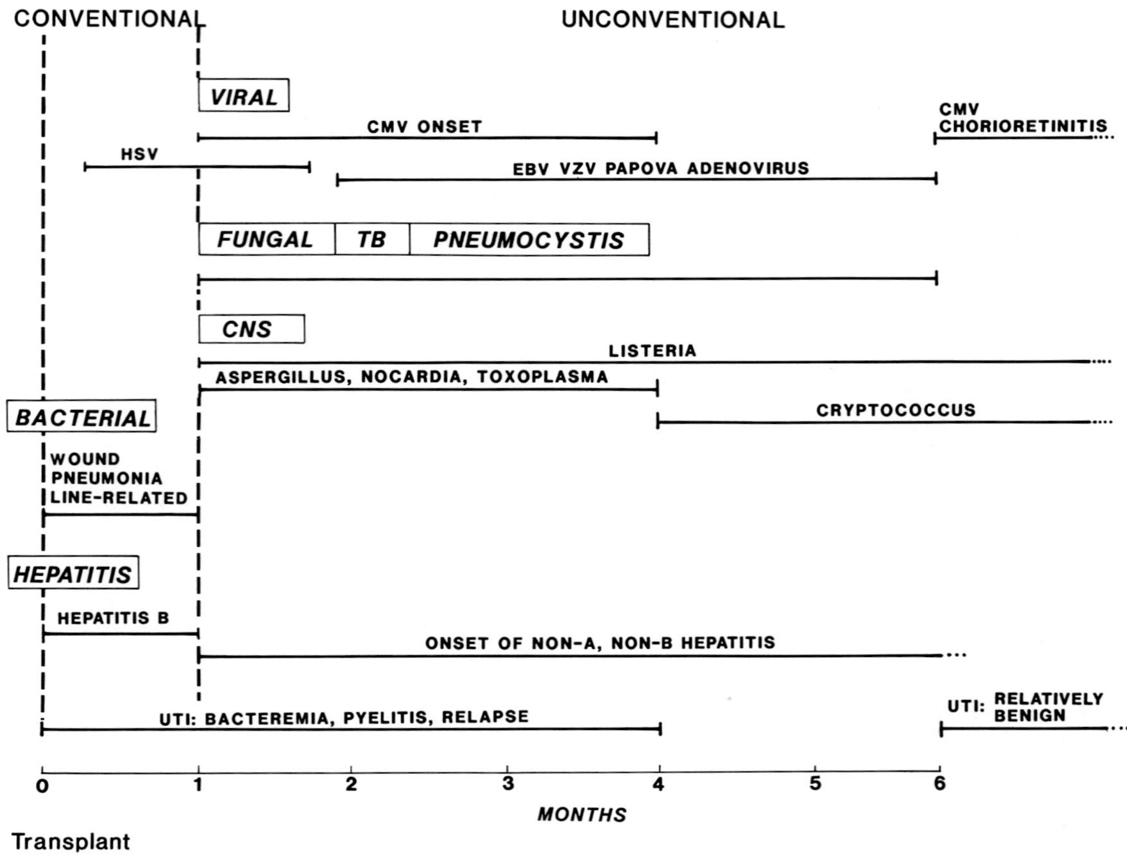

Figure 1 Timetable for the occurrence of infection in the renal transplant patient. (From: Rubin et al. [37]. Used with permission of *American Journal of Medicine*.)

A. Genitourinary Tract

During the first 4 months after renal transplantation, Tolkoff-Rubin et al. reported GU tract infections in 30-40% of recipients [38]. GU tract infection during the first 3 months posttransplantation is frequently associated with overt pyelonephritis, bacteremia, and a high rate of relapse, whereas those infections occurring 6 months or more posttransplant are relatively benign [38]. These early infections are usually associated with parenchymal renal invasion [38]. Tolkoff-Rubin et al. performed a randomized prophylactic antibiotic trial by giving one trimethoprim/sulfamethoxazole (T/S) tablet (160 mg trimethoprim plus 800 mg sulfamethoxazole) daily for 4 months, beginning on the day of Foley catheter removal following transplantation [38]. Of 26 patients, 2 (8%) taking T/S developed urinary tract infection versus 10 of 26 patients (38%) not taking T/S [38]. During this study, mycostatin treatment was initiated after the first 3 of 5 patients given T/S developed oral candidiasis [38]. Another possible concern is enhanced marrow suppression related to treatment with T/S plus azathioprine [38]. The development of T/S-resistant fecal *Escherichia coli* has been reported in RT recipients receiving prophylactic T/S, and one of these recipients also developed bacteremia [39]. Unusual etiologies of pyelonephritis in the RT patient have included *Cryptococcus* [40] and *Legionella* [41].

B. Wound Infections

As one would expect, postsurgical wound infections (WI) usually occur in the first month following renal transplantation [37]. The technical quality of the surgery is extremely important, and such factors as hematoma and urinary fistula formation predispose to the development of WI [42]. Infection may arise from lymphoceles [43]. Unrelated cadaver kidneys and diabetes mellitus were also implicated in the development of WI by Kyriakides et al. [42]. Utilization of Penrose drains have also been implicated in the development of infections [44]. These factors seem to be especially significant in the development of deep infections.

Numerous organisms can be identified in WI, and these include *Staphylococcus aureus* and *epidermidis,* gram-negative bacilli, and fungi [42,44]. These organisms primarily arise from skin structures, the GU tract, and environmental sources. In the report by Kyriakides et al., WI resulted in bacteremia in 37% of cases, mycotic aneurysm formation in 26%, transplant nephrectomy in 55%, and death in 30% [42]. Antibiotic treatment is suggested for the presence of organisms in the urine prior to transplantation [44].

The recognition of a perinephric infectious focus can be difficult, and computed tomographic (CT) scanning can be helpful, especially in identifying gas-containing collections, and can be additive to ultrasonographic studies [43]. The rate of prophylactic antimicrobials is less clearly defined when technical difficulties are kept to a minimum. Initial empiric treatment should be directed against staphylococci and gram-negative bacilli and a Gram stain of appropriate clinical material may assist in the initial assessment.

C. Pulmonary Infections

The renal transplant patient with or without neutropenia who presents with pulmonary infiltration on the chest radiograph always poses a differential diagnostic challenge because of the numerous etiologies that must be considered (Table 1). In the series reported by Ramsey et al., the clinical presentation of primary bacterial pneumonia in renal transplant patients was similar to that seen in a nonimmunosuppressed population [45]. This same series demonstrated that primary pneumonia occurring in the ambulatory setting was frequently caused by gram-positive agents, whereas gram-negative organisms were predominant in nosocomial pneumonia [45].

Practically any agent may be associated with necrosis and cavitation, including *Legionella pneumophila* [46], *Hemophilus influenzae* [47], *S. aureus* [48], *Nocardia* [48], and *Pseudomonas aeruginosa.* One of our patients with a necrotizing *Pseudomonas aeruginosa* infection doubled the size of his pulmonary cavity within 4 days and required immediate surgery. Disseminated pseudomonal or gram-negative bacillary infection may be accompanied by necrotic skin lesions (ecthyma gangrenosum) [49]. A history of COPD or chronic bronchitis might suggest the presence of *H. influenzae,* and every effort should be made to probe possible unusual contacts (e.g., i.e., psittacine birds) and occupational exposures. Recent or distant travel may also have an important relationship to clinical assessment.

A pneumococcal etiology in a RT patient presenting with pneumonitis, after a prolonged absence from the hospital, is a consideration despite other possible exotic etiologies. Ramsey et al. noted that all cases of pneumococcal pneumonia developed at least 5 months removed from the transplant operation [45]. Our two experiences with nosocomial pneumococcal disease in RT recipients occurred in conjunction with direct exposure to roommates with pneumococcal pneumonia. Bourgault et al. reported five cases of pneumococcal bacteremia in asplenic RT recipients, and three of these patients had pneumonia [50]. A majority of pneumococcal pneumonias also occurred in splenectomized renal transplant patients in a study reported by Linnemann et al., and it is known that asplenia appears to affect the severity of pneumococcal disease [51].

Legionella pneumophila pneumonitis must always be considered in the differential diagnosis since therapy with erythromycin is curative [52]. In fact, Haley et al. demonstrated that RT patients were at highest risk for nosocomial *Legionella,* and interestingly, length of hospital stay was not a risk factor [53]. An initial nodular consolidative pneumonia is not uncommon, and increased tempera-

Table 1 Etiologies of Pulmonary Disease (Renal Transplantation)

Bacterial	Pneumococcal, staphylococcal, gram-negative bacillary (including *Hemophilus influenzae, Legionella, Klebsiella, E. coli, Enterobacter, Pseudomonas*), *Nocardia,* polymicrobial, and others
Viral	CMV, Herpes, Varicella zoster, adenovirus
Mycotic	*Candida, Aspergillus, Zygomycetes,* cryptococcal, histoplasmosis, coccidioidal, blastomycotic, *C. glabrata,* and others
Mycobacterial	Mycobacterial tuberculosis, atypical, and others
Parasitical	Pneumocystis, *Toxoplasma, Strongyloides*
Mycoplasma	*M. pneumoniae*
Noninfectious	Pulmonary edema, emboli, radiation, drug therapy, and others

ture is likely [54]. Temperature-pulse dissociation may also be seen [55]. We had a dramatic experience with a RT patient who had a consolidative pneumonia with a hectic fever unresponsive to cephalosporin and aminoglycoside therapy. This patient was afebrile within 48 hr after initiating IV erythromycin. Although the appropriate duration of therapy is unknown, we have generally selected a 3-week treatment course with a daily dose of 2 g erythromycin (the literature supports doses up to 6 g/day or greater) [56]. Relapse has been reported even following more than 2 weeks of erythromycin therapy [46]. Possible sources of *legionella* include water, and this agent has been isolated from shower baths [57]. Rifampin may be utilized in conjunction with erythromycin, and if erythromycin cannot be employed, doxycycline may be substituted [55].

Legionella micadadei (the Pittsburgh agent) has been etiologically linked to pneumonitis in RT patients [58]. The interval from transplantation to the onset of pneumonia was shorter for *L. micadadei* pneumonia than for *L. pneumophila* pneumonia [58]. *Legionella micadadei* has also been isolated from potable water in the hospital setting [58]. Nodular pulmonary infiltrates have been reported with this agent [59]. Erythromycin therapy is generally efficacious [60].

Pneumocystis carinii pneumonia has been rare in our RT group; however, Hardy et al. reported 14 cases over a 19-month period in 156 RT recipients treated with cyclosporin and steroids [61]. This represented a significant increase in this type of pneumonia versus previous RT patients who received azathioprine and steroids [61]. In this series, *Pneumocystis* occurred more frequently in men, 86% of cases had onset of disease 3 or 4 months following transplantation, and all had evidence of CMV infection [61]. Further cases were not described following the institution of trimethoprin/sulfamethoxazole prophylaxis [61]. The radiographic appearance of pneumocystis in the immunocompromised patient is primarily a bilateral diffuse or patchy interstitial infiltrate, and pleural effusion is distinctly uncommon [62]. The cough is primarily nonproductive, and hemoptysis is rare [62]. Current data would suggest that trimethoprim/sulfamethoxazole (15-20 mg/kg per day of trimethoprim) is the preferred initial treatment, although pentamidine is a therapeutic alternative [63]. Careful consideration for posttherapeutic suppressive treatment is suggested [63]. No inanimate environmental reservoir of *Pneumocystis* has been identified [64].

Nocardia asteroides is a soil-borne aerobic gram-positive filamentous rodlike bacterium that on Gram stain is similar to *Actinomyces* and has been reported to cause pneumonia in RT recipients by Lovett et al. [65]. In this reported outbreak, pleuritic pain was common and the radiographic appearance was primarily nodular (usually less than 12 mm in diameter) with cavitation [65]. This organism is slow growing and may take weeks to isolate. Neurological signs and symptoms may be associated with nocardial cerebral abscess formation [66]. Sulfonamide is considered by many investigators to be an essential part of therapy. Relapses, however, have occurred with trimethoprim/sulfamethoxazole treatment [67]. Amikacin has been utilized successfully in a pediatric RT patient with extrapulmonary nocardiosis [68]. Prolonged antimicrobial treatment for months is usually necessary. Whether respiratory isolation may be necessary in pulmonary nocardiosis is an interesting issue raised by Stevens et al. [69].

Ramsey et al. noted that mycotic infections were the most common cause of primary pneumonia in their population [45]. Mycotic pulmonary involvement in RT recipients has been described with numerous agents, including *Cryptococcus, Candida, Aspergillus,* and *Phycomycetes* [70]. Cryptococcal disease is often seen with central nervous system dysfunction with a picture of subacute meningitis [70]. *Candida* pneumonitis may occur with multiple organ involvement [70]. Fluffy white chorioretinal lesions may be noted along with macronodular cutaneous lesions with hematogenous *Candida* infection [71]. Cutaneous biopsy with appropriate straining may reveal this agent [71]. A patient with cultures positive for *Candida* from multiple sites (e.g., urine, sputum, and stool) and clinical deterioration should be strongly suspected of having disseminated candidiasis, which may include pneumonitis. Primary therapy of *Candida* pneumonitis should include amphotericin B and 5-flucytosine. *Aspergillus pneumonitis* can be associated with pleuritic pain and invasion and thrombosis of blood vessels [72]. Pericardial involvement has also been noted in our experience. Environmental sources need to be sought if *A. pneumonitis* is identified, especially if a cluster of cases is documented [72]. Gustafson et al. documented that the single most important risk factor for invasive *Aspergillus* in RT recipients was the average daily dose of corticosteroids [73]. Tissue biopsy is especially important in diagnosing this entity. Amphotericin B is the treatment of choice.

Ramsey et al. reported that the most common form of primary pneumonia during recent surveillance was due to cytomegalovirus [45]. All these cases were identified 1-4 months posttransplant [45]. The onset of disease in these patients was insidious, with several days of fever, malaise, anorexia, fatigue, night sweats, myalgias, and arthralgias ushering in a period of dry cough and tachypnea that heralded the onset of pneumonia [45]. One of our patients developed acute onset of pleuritic pain, which suggested the clinical syndrome of pulmonary infarction. Peterson et al. noted that immunosuppression with cyclosporine plus low-dose prednisone was less likely to predispose patients to the development of CMV-related pneumonia than was a regimen of antilymphocyte globulin, azathioprine, and prednisone in higher dosages [74]. Recipients of kidneys from seropositive donors had more than a threefold greater risk of developing CMV-related pneumonia [74]. Anti-CMV therapy is currently unsatisfactory. Studies, however, continue with a guanosine analog similar to acyclovir [25]. Superinfection is often caused by bacteria, fungi, or protozoa [75].

Other possible etiologies of viral pneumonitis in the RT recipient include herpes simplex, varicella zoster, adenovirus [76], and community-acquired agents, such as influenza A_2 [45]. Mucocutaneous lesions often precede herpetic pneumonia in the compromised host, and investigation for herpetic esophagitis or tracheitis should be made [77]. If one encounters disseminated varicella zoster infection, respiratory isolation may be indicated, especially if pneumonitis is present.

A possible mycobacterial etiology of pneumonitis in the RT patient should always be considered. The estimated incidence of mycobacterial disease in this immunosuppressed population from the literature is low (0-1.3%) [78]. A miliary chest radiographic pattern is not uncommon [79]. More conventional upper lobe infiltrates with or without cavitation may suggest this diagnosis [78]. AFB sputum smears, however, are often not of value [79]. Cutaneous biopsy may be available as an adjunct to other diagnostic procedures [49]. When a mycobacterial isolate is identified from any source, susceptibility studies should be performed. Lichtenstein et al. [78] recommended the following guidelines: (1) All recipients and donors should have tuberculin skin tests and chest x-rays. (2) Isoniazid (300 mg daily) should be given to all tuberculin-reactive donors for several months before surgery if possible (since the transplanted kidney may be a source of infection). (3) A year of isoniazid treatment should be considered for any recipient who has negative skin test results and normal chest x-ray findings and who is receiving a kidney from a living tuberculin-reactive donor or from a cadaveric donor with a history of tuberculosis or a positive tuberculin reaction. (4) Isoniazid should be given for 1 year to any renal transplant recipient who is tuberculin reactive, has a history of tuberculosis, or has chest x-ray findings suggestive of previous tuberculosis. Isoniazid and rifampin are the primary agents employed in the treatment of active disease.

Table 2 Empiric Therapy of Pneumonitis

Erythromycin
Aminoglycoside
Trimethoprim/sulfamethoxazole

Although toxoplasmosis in RT recipients usually presents with neurological findings, pneumonitis may occur [1]. Patients presenting with diarrhea and pneumonitis should be evaluated for *Strongyloides stercoralis,* and patients with this parasite may also experience unexplained and persistent bacteremia with different enteric organisms, which may also be found in sputum cultures [80]. Eosinophilia may be present. Therapy with thiabendazole is usually satisfactory [80].

Pneumonic infiltrate in the RT recipient may also reflect embolization, edema, (secondary to uremia, for example), hemorrhage, fibrosis, vasculitis, and so on. Medications should also be carefully screened to assess possible pulmonary toxicity.

Pulmonary infiltrate in the RT recipient necessitates a sense of urgency, especially if the individual is clinically deteriorating. Table 2 summarizes our initial chemotherapeutic approach to these patients if there is no clue pointing to a viral, mycotic, or mycobacterial etiology. Wilson et al. [49] have recommended initial empiric therapy with a cephalosporin and an antipseudomonal penicillin, in addition to the agents shown in Table 2 [49]. Another important aspect of treatment is to decrease or discontinue (wherever possible) immunosuppressive agents. Careful physical examination is always essential to detect cutaneous lesions, lymph nodes, or retinal lesions (examination by an ophthalmologist is suggested). Cutaneous lesions or lymph nodes may provide a biopsy diagnosis. Sputum examination, bone marrow biopsy, thoracentesis, arthrocentesis, lumbar puncture, and stool examination (for ova and parasites), in addition to blood, urine, and other body fluid cultures, may be especially helpful. Computed tomography of brain may also help to suggest pathogens, like *Nocardia* and *Toxoplasma.* An acridine orange stain, although not specific, may be helpful to recognize microbiologic agents in sputum and body fluids. A serological screening approach has been suggested by Wilson et al. and is represented in Table 3 [49].

Although historical and epidemiological information is sought, diagnosis of pneumonitis in the RT patient often depends on lung biopsy. If the patient is not acutely deteriorating, and bleeding, coagulation and platelet parameters allow, a fiberoptic bronchoscopy with bronchoalveolar lavage and transbronchial brush and forceps biopsy is performed. Any patient who is rapidly deteriorating or developing increasing pulmonary infiltrates merits an immediate open lung biopsy. Wilson et al. reported 95 immunocompromised patients with pulmonary infiltrates who underwent open lung biopsy and noted that a specific etiologic diagnosis was established in 77 (81%) [49]. Open lung biopsy should be aggressively pursued when an etiologic diagnosis is not in hand, and this procedure in our experience is usually reasonably tolerated by most patients. The importance of open lung biopsy cannot be overstressed. Special stains that should be performed on the lung tissue include (1) hematoxylin-eosin, (2) Gram stain, (3) methenamine silver, (4) auramine-rhodamine, (5) periodic acid-Schiff, (6) Direct immunofluorescent *Legionella* stain, (7) Dieterle silver, when indicated, and (8) immunologic stains for herpes simplex and CMV, when indicated. Lung tissue cultures should include (1) bacterial (aerobic and anaerobic), (2) fungal, (3) mycobacterial, (4) viral, (5) *Legionella,* (6) *Mycoplasma,* and (7) *Chlamydia.* Tissue impression smears may be helpful, especially for *Legionella* and *Pneumocystis* recognition [49]. Electron microscopic tissue analysis has occasionally proved beneficial.

An alveolar inflammatory process can be seen in any bacterial pneumonitis, including *Legionella.* Interstitial inflammation can be seen in viral, pneumocystis, mycoplasmal, chlamydial, chemical-induced, and noninfectious related etiologies. The alveoli are usually filled with a proteinaceous material in *Pneumocystis* infection. Since new microbiologic agents continue to be recognized, the physician's interest should only be piqued when a specific etiologic diagnosis is not possible.

D. Central Nervous System Infections

Tilney et al. noted a 44% mortality in a review of RT patients with cerebromeningitis spanning 20 years [81]. In a review by Hooper et al. of central nervous system (CNS) infection in chronically immunosuppressed individuals, the largest number of CNS infections were in RT patients [82]. In this series, *Listeria monocytogenes* (LM), *Cryptococcus neoformans* (CN), and *Aspergillus fumigatus* (AF) CNS infections occurred with equal frequency [82]. In this group of RT recipients, headache and fever were common with LM and CN infection and fever alone with AF infection [82]. Meningismus was noted most frequently with LM involvement [82]. Subacute and chronic CNS disease presentations were the rule with CN, and this tended to occur more than 6 months posttransplant [82]. Neiman et al. noted that RT recipients were particularly prone to develop listeriosis [83]. Of the cases, 23% were described in RT patients, and approximately one-third of these individuals died [83]. Most of these cases were associated with *Listeria* bacteremia, and the cerebrospinal fluid often showed a predominance of polymorphonuclear leukocytes with an increased protein [83]. In nonmeningitic disease, blood cultures were uniformly positive for LM, and the spec-

Table 3 Serological Studies Currently Used at the Mayo Clinic (Organisms Associated with Infections in Immunocompromised Patients)

Organism	Test[a]	Significant result	
		Acute	Convalescent
Bacteria			
Legionella pneumophila (types I-IV) or *micdadei*	Indirect immunofluorescence	$>1:256$	Any fourfold rise
Mycoplasma pneumoniae	Complement fixation	$\geq 1:16$	Any fourfold rise
Viruses			
Cytomegalovirus	IgG anticomplement immunofluorescence	$\geq 1:160$	Any fourfold rise
	IgM indirect immunofluorescence	$\geq 1:10$	–
Chlamydia trachomatis	Complement fixation	$>1:64$	Any fourfold rise
Toxoplasma gondii	IgG indirect immunofluorescence	$\geq 1:1024$	Any fourfold rise
	IgM indirect immunofluorescence	$\geq 1:8$	–

Fungi		
Aspergillus fumigatus, flavus, or *niger*	Immunodiffusion	One or more bands, suggestive of active infection
Blastomyces dermatitidis	Complement fixation	Titers of 1:8 or 1:16, suggestive of active infection; 1:32, highly suggestive of active infection
	Immunodiffusion	Positive–highly suggestive of active infection
Coccidioides immitis	Complement fixation	Titers of ⩾1:2, suggestive of active infection
Cryptococcus neoformans	Latex agglutination (detection of antigen)	Any positive, active infection, although rheumatoid factor can produce false-positive results
Histoplasma capsulatum	Complement fixation	Titers of 1:8 or 1:16, suggestive of active infection; ⩾1:32, highly suggestive of active infection
	Immunodiffusion	M band alone, early infection, late or treated infection, or after skin testing; H band and M band, active infection
Sporothrix schenckii	Latex agglutination	Titers of ⩾1:80, usually, active infection

[a]Serology detects IgG antibody unless otherwise specified.
Source: Wilson et al. [49]. Used with permission of *Mayo Clinic Proceedings.*

trum of CNS involvement ranged from well-localized abscesses to diffuse encephalitis [83].

In this nonmeningitic group, neurological impairment with hemiparesis or cranial nerve involvement with minimal spinal fluid findings was the rule [83]. We have seen this nonmeningitic form of disease presenting as a "stroke syndrome" with hemiparesis. Difficulty in the laboratory identification of this organism can complicate the diagnosis. LM has been misidentified as diphtheroid, streptococcal, and *Corynebacterium* species by a number of laboratories. The clinician must exhibit a high degree of awareness to diagnose the nonmeningitic type of LM infection. Stamm et al. reported an outbreak of listeriosis and suggested that secretion-excretion precautions and respiratory isolation (in the presence of pneumonia) might be appropriate [84]. Intravenous ampicillin or penicillin appears to be effective therapy for CNS disease. The frequency of diagnosed listeriosis among RT recipients appears to be increasing [83]. Since T cells have been shown to be involved in the host defense mechanisms to kill LM [85], utilization of antilymphocyte globulin and cyclosporine may enhance the dissemination of LM to the CNS.

With *C. neoformans* infections of the CNS, common findings of spinal fluid include a lymphocytic pleocytosis and decreased glucose [82]. Spinal fluid cultures are not always positive, but the determination of cryptococcal antigen in the spinal fluid should be positive in all cases. Therapy includes intravenous amphotericin B alone or in combination with oral 5-flucytosine.

AF involvement of CNS may be associated with acute CNS deterioration, including seizures and hemiparesis [82]. Most of these patients have brain abscesses, and the lung is usually the apparent portal of entry [82]. Renal and wound sites, however, have also been indicated [81]. Brain CT scans may be of value in initial assessment. Survival with this condition is rare, but therapy with IV amphotericin B should be attempted [81].

Numerous other agents have been identified causing CNS infection in this group of patients. These agents include *Candida* [82], *Coccidioides* [81], *Phycomycetes* [82], *Strongyloides* [82], *Nocardia* [82], *Polyomavirus* [86], and *Toxoplasma gondii* [82]. *Phycomycetes* involvement should be suspected in any patient with necrosis of palatal or nasal tissues, black, necrotic drainage from these sites, or unexplained visual loss. Immediate surgical intervention for diagnostic and therapeutic reasons is imperative. Intravenous amphotericin B is the primary drug of choice. *Strongyloides* infection may be associated with pulmonary disease and sustained bacteremia [82]. Nocardial CNS involvement is usually associated with pulmonary disease. Papova viruses or polyomaviruses (JC and BK) have been identified in the urine of RT patients [87]. Most JC virus infections appear to be primary, and most BK virus infections appear to result from reactivation [87]. BK virus may be transmitted from transplanted kidneys, and this merits further research [88]. Slowly progressive focal neurological deficits may be noted with hemiparesis with or without aphasia in polyomavirus CNS infections [82]; this is known as progressive multifocal leukoencephalopathy. The CT scan in these patients may reveal an area of decreased density in white matter without mass effect or contrast enhancement [82]. Electron microscopy of brain tissue may also be helpful in suggesting the diagnosis. Ruskin et al. reviewed the manifestations of toxoplasmosis in the compromised host and described predominantly neurological syndromes (including diffuse encephalopathy, meningoencephalitis, and cerebral mass lesions) [89]. Histopathologic screening for the proliferative forms of the parasite from the biopsy specimens of infected organs and electron micrographic analysis may provide a diagnosis [89]. Serological diagnosis (with the Sabin-Feldman dye test, indirect fluorescent antibody test, and others) should also be pursued [90]. Rash, pneumonitis, and myocarditis may be a part of the clinical picture [89]. Sulfadiazine combined with pyrimethamine is the mainstay of treatment [82], and this may have to be continued for months. Vesicular cutaneous lesions (usually initially dermatomal) associated with neurological obtundation should suggest the diagnosis of disseminated varicella zoster infection.

E. Gastrointestinal Infections

Candida species are etiologically linked to acute pseudomembranous candidiasis (thrush) and esophagitis. Oral candidiasis presents with whitish plaques on the mucosal surfaces and can usually be effectively treated with nystatin suspension or tablets.

Odynophagia, dysphagia, and/or substernal pain should alert one to the possibility of esophagitis. Barium swallow may elucidate irregularity of the esophageal mucosa. Etiologic agents that should be a primary consideration include *Candida* and HSV. Endoscopy, esophageal biopsy, and appropriate cultures usually confirm the diagnosis. *Candida* esophagitis can be treated with nystatin suspension, but in some cases modest doses of intravenous amphotericin B may be required [91]. More recently, oral ketoconazole has produced good results [92]. Surveillance for possible ketoconazole-resistant forms is suggested. Ideal therapy for HSV esophagitis is not known; however, primary therapy consists of topical anesthetic agents. If symptoms are progressive or last longer than 2 weeks, a course of antiviral treatment can be utilized.

CMV has also been associated with gastrointestinal disease, although etiologically linked occurrences are much more difficult to prove. Diethelm et al. have described gastrointestinal hemorrhage in association with gastric ulcerations and the presence of inclusion bodies in chief cells [93]. Ulcerative cecal disease has also been seen [94].

V. SPECIAL CONSIDERATIONS

Every effort should be made to assure appropriate screening of the prospective renal donor and to afford appropriate health screening and vaccine protection to the RT recipient. Review of the medical history of the prospective renal donor may identify areas of concern. Serological screening of the renal donor and recipient might include CMV, hepatitis B virus, *Toxoplasma,* polyomavirus, human T-lymphotropic virus type III, and VDRL (Venereal Disease Research Laboratories). Health screening of the donor should include an inquiry regarding a past history or exposure to mycobacterial disease, including intermediate purified protein derivative (PPD) skin test for tuberculin. Health screening of the recipients, in addition to inquiry regarding mycobacterial exposure, should include a thorough dental history and examination, eliciting a history of chronic GU tract infection, especially associated with stone formation and/or obstruction, inquiry regarding previous mycotic and parasitical diseases, and documentation of previous geographic exposures.

Influenza vaccine has been given to RT recipients with good antibody response [95]. Pneumococcal vaccine in RT patients produces lower antibody titers than in healthy controls, but one cannot exclude possible benefit from immunization [96]. The possible advantages of CMV and hepatitis B vaccine have already been discussed.

ACKNOWLEDGMENTS

Special gratitude is extended to Gregory Trudell, Amar Jaglan, Vincent Esposito, Aliza Landy, and Lisa Freitag for preparation of this manuscript.

REFERENCES

1. Peterson, P. K., Ferguson, R., Fryd, D. S., Balfour, H. H., Jr., Rynasiewicz, J., and Simmons, R. L.: Infectious diseases in hospitalized renal transplant recipients: A prospective study of a complex and evolving problem. Medicine (Baltimore) 61:360-372, 1982.
2. Masur, H., Cheigh, J. S., and Stubenbord, W. T.: Infection following renal transplantation: A changing pattern. Rev. Infect. Dis. 4:1208-1219, 1982.
3. Hill, R. B., Jr., Dahrling, B. E., II, Starzi, R. E., and Rifkind, D.: Death after transplantation: An analysis of sixty cases. Am. J. Med. 42:327-334, 1967.
4. Sheil, A. G. R., Kelly, G. E., Storey, B. G., et al.: Controlled clinical trial of antilymphocyte globulin in patients with renal allografts from cadaver donors. Lancet 1:359-363, 1971.
5. Eickhoff, T. C., Olin, D. B., Anderson, R. J., and Schafer, L. A.: Current problems and approaches to diagnosis of infection in renal transplant recipients. Transplant. Proc. 4:693-697, 1972.
6. Fauci, A. S., Dale, D. C., and Balow, J. E.: Glucocorticosteroid therapy: Mechanisms of action and clinical considerations. Ann. Intern. Med. 84: 304, 1976.

7. Waller, M., Pierce, J. C., Lee, H. M., and Levinson, H. J.: Humoral antibody responses following transplantation in man. Transplantation 19:210, 1975.
8. Quadracci, L. J., Ringdan, O., and Krzymanski, M.: The effect of uremia and transplantation on lymphocyte subpopulations. Kidney Int. 10:179, 1976.
9. Britton, S., and Palacios, R.: Cyclosporin A: Usefulness, risks and mechanism of action. Immunol. Rev. 65:5, 1982.
10. Boggs, D. R., and Frei, E., III: Clinical studies of fever and infection in cancer. Cancer 13:1240, 1960.
11. Stossel, T. P.: Phagocytosis. N. Engl. J. Med. 290:833, 1974.
12. Golshan, N., Barker, C. F., and MacGregor, R. R.: Granulocyte function in recipients of renal transplants from live related donors and from cadavers. J. Infect. Dis. 142:876-883, 1980.
13. Peterson, P. K., Balfour, H. H., Jr., Fryd, D. S., Ferguson, R. M., and Simmons, R. L.: Fever in renal transplant recipients: Causes, prognostic significance and changing patterns at the University of Minnesota hospital. Am. J. Med. 71:345-351, 1981.
14. Adler, S. P.: Transfusion-associated cytomegalovirus infections. Rev. Infect. Dis. 5:977-993, 1983.
15. Ho, M., Suwansirikui, S., Dowling, J. N., Youngblood, L. A., and Armstrong, J. S.: The transplanted kidney as a source of cytomegalovirus infection. N. Engl. J. Med. 293:1109-1112, 1975.
16. Naraqi, S., Jackson, G. G., Jonasson, O., and Rubenis, M.: Search for latent cytomegalovirus in renal allografts. Infect. Immun. 19:699-703, 1978.
17. Glenn, J.: Cytomegalovirus infections following renal transplantation. Rev. Infect. Dis. 3:1151-1178, 1981.
18. Rubin. R. H., Russell, P. S., Levin, M., and Cohen, C.: Summary of a workshop on cytomegalovirus infections during organ transplantation. J. Infect. Dis. 139:728-734, 1979.
19. Fiala, M., Payne, J. E., Berne, T. V., et al.: Epidemiology of cytomegalovirus infection after transplantation and immunosuppression. J. Infect. Dis. 132: 421-433, 1975.
20. Luby, J. P., Burnett, W., Hull, A. R., Ware, A. J., Shorey, J. W., and Peters, P. C.: Relationship between cytomegalovirus and hepatic function abnormalities in the period after renal transplant. J. Infect. Dis. 511-518, 1974.
21. Pass, R. F., Long, W. K., Whitley, R. J., et al.: Productive infection with cytomegalovirus and herpes simplex virus in renal transplant recipients. J. Infect. Dis. 137:556-563, 1978.
22. Pass, R. F., Whitley, R. J., Diethelm, A. G., Whetchel, J. D., Reynolds, D. W., and Alford, C. A.: Cytomegalovirus infection in patients with renal transplants: Potentiation by antithymocyte globulin and an incompatible graft. J. Infect. Dis. 142:9-17, 1980.
23. Richardson, P., Colvin, R. B., Cheeseman, S. H., et al.: Glomerulopathy associated with cytomegalovirus viremia in renal allografts. N. Engl. J. Med. 305: 1981.

24. Peterson, P. K., Balfour, H. H., Marker, S. C., Fryd, D. S., Howard, R. J., and Simmons, R. L.: Cytomegalovirus disease in renal allograft recipients: A prospective study of the clinical features, risk factors and impact on renal transplantation. Medicine (Baltimore) 59:283-300, 1980.
25. Shepp, D. H., Dandliker, P. S., De Miranda, P., et al.: Activity of 9-12-hydroxy-1-(hydroxymethyl)ethoxymethylguanine in the treatment of cytomegalovirus pneumonia. Ann. Intern. Med. 103:368-373, 1985.
26. Land, D. J.: Cytomegalovirus immunization: Status, prospects, and problems. Rev. Infect. Dis. 2:449-458, 1980.
27. Luby, J. P., Ramirez-Ronda, C., Rinner, S., Hull, A., and Vergne-Marini, P.: A longitudinal study of varicella-zoster virus infections in renal transplant recipients. J. Infect. Dis. 135:659-663, 1977.
28. Armstrong, J. A., Evans, A. S., Rao, N., and Ho, M.: Viral infections in renal transplant recipients. Infect. Immun. 14:970-975, 1976.
29. Naraqi, S., Jackson, G. G., Jonasson, O., and Yamashiroya, H. M.: Prospective study of prevalence, incidence, and source of herpesvirus infections in patients with renal allografts. J. Infect. Dis. 136:531-540, 1977.
30. Pass, R. F., Whitley, R. J., Whelchel, J. D., Diethelm, A. G., Reynolds, D. W., and Alford, C. A.: Identification of patients with increased risk of infection with herpes simplex virus after renal transplantation. J. Infect. Dis. 140: 487-492, 1979.
31. Elliott, W. C., Houghton, D. C., Bryant, R. E., Wicklund, R., Barry, M. J., and Bennett, W. M.: Herpes simplex type 1 hepatitis in renal transplantation. Arch. Intern. Med. 40:1656-1660, 1980.
32. Wade, J. C., Newton, B., Flournoy, N., and Meyers, J. E.: Oral acyclovir for prevention of herpes simplex virus reactivation after marrow transplantation. Ann. Intern. Med. 100:823-828, 1984.
33. Cheeseman, S. H., Henle, W., Rubin, R. H., et al.: Epstein-Barr virus infection in renal transplant recipients. Ann. Intern. Med. 93(Part 1):39-42, 1980.
34. Hanto, D. W., Frizzera, G., Gajl-Peczalska, K. J., et al.: Epstein-Barr virus-induced b-cell lymphoma after renal transplantation. N. Engl. J. Med. 306: 913-918, 1982.
35. Pirson, Y., Alexandre, G. P. J., and Van Ypersele De Strihou, C.: Long-term effect of HBs antigenemia on patient survival after renal transplantation. N. Engl. J. Med. 296:194-196, 1977.
36. Wolf, J. L., Perkins, H. A., Schreeder, M. T., and Vincenti, F.: The transplanted kidney as a source of hepatitis B infection. Ann. Intern. Med. 91: 412-413, 1979.
37. Rubin, R. H., Wolfson, J. S., Cosimi, A. B., and Tolkoff-Rubin, N. E.: Infection in the renal transplant recipient. Am. J. Med. 70:405-411, 1981.
38. Tolkoff-Rubin, N. E., Cosimi, A. B., Russell, P. S., and Rubin, R. H.: A controlled study of trimethoprim-sulfamethoxazole prophylaxis of urinary tract infection in renal transplant recipients. Rev. Infect. Dis. 4:614-618, 1982.
39. Wells, C. L., Podzorski, R. P., Peterson, P. K., Ramsay, N. K., Simmons, R. L., and Rhame, F. S.: Incidence of trimethoprim-sulfamethoxazole-resistant

enterobacteriaceae among transplant recipients. J. Infect. Dis. 150:699-706, 1984.
40. Hellman, R. N., Hinrichs, J., Sicard, G., Hoover, R., Golden, P., and Hoffsten, P.: Cryptococcal pyelonephritis and disseminated cryptococcosis in a renal transplant recipient. Arch. Intern. Med. 141:128-130, 1981.
41. Dorman, S. A., Hardin, N. J., and Winn, W. C., Jr.: Pyelonephritis associated with *Legionella pneumophila,* serogroup 4. Ann. Intern. Med. 93: 835-837, 1980.
42. Kyriakides, G. K., Simmons, R. L., and Najarian, J. S.: Wound infections in renal transplant wound: Pathogenetic and prognostic factors. Ann. Surg. 182:770-775, 1975.
43. Bia, M. J., Baggish, D., Katz, L., Gonzalez, R., Kliger, A. S., and Rosenfield, A. T.: Computed tomography in the diagnosis of pelvic abscesses in renal transplant patients. JAMA 246:1435-1437, 1981.
44. Hoy, W. E., May, A. G., and Freeman, R. B.: Primary renal transplant wound infections. N.Y. State J. Med. 81:1469-1473, 1981.
45. Ramsey, P. G., Rubin, R. H., Tolkoff-Rubin, N. E., Cosimi, A. B., Russell, P. S., and Greene, R.: The renal transplant patient with fever and pulmonary infiltrates: Etiology, clinical manifestations, and management. Medicine (Baltimore) 59:206-222, 1980.
46. Gump, D. W., Frank, R. O., Winn, W. C., Foster, R. C., Broome, C. V., and Cherry, W. B.: Legionnaires' disease in patients with associated serious disease. Ann. Intern. Med. 90:538-542, 1979.
47. Esler, W. V., and Aber, R. C.: Cavitary pulmonary nodule caused by *Haemophilus influenzae* in a renal transplant recipient. South. Med. J. 75:376-377, 1982.
48. Ludmerer, K. M., and Kissane, J. M.: Cavitary lung disease following renal transplantation. Am. J. Med. 72:145-155, 1982.
49. Wilson, W. R., Cockerill, F. R., III, and Rosenow, E. C., III: Pulmonary disease in the immunocompromised host (second of two parts). Mayo Clin. Proc. 60:610-631, 1985.
50. Bourgault, A. M., Van Scoy, R. E., Wilkowske, C. J., Zincke, H., and Sterioff, S.: Severe infection due to *Streptococcus pneumoniae* in asplenic renal transplant patients. Mayo Clin. Proc. 54:123-126, 1979.
51. Linnemann, C. C., Jr., and First, M. R.: Risk of pneumococcal infections in renal transplant patients. JAMA 241:2619-2621, 1979.
52. Saravolatz, L. D., Burch, K. H., Fisher, E., et al.: The compromised host and legionnaries' disease. Ann. Intern. Med. 90:533-537, 1979.
53. Haley, C. E., Cohen, M. L., Halter, J., and Meyer, R. D.: Nosocomial legionnaires' disease: A continuing common-source epidemic at Wadsworth Medical Center. Ann. Intern. Med. 90:583-586, 1979.
54. Foster, R. S., Winn, W. C., Jr., Marshall, W., and Gump, D. W.: Legionnaires' disease following renal transplantation. Transplant. Proc. 11:93-95, 1979.
55. Meyer, R. D.: *Legionella* infections: A review of five years of research. Rev. Infect. Dis. 5:258-278, 1983.

56. Marshall, W., Foster, R. S., Jr., and Winn, W.: Legionnaire's diseases in renal transplant patients. Am. J. Surg. 141:423-428, 1981.
57. Tobin, J. O., Dunnill, M. S., French, M., et al.: Legionnaire's disease in a transplant unit: Isolation of the causative agent from shower baths. Lancet 2:118-121, 1980.
58. Dowling, J. N., Pasculle, A. W., Frila, F. N., Zaphyr, M. K., and Yee, R. B.: Infections caused by *Legionella Micdadei* and *Legionella pneumophila* among renal transplant recipients. J. Infect. Dis. 149:703-713, 1984.
59. Pope, T. L., Jr., Armstrong, P., Thompson, R., and Donowitz, G. R.: Pittsburgh pneumonia agent: Chest film manifestations. AJR 138:237-241, 1982.
60. Wing, E. J., Schafer, F. J., and Pasculle, A. W.: Successful treatment of *Legionella micdadei* (Pittsburgh pneumonia agent) pneumonia with erythromycin. Am. J. Med. 71:836-840, 1981.
61. Hardy, A. M., Wajszczuk, C. P., Suffredini, A. F., Hakala, T. R., and Ho, M.: *Pneumocystis carinii* pneumonia in renal transplant recipients treated with cyclosporine and steroids. J. Infect. Dis. 149:143-147, 1984.
62. Walzer, P. D., Perl, D. P., Krogstad, D. J., Rawson, P. G., and Schultz, M. G.: *Pneumocystis carinii* pneumonia in the United States. Ann. Intern. Med. 80:83-93, 1974.
63. Young, L. S.: Trimethoprim/sulfamethoxazole in the treatment of adults with pneumonia due to *Pneumocystis carinii.* Rev. Infect. Dis. 4:608-613, 1982.
64. Hughes, W. T.: *Pneumocystis carinii* pneumonia. N. Engl. J. Med. 297: 1381-1383, 1977.
65. Lovett, I. S., Houang, E. T., Burge, S., et al.: An outbreak of *Nocardia asteroides* infections in a renal transplant unit. Q. J. Med. 198:123-135, 1981.
66. Barmeir, E., Mann, J. H., and Marcus, R. H.: Cerebral nocardiosis in renal transplant patients. Br. J. Radiol. 54:1107-1109, 1981.
67. Stamm, A. M., McFall, D. W., and Dismukes, W. E.: Failure of sulfonamides and trimethoprim in the treatment of nocardiosis. Arch. Intern. Med. 143: 383, 1983.
68. Yogey, R., Greenslade, T., Firlit, C. F., and Lewy, P.: Successful treatment of *Nocardia asteroides* infection with amikacin. J. Pediatr. 96:771-773, 1980.
69. Stevens, D. A., Pier, A. C., Beaman, B. L., Morozumi, P. A., Lovett, I. S., and Houang, E. T.: Laboratory evaluation of an outbreak of nocardiosis in immunocompromised hosts. Am. J. Med. 71:928-934, 1981.
70. Gallis, H. A., Berman, R. A., Cate, T. R., Hamilton, J. D., Gunnells, J. D., and Stickel, D. L.: Fungal infection following renal transplantation. Arch. Intern. Med. 135:1163-1172, 1975.
71. Edwards, J. E.: Jr., Lehrer, R. I., Stiehm, E. R., Fischer, T. J., and Young, L. S.: Severe candidal infections. Ann. Intern. Med. 89:91-106, 1978.
72. Burton, J. R., Zachery, J. B., Bessin, R., et al.: Aspergillosis in four renal transplant recipients. Ann. Intern. Med. 77:383-388, 1972.
73. Gustafson, T. L., Schaffner, W., Lavely, G. B., Stratton, C. W., Johnson, H. K.,

and Hutcheson, R. H.: Invasive aspergillosis in renal transplant recipients: Correlation with corticosteroid therapy. J. Infect. Dis. 148:230-238, 1983.
74. Peterson, P. K., Balfour, H. H., Fryd, D. S., Ferguson, R., Kronenberg, R., and Simmons, R. L.: Risk factors in the development of cytomegalovirus-related pneumonia in renal transplant recipients. J. Infect. Dis. 148-1121, 1983.
75. Simmons, R. L., Matas, A. J., Rattazzi, L. C., Balfour, H. H., Jr., Howard, R. J., and Najarian, J. S.: Clinical characteristics of the lethal cytomegalovirus infection following renal transplantation. Surgery 82:537-546, 1977.
76. Keller, E. W., Rubin, R. H., Black, P. H., Hirsch, M. S., and Hierholzer, J. C.: Isolation of adenovirus type 34 from a renal transplant recipient with interstitial pneumonia. Transplantation 23:188-191, 1977.
77. Ramsey, P. G., Fife, K. H., Hackman, R. C., Meyers, J. D., and Corey, L.: Herpes simplex virus pneumonia. Ann. Intern. Med. 97:813-820, 1982.
78. Lichtenstein, I. H., and MacGregor, R. R.: Mycobacterial infections in renal transplant recipients: Report of five cases and review of the literature. Rev. Infect. Dis. 5:216-226, 1983.
79. Lloveras, J., Peterson, P. K., Simmons, R. L., and Najarian, J. S.: Mycobacterial infections in renal transplant recipients. Seven cases and a review of the literature. Arch. Intern. Med. 142:888-892, 1982.
80. Scowden, E. B., Schaffner, W., and Stone, W. J.: Overwhelming strongyloidiasis an unappreciated opportunistic infection. Medicine (Baltimore) 57:527-544,
81. Tilney, N. L., Kohler, T. R., and Strom, T. B.: Cerebromeningitis in immunosuppressed recipients of renal allografts. Ann. Surg. 195:104-109, 1982.
82. Hooper, D. C., Pruitt, A. A., and Rubin, R. H.: Central nervous system infection in the chronically immunosuppressed. Medicine (Baltimore) 61: 166-188,
83. Nieman, R. E., and Lorber, B.: Listeriosis in adults: A changing pattern. Report of eight cases and review of the literature, 1968-1978. Rev. Infect. Dis. 2:207-227, 1980.
84. Stamm, A. M., Dismukes, W. E., Simmons, B. P., et al.: Listeriosis in renal transplant recipients: Report of an outbreak and review of 102 cases. Rev. Infect. Dis. 4:665-682, 1982.
85. Krahenbuhl, J. L., Rosenberg, L. T., and Remington, J. S.: The role of thymus-derived lymphocytes in the in vitro activation of macrophages to kill *Listeria monocytogenes*. J. Immunol. 111:992-995, 1973.
86. Manz, H. J., Dinsdale, H. B., and Morrin, P. A. F.: Progressive multifocal leukoencephalopathy after renal transplantation. Ann. Intern. Med. 75: 77, 1971.
87. Hogan, T. F., Borden, E. C., McBain, J. A., Padgett, B. L., and Walker, D. L.: Human polyomavirus infections with JC virus and BK virus in renal transplant patients. Ann. Intern. Med. 92:373-378, 1980.
88. Andrews, C., Shah, K. V., Rubin, R., and Hirsch, M.: BK papovavirus infec-

tions in renal transplant recipients: Contribution of donor kidneys. J. Infect. Dis. 145:276, 1982).
89. Ruskin, J., and Reminston, J. S.: Toxoplasmosis in the compromised host. Ann. Intern. Med. 84:193-199, 1976.
90. Remington, J. S., and Anderson, S. E.: Diagnosis and treatment of pneumocystosis and toxoplasmosis in the immunosuppressed host. Transplantation Proc. V:1263-1270, 1973.
91. Sherlock, P., Goldstein, M. J., and Eras, P.: Esophageal moniliasis. Mod. Treat. 7(6):1250, 1970.
92. Fazio, R. A., Wickremesinghe, P. C., and Arsura, E. L.: Ketoconazole treatment of candida esophagitis—a prospective study of 12 cases. Am. J. Gastroenterol. 78:261-264, 1983.
93. Diethelm, A. G., Gore, I., Ch'ien, L. T., et al.: Gastrointestinal hemorrhage secondary to cytomegalovirus after renal transplantation. A case report and review of the problem. Am. J. Surg. 131:371, 1976.
94. Sutherland, D. E. R., Chan, F. Y., Foucar, E., et al.: The bleeding cecal ulcer in transplant patients. Surgery 86:386, 1979.
95. Briggs, W. A., Rozek, R. J., Migdal, S. D., et al.: Influenza vaccination in kidney transplant recipients: Cellular and humoral immune responses. Ann. Intern. Med. 92:471-477, 1980.
96. Linnemann, C. C., First, M. R., and Schiffman, G.: Response to pneumococcal vaccine in renal transplant and hemodialysis patients. Arch. Intern. Med. 141:1637-1640, 1981.

7

Kidney Transplantation: Cardiovascular Complications

HERVY H. HINER, JR., and WADI N. SUKI
Baylor College of Medicine and The Methodist Hospital, Houston, Texas

Because of the progressive reduction of mortality associated with renal transplantation, the potential for cardiovascular complication is enhanced. The etiology of the initial renal lesion, immunosuppressive therapy, genetic factors, transplant rejection, and metabolic abnormalities are all possible contributing factors.

In this chapter we will attempt to define the normal hemodynamic parameters in the stable renal transplant recipient and describe the various cardiovascular complications associated with renal transplantation. In addition to the description, we will discuss the probable mortality and morbidity, pathogenesis, preventive measures, and management of each entity.

I. MORTALITY FROM CARDIOVASCULAR COMPLICATIONS

The major cardiovascular causes of death include myocardial ischemia, cerebrovascular accident, cardiac arrest of undetermined etiology, and pulmonary embolism. The European Dialysis and Transplant Registry noted that more than 50% of the deaths were attributed to cardiovascular complications [1].

A U.S. study in 1981 estimated that 40% of all deaths in renal transplant recipients were cardiovascular related. This was a limited study, consisting of 30% of the total renal transplants performed between 1977 and 1980 [2]. However, another study utilizing a smaller number of patients revealed that only 20% of the posttransplant deaths were cardiovascular related. The individuals dying of cardiovascular-related problems were also noted to have a higher mean age at transplantation [3]. The diminished survival in renal transplant recipients with a prior history of end-stage renal disease, secondary to hypertension or diabetes mellitus, is probably related to the greater prevalence of cardiovascular disease associated with these disorders [4].

It is of interest that Kirkman noted cardiovascular-related deaths in only 7 of 33 (21%) individuals dying in 5½ to 20½ years posttransplantation, although hypertension was present in 100 of 204 (49%) transplant recipients greater than 5 years posttransplantation [5].

II. HEMODYNAMICS OF STABLE RENAL TRANSPLANT RECIPIENTS

Left ventricular function in patients with end-stage renal disease may be normal, decreased, or even increased. The majority of patients have normal or increased left ventricular function. This has been associated with anemia, increased heart rate and stroke volume, positive fluid balance, and a left-to-right shunt associated with arteriovenous fistulas. Left ventricular dysfunction has been noted to occur in as many as 25-40% of individuals with end-stage renal disease. This may be related to chronic volume overload, drugs (such as the β blockers), hyperkalemia, acidosis, hypoxemia, possible uremic toxins, asymptomatic ischemic heart disease, and long-standing hypertension [6]. Dialysis appears to benefit patients with depressed left ventricular function. This has been documented with improvement of left ventricular ejection fraction acutely during hemodialysis and following long-term hemodialysis and peritoneal dialysis [6].

In renal transplant recipients, left ventricular function can either decrease or increase posttransplantation [7-9]. This is apparently dependent on the pretransplant left ventricular function. Echocardiographic studies in both children and adults, with normal and increased ejection fractions and cardiac outputs, revealed a reduction in ejection fraction and cardiac output toward normal. In addition to the above, a reduction in left ventricular volume and mass and in heart rate plus a significant increase in hematocrit were noted [7,8].

Lai et al. [9] evaluated 14 individuals with echocardiography and radionuclide ventriculography pre- and posttransplantation. These individuals were presumed to be free of ischemic heart disease. However, 64% of the patients had abnormal left ventricular function. Within the first 2 months posttransplantation, he noted an increase in cardiac index, ejection fraction, and mean velocity of circumferential fiber shortening, indicating inproved ventricular function (Fig. 1). However, there was significant increase in hematocrit or decrease in heart rate. This would imply that individuals with compromised left ventricular function may have improvement in left ventricular function posttransplantation.

The hemodynamic parameters of 24 stable renal transplants were compared in another study by Kim et al. to hemodynamic parameters of 25 normal sub-

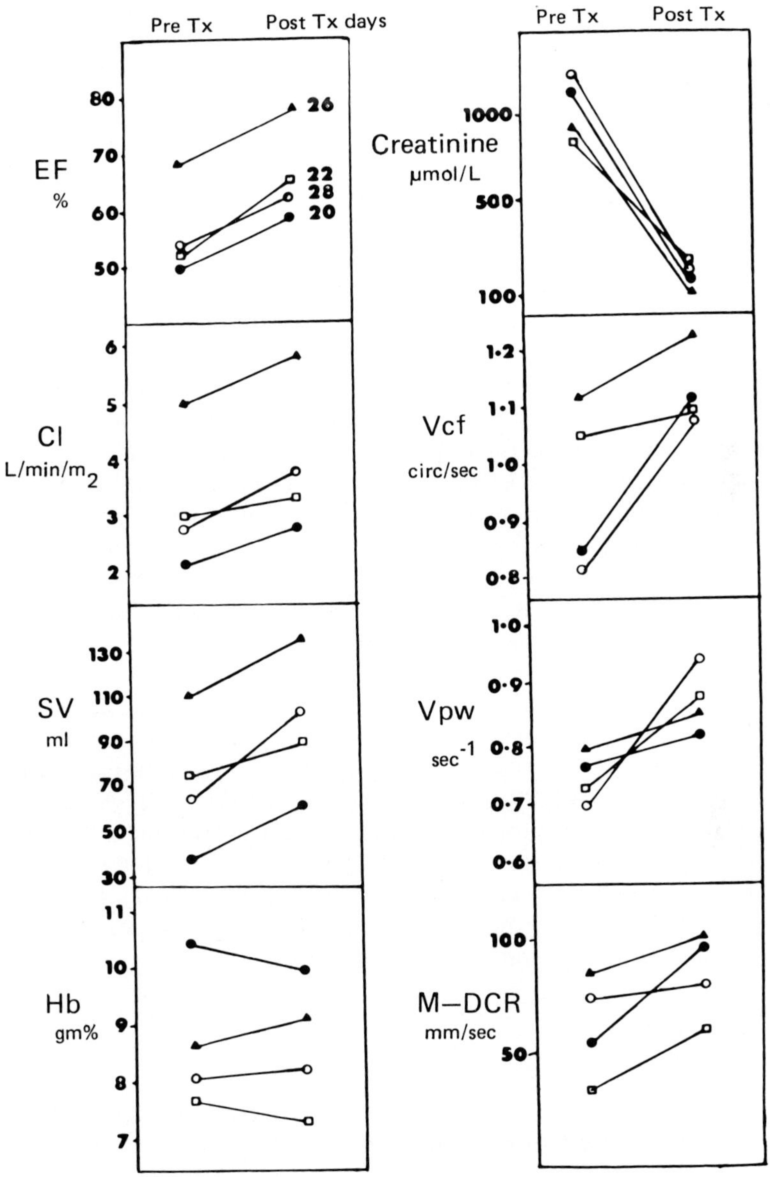

Figure 1 Improvement of the left ventricular function after successful renal transplantation in four transplant recipients. (From Lai, K. N., et al.: Clin. Nephrol. 18(2):74, 1982. Reproduced with permission.

jects [10]. The transplant recipients had a mean serum creatinine concentration of less than 177 μmol/L and a packed red cell volume greater than 30%. The mean cardiac index in both groups were not significantly different [10].

Thus, the changes in myocardial function following transplantation may be quite variable and may reflect the changes in volume status, hematocrit, and uremic environment, with some improvement expected especially when myocardial function had been depressed.

III. HYPERTENSION

Hypertension is the most common cardiovascular complication associated with renal transplantation. The prevalence of hypertension has varied between 20% and 80%. Bachy et al. [11], Rao et al. [12], and Whelton et al. [13] noted a prevalence of approximately 50%, which may be a more accurate estimate. However, the prevalence is probably higher during the first 3 months posttransplantation [14]. Hypertension is also the most common cardiovascular complication in patients with end-stage renal disease, occurring in 80% to 90% of patients with irreversible uremia. Approximately 4 of 5 of these individuals will have a reduction in their blood pressure when treated with salt restriction and ultrafiltration, which is indicative of volume-dependent hypertension.

Depsite the high prevalence of hypertension in renal transplant recipients, there is a marked reduction in the prevalence of hypertension posttransplantation. Rao et al. noted a 40% reduction in the prevalence of hypertension following renal transplantation [12]. When present, hypertension is usually of mild to moderate severity, with blood pressures frequently less than 100 mmHg diastolic. When severe hypertension is present and of new onset, it is frequently secondary to renal artery stenosis. The possible causes of hypertension posttransplantation are numerous (Table 1). However, the genesis of hypertension posttransplantation is probably multifactoral in most situations.

A. Potential Etiologies

1. Acute and Subacute Rejection

The association of hypertension with acute and subacute rejection appears to be variable. Porter et al. noted hypertension in 3 out of 4 individuals with acute rejection [15]. However, Dempster noted only an inconstant association with hypertension [16].

In the four patients of Porter who presented with fever, tachycardia, and decreased renal function, histological examination of the kidney was consistent with acute rejection. However, histological examination, after an apparent second episode of acute rejection, revealed less cellular infiltration and edema of the

Table 1 Potential Causes of Posttransplantation Hypertension

Acute and subacute rejection
Acute tubular necrosis
Steroids
Acute obstruction
Transplant renal artery stenosis
Hypercalcemia
Increased renin production from native kidneys
Genetic predisposition
Chronic rejection
Recurrent de novo glomerulonephritis

kidney with prominent vascular changes. Marked obliterative changes extended from the anastomotic site of the renal artery throughout the interlobar and arcuate arteries [15]. Gunnels et al. later suggested that the acute episodes of hypertension accompanying acute rejection are related to ischemia of the transplant grafts [17]. This was based on the association of reduced renal blood flow and increased tubular reabsorption of water and sodium. The reduction in renal blood flow was considered to be secondary to pressor effects of the renin-angiotension system. He also demonstrated increased peripheral renin activity and increased urinary aldosterone excretion coinciding with hypertension in two transplant recipients with acute rejection [17]. Dempster surmised that the renin-angiotension system played a role in the etiology of hypertension. However, he thought that a reduction in cortical blood flow was the result of increased edema and cellular infiltration secondary to acute rejection. This reduction in cortical blood flow would be the stimulant for increased renin secretion. A lack of correlation among blood pressure, plasma renin activity, and aldosterone excretion suggested the possibility of other causative factors [16]. Other mechanisms included large doses of steroid given during acute rejection and volume overload from exorbitant volume administration.

2. Acute Tubular Necrosis

Acute tubular necrosis (ATN) has been associated with hypertension and usually occurs immediately posttransplantation. The diagnosis of acute tubular necrosis is made by excluding other causes of acute renal failure. In those individuals with ATN, hypertension is most often due to fluid and salt retention. Therefore, the hypertension usually responds to volume removal and sodium restriction [18,19].

Increased plasma renin activity has also been found in individuals with ATN. However, it is unclear whether the increase in plasma renin activity is the result of ATN or other possible underlying mechanisms, such as hemorrhage or sepsis. Roguska et al. obtained serial determinations of peripheral renin activity in 19 transplant recipients, 5 of whom were thought to have ATN, who had only transient hypertension [20]. Even though there was an increase in plasma renin activity compared to controls, the increment was not significant. Therefore, other factors are probably involved in the genesis of hypertension in transplant recipients with ATN.

3. Steroids

The concept of steroids being the major source of hypertension in transplant recipients is controversial. Popovtzer et al. suggested that during acute rejection, the increase in blood pressure may at least be related to renal pressor mechanisms; however, with normal renal function, the high doses of glucocorticoids may play an important role in the development of hypertension [21]. They noted that blood pressure increased early posttransplantation in patients with normal homograft function, yet returned to normal 3-8 weeks after transplantation. The blood pressure correlated closely with the dose of prednisone [21]. Several authors have also noted a positive correlation between the frequency of hypertension and prednisone therapy. Curtis et al. [22], McHugh et al. [23], and Sampson and Albert [24] noted a decrease in the frequency of hypertension in patients converted to alternate-day steroid therapy. Sampson attributed the hypertensive effects of steroids to aldosterone or aldosteronelike metabolites. He was able to demonstrate, in the body, the conversion of ^{14}C-labeled cortisone to aldosterone. Elevated levels of aldosterone in hypertensive transplant recipients was also noted by Sampson. After converting patients to alternate-day steroids, he was able to obtain good correlation between the quantity of aldosterone antagonists and a fall in blood pressure and urinary aldosterone excretion [25]. However, McHugh et al. noted an increase in aldosterone levels with decreased potassium levels and slight elevation in exchangeable sodium in recipients converted to alternate-day therapy [23]. They suggested that alternate-day steroid therapy resulted in less suppression of the pituitary adrenal axis. This would theoretically cause increased production of adrenocorticotropic hormone, resulting in increased aldosterone secretion. These investigators also noted a marked reduction in plasma renin activity after alternate-day therapy. However, no direct correlation could be obtained with plasma renin activity and blood pressure. McHugh theorized that the reduction in plasma renin activity was not due to a reduction in renin production, but to a reduction in output of angiotensinogen by the liver [23]. The production of angiotensinogen is influenced by steroid hormones and has been shown to be increased in conditions of steroid excess, such as Cushing's syndrome, glucocorticoid therapy, and oral contraceptives [26].

Despite the above studies, many long-term studies have failed to show an increase in the dose of steroids in hypertensive recipients compared to normotensive recipients [11-13,27,28]. Consequently, the extremely large doses of steroids given during the initial posttransplant period and during acute rejection potentially contribute to the genesis of early hypertension. Yet, the maintenance doses of steroids probably contribute little to hypertension in stable patients.

4. Acute Ureteral Obstruction

Campese listed ureteral obstruction as a possible cause of acute renal failure and hypertension [18]. Theoretically, hypertension is probably related to salt and water retention. However, the documentation of acute ureteral obstruction as a cause of hypertension in a transplant recipient is scanty at best [18].

5. Transplant Renal Artery Stenosis

The incidence of renal artery stenosis varies from 0.6 to 16% [13,18,29]. Clinical features suggestive of transplant renal artery stenosis include the development of hypertension in a previously normotensive individual or severe exacerbation of pre-existing hypertension [12]. Bruits over the transplanted kidney, plasma renin activity, and selective renal vein renins are not sensitive or specific indicators of transplant renal artery stenosis. The etiology of transplant renal artery stenosis may be mechanically or immunologically related [18]. Transplant renal artery stenosis will be discussed in detail in other sections of the text.

6. Hypercalcemia

Persistent hypercalcemia and significant hyperparathyroidism occur in 20-34% of renal transplant recipients [30-32]. The hypercalcemia appears within the first 6 months of renal transplantation in the majority of cases, but it may appear later. This is dependent on body stores of phosphate, doses of glucocorticoids, the rate of involution of hyperplastic parathyroid glands, and the rapidity with which skeletal resistance to the calcemic action of parathyroid hormone disappears [30].

Hypercalcemia may be transient or persistent. However, persistent hypercalcemia rarely exists for more than 2 years' duration. In most patients, the hypercalcemia is mild, with the serum calcium ranging between 11.0 and 12.0 mg/dL. Only a small number of patients will have a serum calcium greater than 13 mg/dL.

There are several roles calcium could play in the genesis of hypertension. First, hypertension could be related to a reduction in renal function with increased salt and water retention. However, reduction in renal function usually does not occur until serum calcium is greater than 13 mg/dL [33].

Other possible mechanisms include increased myocardial contractility, increased peripheral vascular resistance, and possible enhanced sensitivity of the cardiovascular and the central nervous systems to the effects of the calcium ion in the presence of uremia or uremic toxins [30,34].

Mild hypercalcemia does not pose an immediate threat to renal function and may or may not be a factor in an individual transplant recipient. However, renal function should be followed closely. If renal function deteriorates, in the absence of other causes or renal deterioration, subtotal parathyroidectomy should be considered.

7. Hypertension Associated with Native Kidneys

In transplant recipients who have not had bilateral pretransplant nephrectomies, the incidence of hypertension approaches 80% compared with 40% in recipients who have pretransplant nephrectomies [35,36]. Implying that the transplant recipient's native kidneys are playing a role in the development of posttransplantation hypertension [37,38], Linas et al. [37] attempted to define the role of the renin-angiotensin system in posttransplantation hypertensive patients. Saralasin acetate, an angiotensin II antagonist, was given to 12 hypertensive patients, 6 with only one kidney and 6 with more than one kidney. Saralasin was given in the sodium-repleted and sodium-depleted states. A marked reduction in angiotensin II activity and blood pressure was noted in the salt-depleted group with multiple kidneys after the administration of saralasin, suggesting angiotensin II-dependent hypertension. He also demonstrated, in 4 of 5 patients, greater renal vein renin activity in one or more host kidneys relative to the transplant kidney. Despite this interesting finding, the use of this test in predicting the curability of hypertension after nephrectomy of the host kidney has been disappointing [12,39,40].

8. Genetic Predisposition to Hypertension

Guyton and Bianchi et al. have suggested that the kidney is the culprit in the genesis of hypertension [41,42]. Bianchi et al. were able to transfer hypertension by kidney cross-transplantation between hypertensive and normotensive rats [42]. Later, Guidi et al. attempted to establish a similar occurrence in humans [43]. They correlated the blood pressure of transplant recipients with the blood pressure in donor family members on the premise that the offspring of hypertensive parents will develop hypertension later in life with a greater frequency than will offspring of normotensive parents. Recipients of kidneys from donors with familial hypertension were found to require more antihypertensive medications compared with recipients without familial hypertension (Fig. 2). These findings were noticeable during the first 4 months after transplantation [43].

The mechanism involved in establishing hypertension is unknown. However, the mechanism should be similar to the mechanism involved in the genesis of essential hypertension. It is of interest that Curtis et al. reported remission of essential hypertension in six individuals receiving renal transplant from normotensive donors [44].

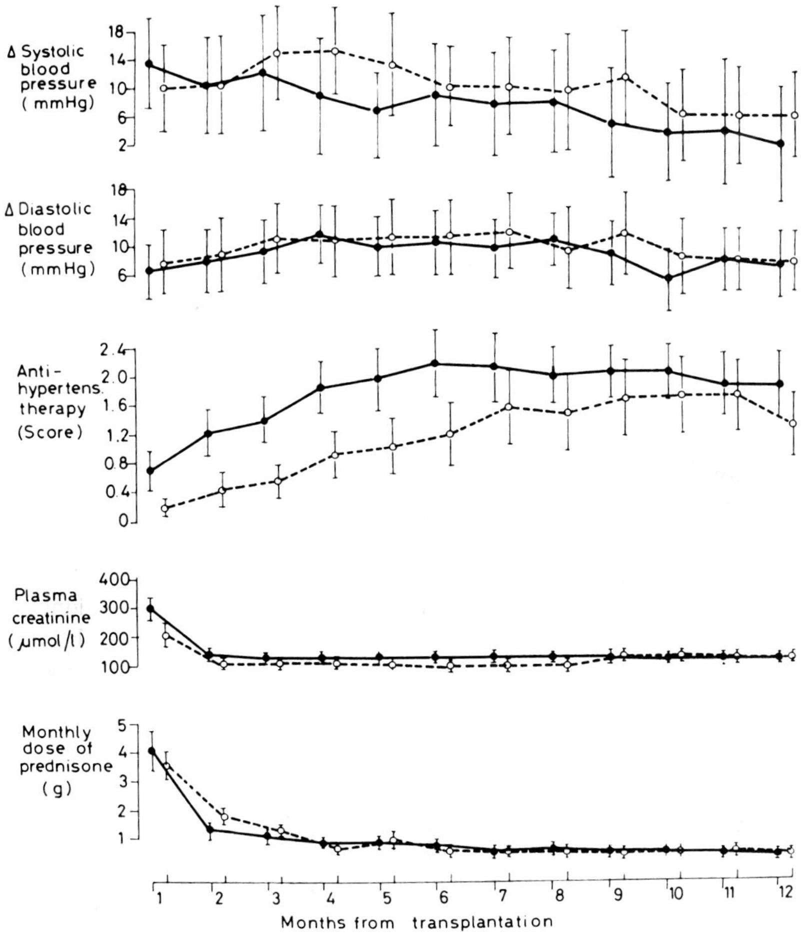

Figure 2 Monthly means of systolic and diastolic blood pressures expressed as the differences from pregrafting blood pressures, plasma creatinine, total dose of prednisone, and monthly dose of antihypertensive drugs expressed as scores in 18 renal transplant recipients from donors with a positive family history for hypertension (●) and in 18 recipients with a negative family history of hypertension (○). No antihypertensive drug, including diuretics, was indicated as 0; 1 point added for each drug given, including diuretic patients with an additional score of 1 point added when the dose of any antihypertensive was more than 4 pills/day. (From Guidi, E., et al.: Nephron 30:318, 1982. Reproduced with permission from S. Karger, AG, Basel.)

9. Chronic Rejection

Several authors have noted a higher mean serum creatinine in hypertensive patients that had no obvious attribution [11,12]. Therefore, this increment was attributed to chronic rejection. Also, several authors have noted an increased prevalence of hypertension in recipients of cadaveric kidneys [13,45,46]. The increased prevalence of hypertension in recipients of cadaveric allografts has also been attributed to the greater frequency of chronic rejection in these individuals.

The pathophysiology of hypertension associated with chronic rejection is unclear. However, Bennett and coinvestigators, with the use of xenon-133 washout technique redemonstrated a reduction in renal and cortical blood flow in 13 hypertensive patients compared with controls (Fig. 3). A total of 11 hypertensive patients underwent renal biopsy, which revealed chronic rejection in 7 patients. The mean renal vein renin activity was markedly elevated in the hypertensive group [47]. However, Grunfeld et al. found normal renal vein renin values in their study [48]. Bennett et al. [47] proposed that renal cortical ischemia was the stimulus for renin production and the development of hypertension. However, the significance of elevated renin levels is unclear.

10. Recurrent De Novo Glomerulonephritis

Late hypertension could possibly be due to recurrent glomerulonephritis. The forms of glomerulonephritis that tend to recur include type II membranopro-

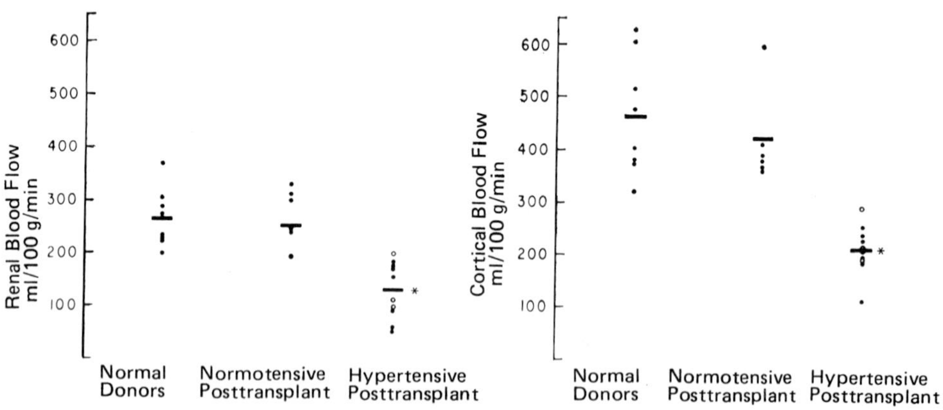

Figure 3 Renal blood flow in normal transplant donors, normotensive posttransplant patients, and hypertensive posttransplant patients. Left, mean renal blood flow rate; right, cortical blood flow rate. Mean values for each group depicted by bar. Asterisk, $P < 0.01$; open circle, transplant artery stenosis. (From Bennet, W. M., et al.: Kidney Int. 6:99, 1974. Reproduced with permission).

liferative glomerulonephritis, IgA nephropathy, focal and segmental glomerulosclerosis, Goodpasture's syndrome, and membranous glomerulonephritis. The documentation of hypertension in reported cases of recurrent disease is often lacking. Nevertheless, this is a potential cause of latent hypertension.

B. Management of Hypertension in the Transplant Recipient

The management of hypertension in patients posttransplantation with relatively normal renal function is practically the same as in individuals with essential hypertension. However, in many patients, hypertension may be refractory to treatment and require special consideration. Transplant recipients with transplant renal artery stenosis, renal insufficiency, and tubular defects associated with potassium abnormalities will also require careful attention.

Transplant recipients taking multiple medications who are refractory to treatment may frequently respond to captopril, which is an angiotensin converting enzyme inhibitor [49-51]. As noted earlier, an overly active renin-angiotensin system has been implicated in the genesis of posttransplantation hypertension. It is therefore conceivable that captopril may be particularly effective in the treatment of posttransplantation hypertension. The saralasin acetate test has been noted to be more sensitive than plasma renin activity as an indicator of renin-dependent hypertension. However, the saralasin acetate test has poor specificity for identification of any one cause of posttransplant hypertension, because of the various causes of renin hypertension [52].

Captopril may also be beneficial in the treatment of non-renin-mediated hypertension. In these individuals, the antihypertensive effect of captopril may be due to its ability to inhibit the breakdown of vasodepressor kinins. Kinin degradation requires normal activity of converting enzymes [52].

Captopril and its metabolites are excreted by the kidney. Many side effects, particularly granulocytopenia and membranous glomerular changes, were noted before it was recognized that doses should be reduced in the presence of impaired renal function and/or combined with other drugs capable of suppressing the bone marrow. Hyperkalemia, requiring discontinuation of captopril, has been reported in a patient with impaired graft function after transplantation [50]. Therefore, white cell count, urine protein, and serum potassium concentration should be monitored closely in transplant recipients receiving this drug.

Curtis et al. described acute reversible loss of renal function when captopril was added to the antihypertensive regimen of four individuals with transplant renal artery stenosis [53]. The renal failure was nonoliguric in nature and was associated with a marked increase in creatinine and blood urea nitrogen, usually after the initial dose. The renal insufficiency in this setting is probably secondary to diminished autoregulation because of the inhibition of angiotensin II formation in the presence of decreased renal blood flow [53].

Minoxidil is a very potent vasodilator and is useful for the treatment of refractory hypertension. Minoxidil acts directly on the arteriolar smooth muscle, causing marked relaxation. Sodium retention can be pronounced, often requiring large doses of loop diuretics. Other side effects include hirsutism and pericardial effusion [54]. Calcium channel blockers, particularly nifedipine, have been used to treat accelerated hypertension but have not been used extensively in the treatment of transplant recipients. However, nifedipine may also cause acute deterioration of renal function in individuals with renal artery stenosis or renal insufficiency. Nifedipine may also interfere with autoregulation by reducing the efficacy of vasoconstrictor hormones in regulation of renal blood flow and glomerular filtration rate, or by inhibiting the compensatory synthesis of vasodilatory prostaglandin E_2 [55].

IV. ATHEROSCLEROTIC COMPLICATIONS

Cardiovascular complications secondary to atherosclerotic cardiovascular disease constitute a major cause of death in renal transplant recipients. Death rates from myocardial infarction and stroke are many times higher than in the normal population [56,57]. These rates are even more pronounced in individuals with a history of prior diabetic nephropathy or hypertensive nephrosclerosis. However, many atheromatous complications may have been the result of atherosclerosis acquired before transplantation, during regular dialysis or before.

A. Myocardial Infarction

Because of improved immunotherapy and medical support of transplant recipients, there is less reluctance in transplanting so-called high-risk patients, such as diabetic patients and older individuals.

Recipients dying of myocardial infarction have a higher mean age and higher mortality. The mean age of individuals dying of myocardial infarction in one study was 50 years [3]. The true incidence of myocardial infarction in transplant recipients is unclear, but it varies between 2 and 11% [58,59]. The variability in incidence is due to differences in the populations studied. These differences include age, location of the study, underlying cause of end-stage renal disease, and pre-existing ischemic heart disease. Likewise, Gunnarson and coinvestigators noted more than a 10-fold greater incidence of myocardial infarction among transplant recipients compared with an age- and sex-matched unselected population [58]. The risk of developing myocardial infarction is greatest for individuals with advanced age who have a history of angina pectoris prior to renal transplantation [58,60]. Mortality also appears to be high in these individuals, with a first infarction mortality of 45% and a mortality of 100% noted within the first year in one study [58].

Braun et al. attempted to identify patients with end-stage renal disease who were at increased risk of developing coronary artery disease [61]. They performed coronary arteriograms in 99 patients on chronic hemodialysis in preparation for renal transplantation. They noted 13 coronary deaths in 23 individuals who died with more than 70% occlusion in one or more coronary vessels compared with none of 27 with less than 70% occlusion. Of the 48 patients receiving renal transplantation, coronary deaths were noted in 2 of 11 individuals dying posttransplantation, with 70% occlusion in one or more coronary vessels, compared to no coronary deaths in recipients with less than 70% occlusion. However, more than three times as many transplants were performed in individuals who had less than 70% occlusion than were done in those with more than 70% occlusion [61].

Survival for diabetic patients receiving renal transplant is less than that of nondiabetic recipients, but is superior to long-term hemodialysis patients. A recent study from the University of Minnesota, involving patients with juvenile-onset diabetes mellitus, noted 43 total deaths. Of these, 28 deaths were cardiovascular related, with 18 deaths secondary to myocardial infarction [62]. Recipients with nephrosclerosis are also at increased risk of developing ischemic heart disease. Mahoney et al. studied 14 patients with end-stage renal disease secondary to essential malignant hypertension [60]. Of 4 patients who had symptoms of ischemic heart disease before transplantation, 3 died of myocardial infarction within 31 months posttransplantation. Also, 2 additional patients developed ischemic heart disease in the 6-year period after renal transplantation.

Therapy for ischemic heart disease in renal transplant recipients is similar to that of the general population. With appropriate preoperative anesthetic, and postoperative management, patients with functioning renal allografts can undergo cardiac surgery without unacceptable morbidity and mortality [63].

B. Occlusive Atherosclerosis

Peripheral and cerebral occlusive disease occurs less frequently than coronary heart disease in transplant recipients. The cumulative incidence of all types of occlusive arterial disease over a 6-year period has been estimated to be 416 per 1000, with 60% of occlusive disease secondary to coronary disease and the remainder due to peripheral and cerebrovascular disease [64]. Of all deaths in renal transplant recipients, 1.8-13% have been the result of cerebrovascular accidents [1,2]. Potential risk factors of occlusive arterial disease include hyperparathyroidism with vascular calcifications, persistent hypertension, excessive smoking, increased serum cholesterol and triglycerides, increased hematocrit, and obesity [64].

Diabetic individuals are particularly prone to the development of peripheral vascular disease. Almost all those with diabetes have some evidence of peripheral vascular disease at the time of transplantation. Vascular disease appears to progress after transplantation, with amputation of digits or extremities in approximately 15% of diabetic recipients. As expected, the incidence of cerebrovascular disease is also increased in these individuals [59,62].

The pathogenesis of atherosclerosis in transplant recipients is probably multifactorial, with its initiation beginning in the predialysis or pretransplant period.

V. VENOUS THROMBOEMBOLISM

Venous thromboembolism is a major problem posttransplantation. Its frequency varies between 0.6 and 21% and may be even higher in diabetic transplant recipients [65,66]. The variability in frequency is due to the definition of the disease and whether the report is a clinical or autopsy study.

Pulmonary embolism is the major cause of venous thromboembolic death. The incidence of pulmonary embolism posttransplantation varies between 3 and 14% and has been noted by some authors to be the second leading cause of death [1,2,66]. Other locations of thromboembolism include the inferior vena cava, renal, femoral, calf, mesenteric, and hemorrhoidal veins.

Renal transplant recipients are probably at greatest risk of developing venous thromboembolism during the first month posttransplantation. However, the risk period may extend up to 1 year, in contrast to other types of surgery, in which it is negligible after 1 month [66]. There are several potential reasons for the increased frequency, which include fibrinolytic inhibition and delayed emptying of the venous system secondary to venous obstruction, caused by hematomas and lymphoceles, and reduced venous blood flow due to polycythemia and portal hypertension [66]. Corticosteroids may enhance factor VIII and reduce plasminogen activator, which would tend to increase the tendency to develop venous thrombosis [67]. However, Arnadottir and Vanrenterghem and their collaborators could not establish an association of steroid therapy with the development of venous thromboembolic disease [66,68]. Recently, Vanrenterghem and coinvestigators studied the frequency of thromboembolic complications in cyclosporine-treated recipients of cadaveric renal allografts. They also compared the results of hemostatic tests in a group of these individuals to those of azathioprine-treated patients and normal controls. In the cyclosporine group, which consisted of 90 patients, 17 thromboembolic complications occurred in 13 patients compared with 1 episode of superficial thrombophlebitis in 90 patients receiving azathioprine. The thromboembolic complications in the cyclosporine group consisted mostly of episodes involving pulmonary embolism. The hemostatic tests revealed enhanced platelet aggregation in the cyclosporine group induced by adenosine-5′-diphosphate (ADP) (Fig. 4). The response to ADP in the cyclosporine patients was closely correlated with the drug levels, implying that a cyclosporine-associated change may be responsible for increased aggregation. Factor VIIIC and fibrinogen were also significantly increased in the cyclosporine group. Both factor VIIIC

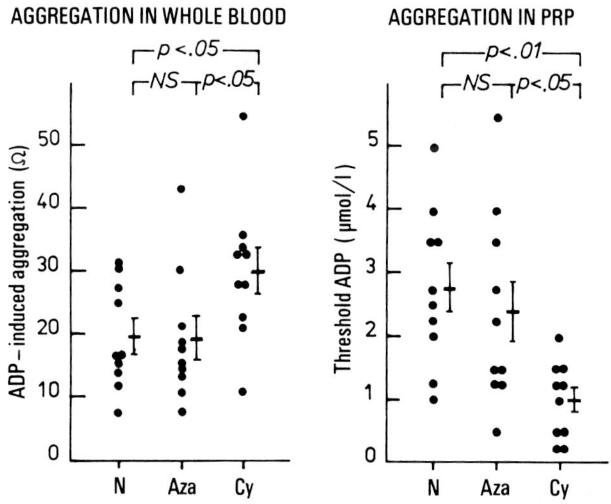

Figure 4 Platelet aggregation in whole blood and platelet-rich plasma in controls and renal transplant recipients receiving azathioprine and cyclosporine. Aggregation was studied about 1 hr after venipuncture in whole blood (impedance aggregometry) stimulated with ADP, 5 μmol/L. Maximum amplitude in ohms (Ω) was calculated. Aggregation studies in PRP are reported as the minimum of the inducer (in μmol/L), which gave a second wave of aggregation. N = normal control; Aza = azathioprine; Cy = cyclosporine; NS = not significant. Bars indicate mean ± SEM. (From Vanrenterghem, Y., et al.: Lancet 1:999, 1985. Reproduced with permission.)

and fibrinogen have been associated with enhanced thrombosis. In contrast, the cyclosporine patients had significantly higher levels of antithrombin III and protein C, which should be protective against venous thromboembolism. The hemostatic tests were obtained several months posttransplantation. If the tests were obtained during the first week posttransplantation, when the occurrence of thromboembolism was greatest, there may have been a greater indication of venous thromboembolism [68].

VI. LIPID ABNORMALITIES IN RENAL TRANSPLANT RECIPIENTS

Lipid abnormalities can result in a predisposition to peripheral atherosclerosis and, more importantly, premature coronary artery disease. Lipid abnormalities exist in patients with end-stage renal disease and in renal transplant recipients. Hypertriglyceridemia is the major lipid abnormality in dialyzed and undialyzed patients with uremia, occurring in 20-70% of those individuals [69]. The lipoprotein pattern is type IV and is characterized by increased very low density lipoproteins (VLDL) [69,70]. This is probably related to decreased postheparin lipolytic activity, which is an indirect measurement of lipoprotein and hepatic lipases. Both enzymes are responsible for the catabolism of triglycerides [69,71]. High-density lipoproteins (HDL), which have been demonstrated to be a protective factor of ischemic heart disease, are also frequently diminished in patients on dialysis [72].

Hyperlipidemia is also very common in renal transplant recipients. The prevalence ranges from 50 to 78%, but it may diminish with increased graft survival [1,73]. The lipid abnormalities may include types IIa and IIb, as well as type IV hyperlipidemia, with types IIb and type IV abnormalities more common [69-71, 73].

HDL cholesterol concentration has been reported to be low, normal, and high. However, most often the HDL cholesterol levels are noted to be low pretransplantation but increase posttransplantation with improved renal function. Yet, HDL cholesterol does not appear to increase after periods of acute rejection or when graft function is not sustained [74]. Successful transplantation has also restored to normal the lipid and protein content of HDL as expressed by an increase in concentration of apolipoprotein A and normalization of the ratio of the HDL cholesterol to apolipoprotein A. This would suggest a reversal of risk factors associated with atherosclerotic cardiovascular disease [74-76].

The pathogenesis of the lipid abnormalities posttransplantation is thought by some to be related to corticosteroid therapy [69,73] but not by others [70,71]. Chan et al. and Ibels et al. noted higher cumulative steroid doses in hyperlipemic than in normolipemic renal allograft recipients [69,73]. Also, a lower prevalence of hyperlipidemia has been reported in patients treated with alternate-day steroid therapy [77]. However, this was not demonstrated by Ponticelli et al. [71]. Nevertheless, insulin resistance and hyperinsulinism associated with the use of corticosteroids has been proposed as a possible mechanism in the pathogenesis of hyperlipidemia in transplant recipients. In acute experimental rats, the rate-limiting enzymes of lipogenesis, acetyl coenzyme A (CoA) carboxylase and free fatty acid synthetase, increase after steroid administration. Furthermore, this increment was preceded by a rise in immunoreactive insulin. No rise in acetyl CoA carboxylase could be demonstrated in alloxan-diabetic rats [69].

Triglyceride clearance mechanisms have also been shown to be impaired in some transplant recipients. Postheparin lipolytic activity has been shown to be diminished in transplant recipients with impaired graft function. This could explain the association between serum creatinine and serum triglyceride concentration [78]. Reduced triglyceride clearance has also been noted in transplant recipients with normal serum creatinine concentration and has been attributed by one author to the suppression of lipoprotein lipase activity by corticosteroids [77]. Drugs may also play a role in the genesis of lipid abnormalities. Hypertriglyceridemia has been associated with estrogens, oral contraceptives, β blockers, and hydrochlorothiazides [79,80]. Jackson and Lee [79] were able to demonstrate a strong correlation between propranolol therapy and an increase in VLDL triglycerides and a decrease in HDL cholesterol in transplant recipients. They also noted increased LDL cholesterol in recipients with greater than 0.5 g of proteinuria in a 24-hr period, which is most often expected when proteinuria is severe.

Because of the association of lipid abnormalities with accelerated atherosclerosis, identification and treatment of the abnormality may be important. Yet, it is unclear whether these abnormalities or the correction of these abnormalities alters the progression of atherosclerosis. Nevertheless, the basic treatment of hyperlipidemia is diet control. Type IV hyperlipidemia may be controlled by weight reduction, limitation of alcohol intake, and reduction in carbohydrate consumption. However, caution must be used to avoid malnutrition. Type II and IV hyperlipidemia may correct by increasing the ratio of polyunsaturated to saturated fat. However, the long-term effects of this diet have not been established [71].

Lipid abnormalities may also be treated with drug therapy. Clofibrate may be used to treat type IV hyperlipidemia. Because clofibrate is metabolized by the kidney, metabolites may accumulate in patients with renal insufficiency. This may result in the elevation of serum creatinine phosphokinase levels and even severe myositis [71,80].

REFERENCES

1. Raine, A. E., and Ledingham, J. G. G.: Cardiovascular complications after renal transplantation. In: Morris, P. J., ed., Kidney Transplantation, London: Grune & Stratton, 1984, p. 470.
2. Rosansky, S. J., and Sugimoto, T.: An analysis of the United States renal transplantation patient population and organ survival characteristics, 1977 to 1980. Kidney Int. 22:685, 1982.
3. Washer, G. F., Schroter, G. J., and Starzl, T. E.: Causes of death after kidney transplantation. JAMA 250:49, 1983.
4. Vollmer, W. M., Wahl, P. A., and Blagg, C. R.: Survival with dialysis and transplantation in patients with end stage renal disease. N. Engl. J. Med. 308: 1553, 1983.
5. Kirkman, R. L., Strom, T. B., and Tilney, N. L.: Late mortality and morbidity in recipients of long term renal allografts. Transplantation 34:347, 1982.
6. Ayus, J. C., Frommer, J. P., and Young, J. B.: Cardiac and circulatory abnormalities in chronic renal failure. Semin. Nephrol. 1:112, 1981.
7. Cueto-Garcia, L., Herrera, J., and Arriaga, J.: Echocardiographic changes after

successful renal transplantation in young non-diabetic patients. Chest 83: 56, 1983.
8. O'Regan, S., Douste-Blazy, M. Y., and Ducharme, G.: Renal transplantation and cardiac function in pediatric patients. Clin. Nephrol. 17:237, 1982.
9. Lai, K. N., Barnden, L., and Mathew, T. H.: Effect of renal transplantation on left ventricular function in hemodialysis patients. Clin. Nephrol. 18:74, 1982.
10. Kim, K. E., Bates, O., and Lyons, P.: Haemodynamics of stable renal transplant recipients. Clin. Sci. 59:377' 1980.
11. Bachy, C., Alexandre, G. J., and Van Ypersele de Strihou, C.: Hypertension after renal transplantation. Br. Med. J. 2:1287, 1976.
12. Rao, T. K. S., Gupta, S. K., and Butt, K. H.: Relationship of renal transplantation to hypertension in end-stage renal failure. Arch. Intern. Med. 138: 1236, 1978.
13. Whelton, P. K., Russel, R. P., and Harrington, D. P.: Hypertension following renal transplantation. JAMA 241:1128, 1979.
14. Bachy, C. H., Van Ypersele de Strihou, C., and Alexandre, G. J.: Hypertension after renal transplantation. Proc. Eur. Dial. Transplant. Assoc. 12:461, 1976.
15. Porter, K. A., Thompson, W. B., and Owen, K.: Obliterative vascular changes in four human kidney homotransplants. Br. Med. J. 2:639, 1963.
16. Dempster, W. J.: Hypertension and acute rejection processes in allotransplanted kidneys. Br. J. Exp. Pathol. 51:149, 1970.
17. Gunnels, J. C., Stickel, O. L., and Robinson, R. R.: Episodic hypertension associated with positive renin assays after renal transplantation. N. Engl. J. Med. 274:543, 1966.
18. Campese, V. M.: Discussion; in Feinstein, E. I., Hypertension in a renal transplant recipient. Am. J. Nephrol. 4:262, 1984.
19. Malekzadeh, M. H., Brennan, L. P., and Payne, V. C.: Hypertension after renal transplantation in children. J. Pediatr., 86:370, 1975.
20. Roguska, J., Del Greco, F., and Simon, N. M.: Serum renin activity in human renal homotransplantation. Nephron 8:289, 1971.
21. Popovtzer, M. M., Pinnggera, W., and Katz, F. H.: Variations in arterial blood pressure after kidney transplantation. Circulation 47:1297, 1973.
22. Curtis, J. J., Gala, J. H., and Kotchen, T. A.: Prevalence of hypertension in a renal transplant population on alternate day steroid therapy. Clin. Nephrol. 5:123, 1976.
23. McHugh, M. E., Tanboga, H., and Wilkinson, R.: Alternate day steroids and blood pressure control after renal transplantation. Proc. Eur. Dial. Transplant. Assoc. 17:496, 1980.
24. Sampson, D., and Albert, D. J.: Alternate day therapy with methylprednisolone after renal transplantation. J. Urol. 109:345, 1973.
25. Sampson, D.: Hypertension after renal transplantation. Transplant. Proc. 7(Suppl. 1):691, 1975.
26. Krakoff, L. R., and Mendlowitz, M.: Plasma renin activity and plasma renin

substrate in hypertension associated with steroid excess. Clin. Sci. Mol. Med. 45:2955, 1973.
27. Pollini, J., Guttman, R. D., and Beaudoin, D. D.: Late hypertension following renal allotransplantation. Clin. Nephrol. 11:202, 1978.
28. Hamilton, D. V., Carmichael, D. S., and Evans, D. B.: Hypertension in renal transplant recipients on cyclosporin A and corticosteroids and azathioprine. Transplant. Proc., 14:597, 1982.
29. Rijksen, J. F. W. B., Koolen, M. I., and Walaszewski, J. E.: Vascular complications in 400 consecutive renal allotransplants. J. Cardiovasc. Surg. 23:91, 1982.
30. Chatterjee, S. W., Friedler, R. M., and Berne, T. V.: Persistent hypercalcemia after successful renal transplantation. Nephron 17:1, 1976.
31. Schwartz, E. H., David, D. S., and Riggio, R. R.: Hypercalcemia after renal transplantation. Am. J. Med. 49:42, 1970.
32. Giess, W. P., Popovtzer, M. M., and Cormen, J. L.: The diagnosis and treatment of hyperparathyroidism after renal homotransplantation. Surg. Gynecol. Obstet. 137:997, 1973.
33. David, D. S., Sukai, S., and Brennan, B. L.: Hypercalcemia after renal transplantation. N. Engl. J. Med. 289:398, 1973.
34. Weidmann, P., Massry, S. G., and Coburn, J. W.: Blood pressure effects of acute hypercalcemia. Studies in patients with chronic renal failure. Ann. Intern. Med. 76:741, 1972.
35. Cohen, S. L.: Hypertension in renal transplant recipients: Role of bilateral nephrectomy. Br. Med. J. 3:78, 1973.
36. Coles, G. A., Crosby, D. L., and Jones, G. R.: Hypertension following cadaveric renal transplantation. Postgrad. Med. J. 48:399, 1972.
37. Linas, S. L., Miller, P. D., and McDonald, K. M.: Role of the renin-angiotensin system in post-transplantation hypertension in patients with multiple kidneys. N. Engl. J. Med. 298:1440, 1978.
38. Grunfeld, J. P., Kleinknecht, D., and Moreau, J. F.: Permanent hypertension after homotransplantation in man. Clin. Sci. Mol. Med. 48:391, 1975.
39. Gupta, S. W., Rao, T. K. S., and Butt, N. M. H.: Renal artery stenosis in renal transplant recipients. Proc. Clin. Dial. Transplant. Forum 6:162, 1976.
40. Ribot, S., and Byrd, L.: Post-renal transplant hypertension. N. Engl. J. Med. 294:342, 1976.
41. Guyton, A. C.: Arterial Pressure and Hypertension, Philadelphia: W. B. Saunders, 1980, p. 457.
42. Bianchi, G., Cusi, D., and Guidi, E.: Renal hemodynamics in human subjects and in animals with genetic hypertension during the prehypertensive stage. Am. J. Nephrol. 3:73, 1983.
43. Guidi, E., Bianchi, G., and Dallosta, V.: Influence of familial hypertension of the donor on the blood pressure and antihypertensive therapy of kidney graft recipients. Nephron 30:318, 1982.
44. Curtis, J. J., Luke, R. G., and Dustan, H. P.: Remission of essential hypertension after renal transplantation. N. Engl. J. Med. 309:1009, 1983.

45. Goldman, R., Meredith, W. T., and Reeve, C. E.: Blood pressure levels and hypertension in patients surviving renal homotransplantation at least one year. Read before the Fourth International Congress of Nephrology, Stockholm, June 22-27, 1969.
46. Jacquot, C., Idatte, J. M., and Bedrossian, J.: Long-term blood pressure changes in renal homotransplantation. Arch. Intern. Med. 138:233, 1978.
47. Bennett, W. M., McDonald, J. W., and Lawson, R. K.: Post-transplant hypertension: Studies of cortical blood flow and the renal pressor system. Kidney Int. 6:99, 1974.
48. Grunfeld, J. P., Kleinchnecht, D., and Moreau, J. F.: Permanent hypertension after renal homotransplantation in man. Clin. Sci. Mol. Med. 48:391, 1973.
49. Venkatachalam, K., and Kosanovich, J. M.: Captopril in hypertension after renal transplantation. Clin. Nephrol. 19:265, 1983.
50. Hamilton, D. V., Evans, W. B., and Maidment, G.: Captopril for refractory hypertension in patients with chronic renal failure and renal transplantation. J. R. Soc. Med. 74:357, 1981.
51. Herlitz, H., Ahlmen, J., and Aurell, M. D.: Captopril in hypertension after renal transplantation. Lancet 2:1366, 1983.
52. Zawada, E. T., Green, S. J., and Johnson, M. D.: Saralasin acetate test in renal transplant hypertension. Arch. Intern. Med. 144:65, 1984.
53. Curtis, J. J., Luke, R. G., and Welchel, A. G.: Inhibition of angiotensin-converting enzyme in renal transplant recipients with hypertension. N. Engl. J. Med. 308:377, 1983.
54. Sullivan, J. M., and Johnson, J. B.: The management of hypertension in patients with renal insufficiency. Sem. Nephrol. 3:40, 1983.
55. Diamond, J. R., Cheung, J. Y., and Fang, L. S. T.: Nifedipine induced renal dysfunction, alterations in renal hemodynamics. Am. J. Med. 77:905, 1984.
56. Nicholls, A. J., Catto, G. R. D., and Edwards, N.: Accelerated atherosclerosis in long term dialysis and renal transplant patients: Fact or fiction. Lancet 1:276, 1980.
57. Brunner, F. P., Brynger, H., and Chantler, C.: Combined report on regular dialysis and transplantation in Europe, IX, 1978. Proc. Eur. Dial. Transplant. Assoc. 16:3, 1979.
58. Gunnarsson, R. L., Lofmark, R., and Nordlander, O.: Acute myocardial infarction in renal transplant recipients: Incidence and prognosis. Eur. Heart J. 5:218, 1984.
59. Najarian, J. S., Simmons, R. L., and Kjellstrand, C. M.: Kidney transplantation for the uremic diabetic patient. Surg. Gynecol. Obstet. 144:682, 1977.
60. Mahony, J. F., Ibels, L. S., and Sheil, R.: Renal transplantation. Effect on the ischemic heart disease of essential malignant hypertension. JAMA 235:2318, 1976.
61. Braun, W. E., Phillips, D., and Vidt, D. G.: Coronary arteriography and coro-

nary artery disease in 99 diabetic and non-diabetic patients on chronic hemodialysis or renal transplant programs. Transplant. Proc. 13:128, 1981.
62. Najarian, J. S., Sutherland, D. E. R., and Simmons, R. L.: Ten-year experience with renal transplantation in juvenile onset diabetics. Ann. Surg. 190: 487, 1979.
63. Bolman, R. M., Molina, J. E., and Levine, B.: Cardiac operations in patients with functioning renal allografts. J. Thorac. Cardiovasc. Surg. 88:537, 1984.
64. Ibels, L. S., Stewart, J. H., and Mahony, F. C.: Occlusive arterial disease in uraemic and hemodialysis patients and renal transplant recipients. Q. J. Med. 46:197, 1977.
65. Rao, V. K., Smith, E. J., and Alexander, J. W.: Thromboembolic disease in renal allograft recipients. Arch. Surg. 111:1086, 1976.
66. Arnadottir, M., Bergentz, S., and Bergqvist, D.: Thromboembolic complications after renal transplantation: A retrospective analysis. World J. Surg. 7: 757, 1983.
67. Jjungquist, U., Bergentz, S. E., and Leandoer, L.: Coagulation and fibrinolysis after renal transplantation. Scand. J. Urol. Nephrol. 3:23, 1969.
68. Vanrenterghem, Y., Roels, L., and Lervt, T.: Thromboembolic complications and haemostatic changes in cyclosporin-treated cadaveric kidney allograft recipients. Lancet 1:999, 1985.
69. Chan, M. K., Zachariah, V., and Moorhead, J. F.: Lipid abnormalities in uremia, dialysis, and transplantation. Kidney Int. 19:625, 1981.
70. Ibels, L. S., Simons, L. S., and King, K. D.: Studies on the nature and causes of hyperlipidemia in uraemia, maintenance dialysis, and renal transplantation. Q. J. Med. 44:601, 1975.
71. Ponticelli, C., Barbi, G., and Cantaluppi, A.: Lipid abnormalities in maintenance dialysis patients and renal transplant recipients. Kidney Int. 13:S72, 1978.
72. Bagdade, J. D., and Albers, J. J.: Plasma high-density lipoprotein concentrations in chronic hemodialysis and renal transplant patients. N. Engl. J. Med. 296:1436, 1977.
73. Ibels, L. S., Alfrey, A. C., and Weil, R.: Hyperlipidemia in adult, pediatric, and diabetic renal transplant recipients. Am. J. Med. 64:634, 1978.
74. Savdie, E., Gibson, J. C., and Stewart, J. H.: High density lipoprotein in chronic renal failure and after renal transplantation. Br. Med. J. 1:928, 1979.
75. Gibson, J. C., Savdie, E., and Simons, L. A.: High density and low density lipoproteins in chronic renal failure before and after renal transplantation. Aust. N.Z. J. Med. 9:136, 1979.
76. Goldstein, S., Duhamel, G., and Laudat, M. H.: Plasma lipids, lipoproteins and apolipoprotein AI, AII, and B in renal transplanted children: What risk for accelerated atherosclerosis? Nephron 38:87, 1984.
77. Bagdade, J. D., Yee, E., and Albers, J.: Impaired triglyceride removal: A mechanism for steroid-induced lipemia. Clin. Res. 134A, 1975.
78. Ibels, L. S., Reardon, M. F., and Nestle, P. J.: Plasma post-heparin lipolytic activity in uremic and hemodialysis patients and renal allograft recipients. J. Lab. Clin. Med. 87:648, 1976

79. Jackson, J. M., and Lee, H. A.: The role of propranolol therapy and proteinuria in the etiology of post-renal transplantation hyperlipidemia. Clin. Nephrol. 18:95, 1982.
80. Schaeffer, E. J.: Discussion; In Flier, J. S., Management and pathogenesis of lipoprotein disorders. N. Engl. J. Med. 312:1300, 1985.

8

Kidney Transplantation: Mineral Metabolism Complications

KHASHAYAR SAKHAEE and J. HAROLD HELDERMAN
University of Texas Health Science Center at Dallas, Southwestern Medical School, Dallas, Texas

Renal transplantation is performed to reverse the uremic syndrome and those physiological consequences of uremia which have caused disease. Renal osteodystrophy is an important consequence of uremia and may profoundly limit the attainment of a normal life for some renal transplant recipients. During the uremic state, two important pathogenic factors in the development of renal osteodystrophy are a disturbance in vitamin D metabolism and parathyroid stimulation, a consequence of hypocalcemia related directly to the failing kidney and indirectly to altered vitamin D metabolism. Indeed the concentration of 1,25-dihydroxy vitamin D, the active metabolite, is significantly reduced in end-stage renal failure and is very low or undetectable in the anephric state [1-4]. Other causes of hypocalcemia responsible for secondary stimulation of the parathyroid gland in a setting of chronic renal failure include renal phosphate retention and increased complexing of circulating calcium [5,6].

It is apparent that deranged vitamin D metabolism and secondary hyperparathyroidism play critical roles in the development of uremic osteomalacia and osteitis fibrosa. When renal transplantation was first introduced into common medical practice, restoration of renal function was expected to eliminate many of the pathogenetic factors responsible for the development of the renal osteodystrophy [4]. Complicating an understanding of the truth of these expectations has been limited data pertaining to the actual effects of successful renal transplantation on mineral metabolism [7,8]. In this chapter, we explore in detail the various aspects of altered mineral metabolism and the impact of successful renal transplantation on these alterations. Other details of posttransplant bone and joint complications may be found in Chapter 10.

I. HYPERCALCEMIA AFTER RENAL TRANSPLANTATION

That successful renal transplantation does not improve all aspects of altered mineral metabolism is demonstrated by the frequent occurrence of hypercalcemia after transplant, as reported initially by McPhaul et al. [9]. More than 85% of patients receiving a renal allograft have been shown to be hypercalcemic at some point in their postoperative course. As transplantation becomes more successful and as transplant physicians become more aware of the issues of mineral metabolism, one might have assumed that posttransplant hypercalcemia would be a diminishing problem. The opposite is true. Although posttransplant hypercalcemia is still encountered and is a clinical problem, its etiologic nature has changed significantly [8]. One of the goals of this chapter will be to define the various etiologic factors that may produce hypercalcemia and to point out the secular trends in the development of this complication.

Three distinct stages in the evolution of hypercalcemia may be discerned, although the transition between the distinct stages has been gradual and unevenly displayed in different transplant centers. In the earliest reports, hypercalcemia was frequently severe enough to be cited as the rationale for urgent parathyroidectomy [10-14]. The first stage, then, is an acute, severe perioperative hypercalcemia. With more experience, it became clear that in most cases of this variety of hypercalcemia, the serum calcium returned toward normal within a few weeks or months, abrogating the perceived requirement for immediate or urgent parathyroidectomy [15-17]. Interestingly, often hypercalcemia did not completely return to normal with time, leading to the appreciation of the presence or persistence of a more chronic variety of hypercalcemia [18-23].

Several mechanisms are responsible for posttransplant hypercalcemia. The factors that play an important role in development of posttransplant hypercalcemia [24] are: (1) slow resolution of hyperparathyroidism; (2) phosphorus depletion; (3) vitamin D therapy and metabolism; (4) steroid therapy; and (5) magnesium deficiency. These mechanisms are variably at play depending on the temporal relationship between the transplant event and the hypercalcemia. In this chapter we shall first examine severe perioperative hypercalcemia and then discuss the more persistent chronic hypercalcemia, taking into account the various mechanisms just listed.

II. EARLY, SEVERE HYPERCALCEMIA AFTER TRANSPLANTATION

In the infancy of renal transplantation, it was not uncommon to encounter hypercalcemia of the magnitude of 14 mg/dl within a few weeks or months postoperative. In this setting, parathyroidectomy was usually the outcome, often performed as an urgent operation [14]. Hypercalcemia after transplantation has become a rarity because physicians have learned to pay more particular attention to aspects of mineral metabolism during the dialytic period. A wide range of strategies have been employed to better control the stimulation of the parathyroid gland during the uremic phase, such as the use of higher calcium levels in dialysate, more palatable phosphate-binding agents, and the wide therapeutic use of various vitamin D metabolites. These measures taken together have reduced the magnitude of the stimulation of the parathyroid gland, thus reducing parathyroid hormone (PTH) stimulation present to cause hypercalcemia, once normal renal excretory and hormonal functions have been restored by successful renal transplantation.

Despite this increased awareness of aspects of mineral metabolism of uremia, milder forms of hypercalcemia in the perioperative period are still often encountered, the result of a normal calcemic response to PTH that is still elevated, a reciprocal response to hypophosphatemia related to antacid use, PTH excess, and/or an intrinsic tubular phosphate leak and restoration of dihydroxy vitamin D synthesis of 1,25-dihydroxy vitamin D (Table 1). Despite these contributing factors in early transplant hypercalcemia, the most important etiologic factor appears to be the slow fall in excess PTH secretion related to the overstimulated parathyroid glands with their exuberant size and blood supply, which needs a period of normal signals to reset the "calcium stat" [25].

The secular trend in management of perioperative hypercalcemia has been to eschew urgent parathyroidectomy, to tolerate mild hypercalcemia early after transplant with expectations of glandular involution in the absence of stimuli to foster secondary hyperparathyroidism, and to adjust the other factors that may have contributed to early hypercalcemia (Table 1).

Although the persistence of secondary hyperparathyroidism is the leading cause of perioperative hypercalcemia, it is wise to examine briefly the other mechanisms that may lead to hypercalcemia (Table 1), attention to which may reduce the occurrence and/or severity of this finding. Reciprocal hypercalcemia follows phosphate depletion most frequently as a consequence of incidental phosphate binding by antacids administered ostensibly to reduce the role of postoperative peptic ulceration [15] (Fig. 1). In our own clinic, encountering perioperative hypophosphatemia often can be explained by routine postoperative antacid use, which we have now abandoned. Moreover, persistent secondary hyperparathyroidism will contribute importantly to the hypercalcemic effect of hypophosphatemia associated with this oral antacid treatment. As antacids are less frequently prescribed routinely for transplant recipients, this problem in many centers has, and in all others should, be overcome. Antacid therapy also produces magnesium depletion, which itself may contribute to the phosphaturia [26], hypophosphatemia, and hypercalcemia. Second, tapering glucocorticoid medication used to prevent allograft rejection may be another contributing factor to posttransplant hypercalcemia. In some, it has been felt that hypercalcemia had been the result of protocols calling for too rapid a reduction in the dose of cor-

Table 1 Mechanisms of Hypercalcemia After Renal Transplantation

Transient	
1.	Delayed restoration of normal homeostasis
2.	Phosphate depletion
3.	Mobilization of soft tissue calcification
4.	Corticosteroid withdrawal
5.	Unmasking of vitamin D intoxication

Source: From Parfitt [8]. Reprinted with permission of S. Karger AG.

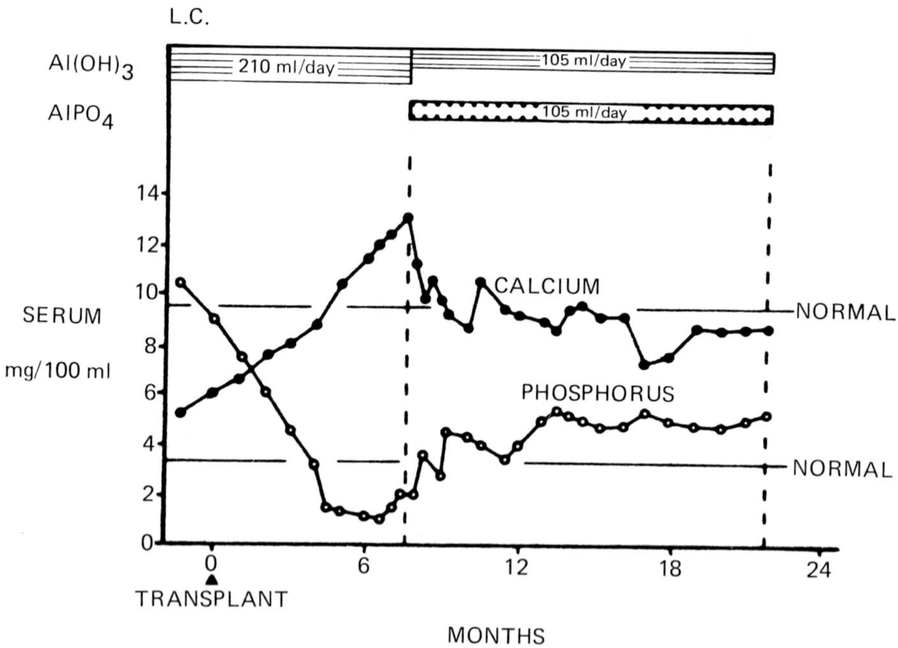

Figure 1 Course of a patient with transient posttransplant hypercalcemia due to iatrogenic phosphate depletion. Note the very large dose of Amphogel and the slow fall in plasma phosphate, suggesting mobilization of extraskeletal calcification. (From Alfrey et al. [15]. Reprinted with permission of *New England Journal of Medicine.*)

Table 2 Frequency of Transient and Persistent Hypercalcemia After Renal Transplantation (RT) in Different Series

			Transient		Persistent		
Authors	Year	RT (*n*)	*n*	%	*n*	%	Duration
Alfrey et al.	1968	175	7	4.0	2	1.1	?
Humpers et al.	1969	150	18	12.0	4	2.7	?
David et al.	1973	64	12	18.7	10	15.6	1-3 years
Pierides et al.	1974	70	9	12.9	11	15.7	1-4 years
Chatterjee et al.	1976	60	0	0	16	26.7	1-6 years
Pieper et al.	1977	42	12	28.6	12	28.6	>3 years
Christensen and Nielsen	1977	188	9	4.8	17	9.0	1-4 years
Henry Ford Hospital	1980	77	4	5.2	9	11.7	1-9 years

Source: From Parfitt [8]. Reprinted with permission of S. Karger AG.

ticosteroid [27]. Although glucocorticoids do not generally influence the hypercalcemia of hyperparathyroidism in the nonuremic patient, hypercalcemia is a well-known feature of steroid withdrawal after adrenalectomy for Cushing syndrome and of acute adrenal insufficiency in Addison disease [28]. More assiduous attention to the appropriate tempo of steroid taper or the use of low-dose steroids early after transplant in the cyclosporine era has rendered this feature of hypercalcemia a rarity.

As one can see, attention to at least several of these conditions that have contributed to the transient perioperative hypercalcemia in the past has reduced in great measure the incidence of transient perioperative hypercalcemia. Perusal of a series from the perspective of time supports this point. Clearly, the reports of such incidents after 1976 have markedly declined (Table 2).

III. LATE, PERSISTENT POSTTRANSPLANT HYPERCALCEMIA

Hypercalcemia lasting longer than 1 year after successful renal transplantation may be defined as "persistent" [29] and has been increasingly recognized in the last 10 years. In a recent survey of 496 cases of hypercalcemia detected by routine biochemical screening [30], in general, 10% of the cases were found in renal transplant recipients, with 22 of these 47 cases (47%) persisting for more than 1 year. A second series reported recovery from hypercalcemia as many as 6-7 years after successful renal transplantation [23,31]. Since this form of transplant hypercalcemia can be ascribed to persistent hyperparathyroidism in great measure, we will review, in some detail, parathyroid function after rental transplantation.

The true prevalence of persistent hyperparathyroidism after renal transplantation has been reported to occur in as little as 5% to as many as 85% of long term survivors of renal transplantation [19,22,32]. Precise diagnosis usually depends on simultaneous measurement of serum total and ionized calcium, parathyroid hormone levels, serum inorganic phosphorus and magnesium concentrations, fasting urinary calcium loads, and urinary cAMP excretion rates. At times, the diagnosis may be difficult to make, so that maneuvers designed to stimulate or inhibit the parathyroid gland are often required to demonstrate an occult variety of hyperparathyroidism. Persistent hyperparathyroidism is not a trivial matter, as it has been implicated in the pathogenesis of persistent metabolic bone disease after transplantation, gastrointestinal disorders including peptic ulcer disease, neuropsychiatric disturbances, obliterative arteriolosclerosis, and hypertension posttransplant, which may complicate otherwise successful renal transplant events [25].

Despite the expectation and perhaps the measurements in early studies that suggested that serum PTH returned to normal within 4-6 months of surgery provided the creatinine clearance was greater than 60 ml/min [33], the majority of recent studies that carefully measured PTH led to the conclusion that persistent hyperparathyroidism may be a more important problem in the well-functioning kidney [25]. Pletka et al. [34] and David et al. [35], for example, report elevated PTH levels and hypercalcemia in allograft recipients with normal renal function (>60 ml/min) up to 4 years after surgery. Kleerekoper et al. [36] not only corroborated these two studies but demonstrated further that in some patients, persistent elevations of PTH may last for a considerable period of time posttransplant.

Earlier in this chapter we have discussed some of the mechanisms that might lead to hyperparathyroidism present immediately after surgery. It is important to the argument and the discussion now to examine some of the mechanisms that may be at play to persistently stimulate the parathyroid gland after successful allograft replacement. Three distinct explanations have been suggested in the literature to explain this phenomenon: (1) a continued effect of steroid treatment used as immunosuppressive on calcium absorption from the gut [37]; (2) the continued slow rate of parathyroid gland involution, which may take years [24,25]; or (3) a renal calcium leak, a new finding recently described in renal allograft recipients at the University of Texas program in Dallas [4].

Persistent excess PTH, a consequence of resetting of the "calcium stat" after transplant, is an often-stated biological principle which has some basis in experimental fact. The inverse, nonlinear relationship between the level of serum ionized calcium and PTH secretion seen in normals may also be detected in postrenal transplants (Figs. 2 and 3) [25,28]. This relationship dictates that there is basal secretion of some PTH not suppressible by progressive hypercalcemia, the calcium set point or "calcium stat." This calcium independent

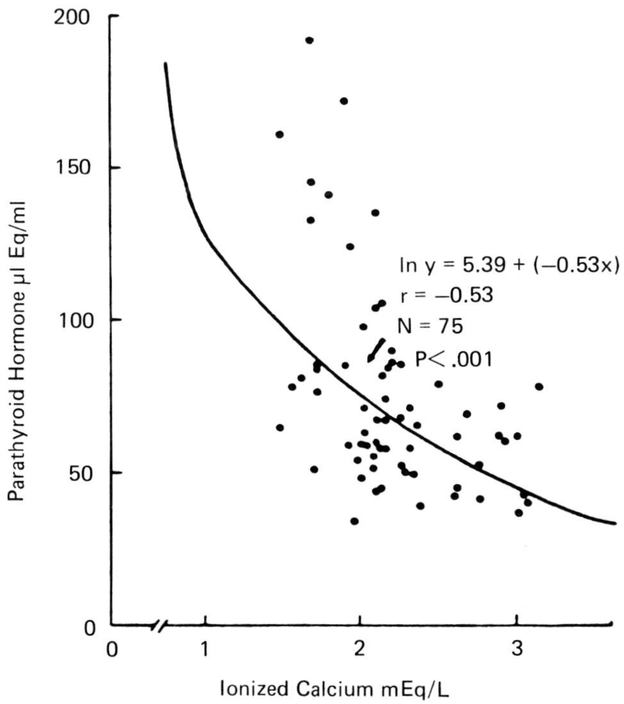

Figure 2 Relation of serum Ca and PTH levels determined simultantously during CA and EDTA infusion in normal subjects. (From McCarron et al. [25]. Reprinted with permission of Americal Society of Clinical Nutrition.)

fraction of parathyroid cell synthetic function previously noted in vitro and in animal studies can be shown to be present in humans as well [39-42]. Ionized calcium, then, exerts its greatest regulatory effect on PTH secretion over a narrow range. In the renal transplant recipient the calcium-independent phase of the relationship appears to be set at a higher level of PTH release than in the normal. Although the calcium stat is set at this higher set-point than in the normal individual (Fig. 4), the gland remains equally responsive to acute changes in serum ionized calcium (Fig. 3), so that parathyroid gland function is not autonomous after successful renal transplantation in great measure. One can conclude from this that, for most patients, the notion of tertiary or autonomous parathyroid gland function, often called tertiary hyperparathyroidism, does not exist [25]. The sensitivity of the hyperplastic parathyroid gland to serum ionized calcium in the transplant recipient is virtually normal (Fig. 4). The simplest explanation of the excessive PTH secretion seen after successful allograft placement relates

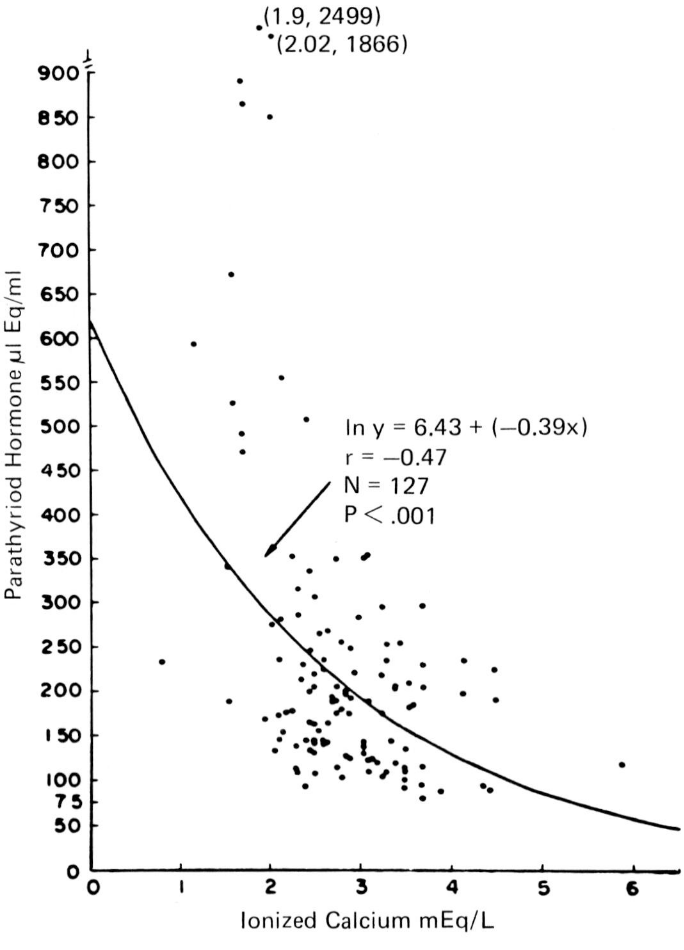

Figure 3 Relation of serum Ca and PTH levels determined simultaneously during Ca and EDTA infusion in hyperparathyroid transplant recipients. (From McCarron et al. [25]. Reprinted with permission of American Society of Clinical Nutrition.)

to increased gland mass, the resetting of the calcium stat, and not to altered sensitivity of the parathyroid cell to calcium stimuli or to abnormal degradation of the hormone in plasma space.

The stimulatory relationship between ionized calcium and PTH has both diagnostic and therapeutic implications for the approximate management of posttransplant hyperparathyroidism. The sigmoid nature of the relationship indicates

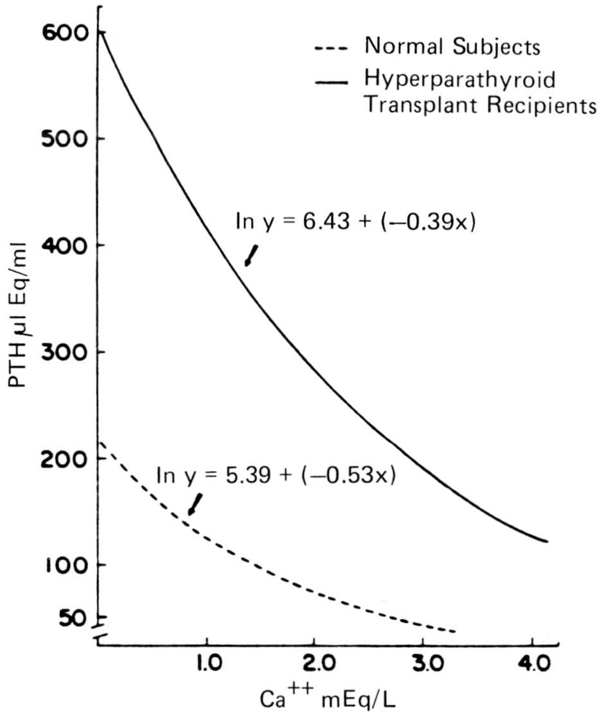

Figure 4 Comparison of the serum Ca-PTH relationships in normal subjects and hyperparathyroid transplant recipients. (From McCarron et al. [25]. Reprinted with permission of Americal Society of Clinical Nutrition.)

that even minimal increases in total serum calcium, and ultimately PTH levels, are likely to reflect significant residual parathyroid hyperplasia [38]. It may be important to discern those patients at greatest risk of having significant peritransplant hypercalcemia by delineating the magnitude of increased parathyroid gland mass. To do so must require provocative maneuvers designed to maximally stimulate and maximally suppress the calcium independently of parathyroid gland function in the transplant recipient. These tests might provide some estimate of gland mass and a reference standard by which the long-term effects of either surgical or medical management may be judged as well as the anticipation of problems in the peritransplant period.

A second clinical lesson that flows from an understanding of the relationship between calcium and PTH in the transplant recipient relates to attempts to maintain an "optimal" serum calcium concentration in the transplant patient. Vigorous attempts to reduce the serum calcium below what this optimal serum calcium concentration may be, usually by institution of oral phosphate therapy, may only serve to further stimulate PTH secretion. Yet, maintenance of hypercalcemia above optimal levels permits the excess parathyroid gland function to be manifest leading to continued or even worsened uremic osteodystrophy despite the working allograft. Since the goal in management of altered mineral metabolism in the transplant patient is to permit healing of renal osteodystrophy and/or to prevent further bone damage, it is imperative that radiographic and special measurements of bone density and health be a routine part of the management of the transplant recipient. In occasional patients, the optimal serum calcium concentration will be difficult to ascertain. In an additional smaller group of these patients, persistent or worsening bone disease demonstrates inability to tolerate hypercalcemia or excessive basal secretions of PTH. In this quite small group, definitive therapy should be directed at reduction of gland mass, which can be accomplished rapidly only by surgical intervention.

IV. PHOSPHATE DEPLETION

In addition to understanding the relationship between calcium and PTH elaboration in the transplant patient, it is essential that one understands the role that phosphate metabolism plays in maintaining persistent hyperparathyroidism many years after successful allograft placement. Hypophosphatemia is a prominent element in the metabolic patterns that are exhibited by many successful transplant recipients. The etiology of hypophosphatemia is multifactorial. The perioperative hypophosphatemia is often thought to be a consequence of secondary hyperparathyroidism able to exert its effects on tubular rejection of phosphorus in an allograft with reasonable glomerular filtration rate [43]. Additionally, patients are often consuming antacids either as a preventive measure for peptic ulceration or following failure to discontinue phosphate-binding agents as the transplanted kidney begins to function [15]. The reduction of phosphorus absorption [44-46] from the gut will compound the renal loss of phosphorus, deepening the level of hypophosphatemia. Attention to the antacid issue eliminates this confounding etiologic factor, and early use of neutral oral phosphate salts will ameliorate phosphate depletion and aid in bone healing [47].

Hypophosphatemia is also observed in the late, more stable posttransplant period even when renal function is excellent ($>$70 ml/min) [48,49]. This late hypophosphatemia is thought to be due, in part, to a reduced rate of renal tubular reabsorption, as assessed by the fraction of filtered phosphorus excreted in the urine or by the maximal reabsorptive rate during phosphate infusions (Table 3) [48,49]. In some patients, this tubular rejection of phosphorus is not necessarily due alone to excess PTH, which we have shown should be an expected

Table 3 Renal Phosphate Handling In Normal Subjects and Transplant Recipients[a]

Patients	C_{Cr} (ml/min)	P_{PO_4}[b] (mg/dl)	TR_{PO_4} (%)	Tm_{PO_4}/GFR (mg/dl)	P_{iPTH} (μl/Eq/ml)
Normal (n = 7)	131 ± 8	3.7 ± 0.1	90 ± 2	3.5 ± 0.2	6 ± 1
Transplant recipients (n = 73)	68 ± 4[c]	3.0 ± 0.1[c]	67 ± 2[c]	3.0 ± 0.1[c]	32 ± 4[c]
Hypophosphatemic recipients (P_{PO_4} < 2.5) (n = 23)	82 ± 8[c,d]	2.1 ± 0.1[c,d]	63 ± 7[c]	1.4 ± 0.2[c,d]	30 ± 7[c]

[a]Results are the mean ± SEM. C_{Cr}, creatinine clearance; P_{PO_4}, plasma phosphate; TR_{PO_4}, tubular reabsorption of phosphorus; Tm_{PO_4}/GFR, renal phosphate threshold by nomogram; P_{iPTH}, plasma immunoreactive PTH.
[b]Normal range of P_{PO_4} is 3.0-5.0 mg/dl.
[c]$p < 0.005$ versus normal.
[d]$p < 0.05$ versus whole transplant recipient group.
Source: From Rosenbaum et al. [50]. Reprinted with permission of Springer Verlag.

feature of these patients. Slatopolsky and his colleagues [50] have demonstrated, in a group of hypophosphatemic transplant recipients, a failure to decrease phosphate excretion even when PTH was suppressed by calcium infusions, suggesting that for some individuals there remains a specific renal tubular transport defect responsible for the development of, maintenance of, or worsening of hypophosphatemia. Persistent hyperparathyroidism and a renal leak of phosphorus taken together do not explain all of the hypophosphatemia that is seen in a successful allograft. This leads to an exploration of other aspects of mineral metabolism in the transplant recipient. Disordered intestinal phosphate absorption [51-53] has been found in these patients and raises questions concerning the repair of vitamin D metabolism [54-57], about which we shall have something more to say later. Finally, it is important to recall that magnesium deficiency [24], which may be associated with a renal tubular transport defect or a primary problem, will worsen phosphaturia, deepen hypophosphatemia, and thus lead to hypercalcemia.

Hypophosphatemia in its own right, as we have shown, will contribute significantly to hypercalcemia in patients who have persistent secondary hyperparathyroidism. Taken together, total body phosphorus depletion and elevated PTH hormone levels lead to important clinical consequences. In our patients, severe bone pain in a successful transplant may be related to this constellation of deranged mineral metabolism. We have also seen pseudo fractures related to osteomalacia. Others have found similar syndromes relating hypophosphatemia [58] to bone pain, weakness, anorexia, and numbness as well as persistent renal osteodystrophy.

V. MAGNESIUM DEFICIENCY AFTER RENAL TRANSPLANTATION

Hypomagnesemia, when measured, appears to be universal after successful renal transplantation [24]. Factors that predispose the transplant patients to magnesium depletion include protein caloric malnutrition in the pretransplant and immediate posttransplant periods [59]. Hypercalcemia [60] induces renal magnesium loss reduction in renal tubular reabsorption of magnesium, steroid therapy [61], and posttransplant diuresis [60]. Theoretically, magnesium depletion might induce hypercalcemia in the posttransplant period by decreasing serum calcium [24] and thus stimulating PTH secretion by hyperplastic glands.

VI. VITAMIN D METABOLISM

Although this chapter has concentrated heavily on describing and understanding persistent hyperparathyroidism in a successful transplant, the uncovering of deranged intestinal absorption of calcium begs the question concerning the integrity of vitamin D metabolism in the working allograft [4,51-56]. In the uremic state, one can easily measure a deficiency of 1,25-dihydroxy vitamin D [4]. In attempt-

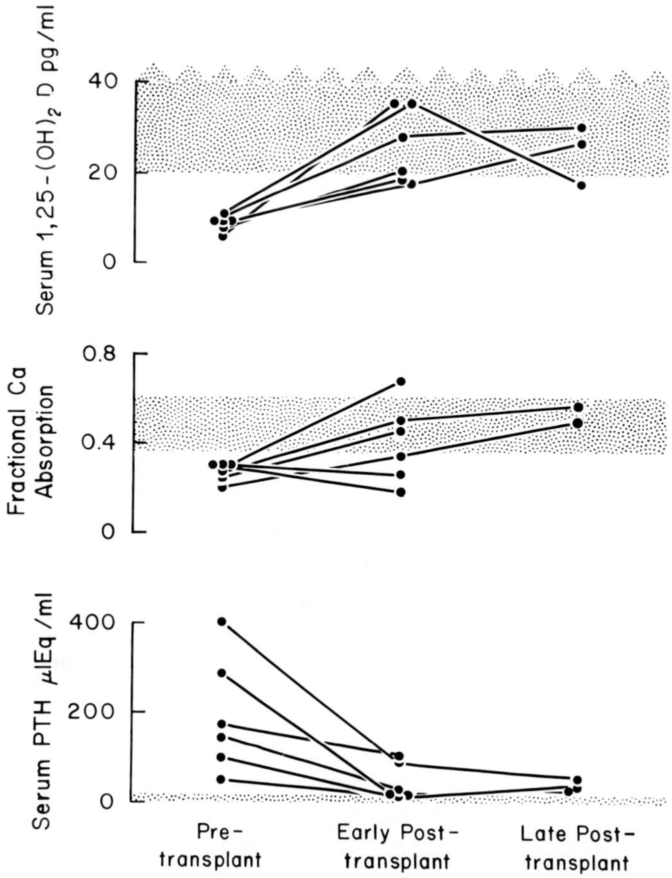

Figure 5 Effect of renal transplantation on serum concentrations of $1,25(OH)_2D$, PTH, and fractional intestinal Ca absorption in patients with end-stage renal disease. Each line represents a study in a separate patient. The shaded area denotes the normal range. (From Sakhaee et al. [4]. Reprinted with permission of S. Karger AG.)

ing to understand the impact of successful transplantation on vitamin D metabolism, our laboratory has measured the active metabolite in the uremic patient about to receive a transplant and confirmed this often reported finding [4]. The metabolic consequence of diminished 1,25-dihydroxy vitamin D was a significant reduction of intestinal calcium absorption (Fig. 5) in our own patients. This diminished intestinal calcium absorption, leading to potential hypocalcemia, is one independent means by which the parathyroid gland is stimulated in uremia along with the independent effect of renal phosphate retention, a consequence of the impairment in renal excretory function.

Many of these derangements in vitamin D metabolism and intestinal calcium absorption were shown to be ameliorated after successful renal transplantation (Fig. 5) in our patients [4]. At an early posttransplantation period, patients as a group show a significant rise in serum 1,25-dihydroxy vitamin D coupled with the expected increase in the fractional intestinal calcium absorption toward, but not, normality. This improvement in vitamin D metabolism leading to enhancement in calcium absorption reduces one means of parathyroid gland stimulation which allows serum PTH to decrease toward normal. A falling PTH, a rising active vitamin D, and the return toward a normal calcemic response to exogenously administered PTH (Table 4), all taken together, demonstrate that successful renal transplantation does lead toward normalization of those disordered parameters of bone metabolism which characterize uremia. Nevertheless, it is important to point out that in several patients with excellent transplant function, serum 1,25-dihydroxy vitamin D and thus fractional intestinal calcium absorption remain subnormal. Furthermore, some patients remained hypercalciuric as a result of urinary calcium exceeding absorbed calcium, indicative of negative calcium balance [4]. The patients who demonstrate this negative calcium balance are among those with the highest doses of steroid, which may be one explanation for this finding. Importantly, from this group may be taken those patients with the most profound, persistent secondary parathyroidism.

Because it is tantalizing to suggest that glucocorticoids used to maintain the allograft may play an important role in the persistence of disordered mineral metabolism, it is reasonable to examine the mechanism by which glucocorticoids may inhibit intestinal calcium transport in general and in these patients in particular. Many authors have suggested that glucocorticoids [37,62] might, in themselves, alter vitamin D metabolism. This contention is supported by the measurements of subnormal serum 1,25-dihydroxy vitamin D in transplant patients receiving the largest doses of glucocorticoids [4]. It is also possible that glucocorticoids affect liver synthesis of 25-hydroxy vitamin D [37,62], which unfortunately was not measured in our study. Alternatively, glucocorticoids have been shown to have, and may have had in these patients, a direct effect to impair calcium movement across the gut [37].

Further supporting the notion that high-dose glucocorticoid use early in transplantation contributes importantly to disordered mineral metabolism is the finding in our center that patients at 2 years after successful allograft placement have further normalization in vitamin D metabolism, intestinal calcium absorption, and calcemic response to PTH (Fig. 5). Importantly, serum PTH was persistently elevated in all these patients despite adequate endogenous creatinine clearance, indicative in some measure of persistent parathyroid gland stimula-

Table 4 Laboratory Presentation in Patients Before and After Renal Transplantation

	Before transplantation (n = 6)	After transplantation: Early (n = 6)	After transplantation: Late (n = 3)
Serum			
Ca, mg/dl	9.51 ± 0.85	9.63 ± 0.34	9.82 ± 0.32*
P, mg/dl	5.55 ± 1.96***	2.96 ± 0.95**	2.71 ± 0.31
Mg, mg/dl	2.87 ± 0.20***	2.13 ± 0.24***	2.31 ± 0.05*
Alk Φ, IU/l	83.5 ± 34.6	98.8 ± 30.4	84.0 ± 20.9
PTH, μlEq/ml	188 ± 132***	42 ± 37**	44 ± 12*
1,25(OH)$_2$D, pg/ml	8.7 ± 1.5**	26.3 ± 8.4***	24.7 ± 7.8*
Urine			
Ca, mg/day	–	159 ± 117	197 ± 106
P, mg/day	–	866 ± 204	634 ± 119
Hydroxyproline, mg/day	–	26.7 ± 8.6	18.2 ± 7.8
Fasting Ca, mg/100 ml GF	–	0.124 ± 0.127	0.123 ± 0.086
Cr clearance, ml/min	–	65.0 ± 17.9	93.3 ± 8.7
Fractional Ca absorption	0.263 ± 0.048***	0.402 ± 0.175*	0.529 ± 0.034**
Calcemic response following infusion of PTH extract, Δpg/ml	0.45 ± 0.21	1.03 ± 0.18***	1.47 ± 0.45*
1,25(OH)$_2$D response following infusion of PTH extract, Δpg/ml	1.3 ± 2.3	15.2 ± 9.7**	–

Values are mean ± SD. Statistical significance of difference between pre- and posttransplantation periods determined by the paired t test are noted by: *$p < 0.05$, **$p < 0.02$, ***$p < 0.005$. Normal values in our laboratory are: serum Ca, 8.5-10.5 mg/dl; P, 2.5-4.5 mg/dl; Mg, 1.7-2.4 mg/dl; Alk Φ, 30-115 IU/L; PTH, <30 μ.Eq/ml; 1,25(OH)$_2$D, 20-50 pg/ml; urinary Ca, 1000-200 mg/day; fasting Ca excretion, <0.11 mg/100 ml GF; hydroxyproline, 6-40 mg/day; fractional intestinal Ca absorption, 0.49 ± SD 0.06.

Source: From Sakhaee et al. [4]. Reprinted with permission of S. Karger AG.

tion, as detailed previously [4,63]. Persistence of hypercalciuria and negative calcium balance has suggested to us that late stimulation of parathyroid gland function in many patients may be related to an intrinsic renal defect [64-68] not only in phosphate transport but in calcium transport by the kidney. A primary calcium leak would lead to negative balance and thus to persistent stimulation of the gland [4]. The renal leak of calcium, if untreated, may be a risk factor for the development of bone disease [69,70] and nephrolithiasis [4,71, 72], as has been previously reported by us in a group of patients with postmenopausal osteoporosis [73]. However, the etiology of renal stone formation might not be due only to hypercalciuria [4], since hyperuricosuria concomitant with Fanconi syndrome [67,68] and hypocitraturia due to metabolic acidosis [74,75] might play an important role in stone formation and bone disease [76].

VII. CONCLUSION

Successful renal transplantation improves, but does not completely correct, the abnormalities in mineral metabolism encountered in chronic renal disease. Adjustment in clinical practice after successful renal transplantation may improve significantly factors that have worsened some aspects of deranged mineral metabolism. The use of very-low-dose steroids in the cyclosporine era may ameliorate the potential disordered intestinal calcium absorption and vitamin D metabolism that we have described [4,37,62]. Further attention to antacid therapy and magnesium depletion in the perioperative period with vigorous treatment of hypophosphatemia also may ameliorate features of this problem. An attempt to characterize parathyroid gland mass pretransplant will help point to those patients most at risk for having problems with mineral metabolism in the successful posttransplant period [25]. In these patients in particular and all recipients in general, an attempt to find the optimal level of serum calcium should be made in order to permit healing of renal osteodystrophy on the one hand with the least stimulation of the parathyroid gland on the other [25,29]. Intrinsic renal leaks of phosphorus and/or calcium may be the culprits in the persistence of clinically important altered mineral metabolism and can potentially be treated by phosphorus or hydrochlorothiazide replacement [4,50,73]. Finally, in a rare patient, optimal levels of serum calcium cannot be found or maintained, or bone disease worsens forcing one to resort to surgical intervention [29]. Only by such assiduous attention to matters of mineral metabolism in the pre- and posttransplant periods can the transplant physician complete his task of normalizing the life of a uremic individual by the transplant.

REFERENCES

1. Brumbaugh, P. F., Haussler, D. H., Bressler, R., and Haussler, M. R.: Radioreceptor assay for 1α,25-dihydroxyvitamin D_3. Science 183:1089-1091, 1974.
2. Portale, A. A., Booth, B. E., Tsai, H. C., and Morris, J. R.: Reduced plasma concentration of $1,25(OH)_2D$ in children with moderate renal insufficiency. Kidney Int. 21:627-632, 1982.
3. Haussler, M. R., and McCain, T. A.: Circulating 1,25-dihydroxyvitamin D in health and disease. Clin. Res. 26:128A, 1978 (abstract).
4. Sakhaee, K., Brinker, K., Helderman, J. H., Bengfort, J. L., Nicar, M. J., Hull, A. R., and Pak, C. Y. C.: Disturbances in mineral metabolism after successful renal transplantation. Mineral Electrolyte Metab. 11:167-172, 1985.
5. Bricker, N. S.: On the pathogenesis of the uremic state. An exposition of the "trade off hypothesis." N. Engl. J. Med. 286:1093-1100, 1972.
6. Massry, S. G., Ritz, E., and Verberckmoes, R.: Role of phosphate in the genesis of secondary hyperparathyroidism of renal failure. Nephron 18:77-81, 1977.
7. Cundy, T., Kanis, J. A., Heynen, G., Morris, P. J., and Oliver, D. O.: Calcium metabolism and hyperparathyroidism after renal transplantation. Q. J. Med. 205:67-78, 1983.
8. Parfitt, A. M.: Hypercalcemic hyperparathyroidism following renal transplantation: Differential diagnosis, management, and implications for population control in the parathyroid gland. Mineral Electrolyte Metab. 8:92-112, 1982.
9. McPhaul, J. J., McIntosh, D. A., Hammand, W. S., and Park, O. K.: Autonomous secondary (renal) parathyroid hyperplasis. N. Engl. J. Med. 217:1342, 1964.
10. Wilson, R. E., Bernstein, D. S., Murray, J. E., and Moore, F. D.: Effects of parathyroidectomy and kidney transplantation on renal osteodystrophy. Am. J. Surg. 110:384-393, 1965.
11. McIntosh, D. A., Peterson, E. W., and McPhaul, J. J.: Autonomy of parathyroid function after renal homotransplantation. Ann. Intern. Med. 65: 900-907, 1966.
12. Hume, D. M., Lee, H. M., Williams, G. M., White, H. J. O., Ferre, J., Wolf, J. S., Prout, G. R., Slapak, M., O'Brien, J., Kilpatrick, S. J., Jauffman, H. M., Jr., and Cleveland, R. J.: Comparative results of cadaver and related donor renal homografts in man, and immunologic implications of the outcome of second and paired transplants. Ann. Surg. 164:352, 1966.
13. Latimer, R. G., Renning, J., Stevens, L. E., Northway, J. D., and Reemtsma, K.: Tertiary hyperparathyroidism following successful renal allografting. Ann. Surg. 172:137-141, 1970.
14. Schwartz, G. H., David, D. S., Riggio, R. R., Saville, P. D., Whitsell, J. C.,

Stenzel, K. H., and Rubin, A. L.: Hypercalcemia after renal transplantation. Am. J. Med. 49:42-51, 1970.
15. Alfrey, A. C., Jenkins, D., Groth, C. G., Schorr, W. S., Gecelter, L., and Ogden, D. A.: Resolution of hyperparathyroidism, renal osteodystrophy and metastatic calcification after renal homotransplantation. N. Engl. J. Med. 279:1349-1356, 1968.
16. Hampers, C. L., Katz, A. I., Wilson, R. E., and Merrill, J. P., Calcium metabolism and osteodystrophy after renal transplantation. Arch. Intern. Med. 124: 282-291, 1969.
17. Johnson, J. W., Hattner, R. S., Hampers, C. L., Bernstein, D. S., Merrill, J. P., and Sherwood, L. M.: Secondary hyperparathyroidism in chronic renal failure. Effects of renal homotransplantation. JAMA 215:478-480, 1971.
18. Buck, B. A., and Robertson, R. D.: Indications for parathyroidectomy in advanced renal disease. Surg. Gynecol. Obstet. 133:218-224, 1971.
19. Geis, W. P., Popovtzer, M. M., Corman, J. L., Halgrimson, C. G., Groth, C. G., and Starzl, T. E.: The diagnosis and treatment of hyperparathyroidism after renal homotransplantation. Surg. Gynecol. Obstet. 137:997-1010, 1973.
20. Cerilli, J., Limbert, J. G., Ferris, T. F., and Tzagournis, M.: Subtotal parathyroidectomy for tertiary hyperparathyroidism thirty-two months after renal transplantation. Am. J. Surg. 125:636-638, 1973.
21. Wilson, R. E., and Roth, S. I.: Case records of the Massachusetts General Hospital: Case 13-1974. N. Engl. J. Med. 190:793, 1974.
22. Chatterjee, S. N., Friedler, R. M., Berne, T. V., Oldham, S. B., Singer, F. R., and Massry, S. G.: Persistent hypercalcemia after successful renal transplantation. Nephron 17:1-7, 1976.
23. Christensen, M. S., Nielsen, H. E., and Torring, S.: Hypercalcemia and parathyroid function after renal transplantation. Acta Med. Scand. 102:35-39, 1977.
24. Schwartz, A. H., David, S., Ribco, R. R., Saville, P. D., Whitsell, T. C., Stenzel, K. H., and Rubin, A. L.: Hypercalcemia after renal transplantation. Am. J. Med. 49:42-51, 1969.
25. McCarron, D. A., Bennet, W. M., Muther, R. S., Barry, J. M., and Krutzik, S.: Post-transplantation hyperparathyroidism: demonstration of retained control of parathyroid function by ionized calcium. Am. J. Clin. Nutr. 33:1536-1540, 1980.
26. Ginn, H. E., and Shanbour, L. L.: Phosphaturia in magnesium-deficient rats. Am. J. Physiol. 212:1347, 1967.
27. Herdman, R. C., Michael, A. F., Vernier, R. L., Kelly, W. D., and Good, R. A.: Renal function and phosphorus excretion after human renal homotransplantation. Lancet 1:121-124, 1966.
28. Parfitt, A. M., and Kleerekoper, M.: Clinical disorders of calcium, phosphorus and magnesium metabolism. In: Maxwell and Kleeman, eds., Clinical Disorders of Fluid and Electrolyte Metabolism, 3rd ed., New York: McGraw-Hill, 1980, pp. 947-1152.
29. Parfitt, A. M.: Hypercalcemic hyperparathyroidism following renal trans-

plantation: differential diagnosis, management, and implications for cell population control in the parathyroid gland. Mineral Electrolyte Metab. 8: 91-112, 1982.

30. Fisken, R. A., Heath, D. A., and Bold, A. M.: Hypercalcemia–A hospital survey. Q. J. Med. 196:405-418, 1980.
31. Christensen, M. S., and Nielsen, H. E.: The clinical significance of hyperparathyroidism after renal transplantation. Scand. J. Urol. Nephrol. Suppl. 42:130-133, 1977.
32. Pieper, R., Alveryd, A., Lundgren, G., Collste, H., Magnusson, G., Svahn, T., and Groth, C. G.: Secondary hyperparathyroidism and its sequelae in renal transplant recipients. Long-term findings in a series of conservatively managed patients. Scand. J. Urol. Nephrol. Suppl. 42:144-148, 1977.
33. Johnson, W. J., Goldsmith, R. S., Beabout, J. W., Jowsey, J., Kelly, P. J., and Arnaud, C. D.: Prevention and reversal of progressive secondary hyperparathyroidism in patients maintained by hemodialysis. Am. J. Med. 56:827-832, 1974.
34. Pletka, P. G., Strom, T. B., Hampers, C. L., Griffiths, H., Wilson, R. E., Bernstein, D. S., Sherwood, L. M., and Merrill, J. P.: Secondary hyperparathyroidism in human kidney transplant recipients. Nephron 17:371-381, 1976.
35. David, D. S., Sakai, S., Brennan, B. L., Riggio, R. A., Cheigh, J., Stenzel, K. H., Rubin, A. L., and Sherwood, L. M.: Hypercalcemia after renal transplantation. Long-term follow-up data. N. Engl. J. Med. 289:398-401, 1973.
36. Kleerekoper, M., Ibels, L. S., Ingham, J. P., McCarthy, S. W., Mahoney, J. F., Stewart, J. H., and Posen, S.: Hyperparathyroidism after renal transplantation. Br. J. Med. 3:690-682, 1975.
37. Hahn, T. J., Halstead, L. R., Teitelbaum, S. L., and Hahn, B. H.: Altered mineral metabolism in glucocorticoid-induced osteopenia. J. Clin. Invest. 64:655-665, 1979.
38. McCarron, D. A., Muther, R. S., Lenfesty, B., and Bennet, W. M.: Parathyroid function in persistent hyperparathyroidism: Relationship to gland size. Kidney Int. 22:662-670, 1982.
39. Blum, J. W., Mayer, G. P., and Potts, J. T.: Parathyroid hormone responses during spontaneous hypocalcemia and induced hypercalcemia in cows. Endocrinology 95:84-92, 1974.
40. Mayer, G. P., Habener, H. F., and Potts, H. R., Jr.: Parathyroid hormone in vivo. Demonstration of a calcium-independent, non-suppressible component of secretion. J. Clin. Invest. 57:678, 1976.
41. Keaton, J. A., Barton, J. A., Moore, M. P., Gruel, J. B., and Mayer, G. P.: Altered parathyroid response to calcium in hypercalemic neonatal calves. Endocrinology 103:2161-2167, 1978.
42. Mayer, G. P., and Hurst, J. G.: Sigmoidal relationship between parathyroid hormone secretion rate and plasma calcium concentrations in calves. Endocrinology 102:1036-1042, 1978.
43. Herdman, R., Vernier, R. L., Michael, A. F., Kelly, W. P., and Good, R. A.:

Renal Function and phosphorus excretion after human renal homotransplantation. Lancet 1:121-123, 1966.
44. Stanbury, S. W.: Bone disease in uremia. Am. J. Med. 44:714-724, 1968.
45. Coburn, J. W., Brickman, A. S., Hartenbower, D. L., and Norman, A. W.: Intestinal phosphate absorption in normal and uremic man: effects of 1,25-$(OH)_2$ vitamin D_3 and 1-α(OH)-vitamin D_3. Adv. Exp. Med. Biol. 81:549-557, 1977.
46. Peacock, M., Aaron, J. E., and Walker, G. S.: The effect of plasma phosphate on the action of 1-α-hydroxyvitamin D_3 in hemodialysis patients. Adv. Exp. Med. Biol. 81:559-570, 1977.
47. Rasmussen, H., and Bordier, P.: Vitamin D and bone. Metab. Bone Dis. Related Res. 1:7-13, 1978.
48. Ward, H. N., Pabico, R. C., McKenna, B. A., and Freeman, R. B.: The renal handling of phosphate by renal transplant patients: correlation with serum parathyroid hormone, cyclic 3′,5′-adenosine monophosphate urinary excretion, and allograft function. Adv. Exp. Med. Biol. 81:173-181, 1977.
49. Moorehead, J. F., Ahmed, K. Y., Varghese, Z., Wills, M. R., Baillod, R. A., and Tatler, G. L. V.: Hypophosphataemic osteomalacia after cadaveric renal transplantation. Lancet 1:694-697, 1974.
50. Rosenbaum, R. W., Kruska, K. A., Krokar, A., Anderson, C., and Slatopolsky, E.: Decreased phosphate reabsorption after renal transplantation. Evidence for a mechanism independent of calcium and parathyroid hormone. Kidney Int. 19:568-578, 1981.
51. Peacock, M., Nordin, B. E. C., Gallagher, J. C., and Varnavides, C.: Action of 1-α-hydroxyvitamin D_3 in man. In: Norman, A. W., Schafer, K., Grigoleit, H. G., Herrath, D. V., and Ritz, E., eds., Vitamin D and Problems Related to Uremic Bone Disease, Berlin: de Gruyter, 1975, pp. 611-618.
52. Farrington, K., Varghese, Z., Newman, S. P., Ahmed, K. Y., Fernanco, O. N., and Moorhead, J. F.: Dissociation of absorptions of calcium and phosphorus after successful cadaveric renal transplantation. Br. Med. J. 1:712-714, 1979.
53. Gennari, J. C., Bernini, M., Nardi, P., and Fusi, L.: Dissociation of absorption of calcium and phosphate in different pathophysiological states in man. In: Massry, S. G., Maschio, G., and Ritz, E., eds., Phosphate and Mineral Metabolism, New York: Plenum Press, 1984, pp. 195-204.
54. Williams, G. A., Bowser, E. N., Henderson, W. J., and Uzgiries, V.: Effects of vitamin D and cortisone on intestinal absorption of calcium in the rat. Proc. Soc. Exp. Biol. Med. 106:664-666, 1961.
55. Lukert, C. P., Stanbury, S. W., and Mawer, E. G.: Vitamin D and intestinal transport of calcium: Effects of prednisolone. Endocrinology 93:718-722, 1973.
56. Favus, M. J., Walling, M. W., and Kimberg, D. V.: Effects of 1,25-dihydroxycholecalciferol on intestinal calcium transport in cortisone-treated rats. J. Clin. Invest. 52:1680-1685, 1973.
57. Fallagher, J. C., Aaron, J. E., Horsman, A., Wilkinson, R., and Nordin. B. E. C.: Corticosteroid osteoporosis. Clin. Endocrinol. Metab. 2:355-368, 1973.

58. Lotz, M., Zisman, E., and Bartter, F. C.: Evidence for a phosphorus-depletion syndrome in man. N. Engl. J. Med. 278-409, 1968.
59. Wacker, W. E. C., and Parisi, A. F.: Magnesium metabolism. N. Engl. J. Med. 278:658, 712, 772, 1968.
60. MacIntyre, I.: Magnesium metabolism. Adv. Intern. Med. 13:143, 1967.
61. Massry, S. G., Coburn, J. W., Chapman, L. W., and Kleeman, C. R.: The effect of long-term desoxycorticosterone acetate administration on the renal excretion of calcium and magnesium. J. Lab. Clin. Med. 71:212, 1968.
62. Klein, R. G. S., Arnaud, S. B., Gallagher, J. C., Deluca, H. F., and Riggs, B. L.: Intestinal calcium absorption in exogenous hypercortisolism. Role of 25hydroxyvitamin D and corticoid dose. J. Clin. Invest. 60:253-259, 1977.
63. Arnaud, C. D.: Hyperparathyroidism in renal failure. Kidney Int. 4:89-95, 1973.
64. Gyory, A. Z., Stewart, J. H., George, C. R. P., Tiller, D. J., and Edwards, K. D. G.: Renal tubular acidosis, acidosis due to hyperkalaemia, hypercalcaemia, disordered citrate metabolism and other tubular dysfunctions following human renal transplantation. Q. J. Med. 150:231-254, 1968.
65. Better, O. S.: Tubular dysfunction following kidney transplantation. Nephron 25:209-213, 1980.
66. Ferguson, R. K., Reed, D. M., Barber, K. G., Bannett, A. D., and Raja, R. M.: Sodium-losing nephropathy and nephrocalcinosis after transplantation. Am. J. Kidney Dis. 15:206-210, 1985.
67. Freidman, A., and Chesney, R.: Fanconi's syndrome in renal transplantation. Am. J. Nephrol. 7:45-47, 1981.
68. Dadirvaziri, N., Nellans, R. E., Brueggmann, R. M., Barton, C. H., and Martin, D. C.: Renal tubular dysfunction in transplanted kidneys. South. Med. J. 72:530-534, 19xx.
69. Gottlieb, M. N., Stephe, M. K., Laurie, E. G., Griffiths, H. J., Denzora, J. K., Strom, T., Lazarus, M., Tilney, N. L., and Merrill, J. P.: A longitudinal study of bone disease after successful renal transplantation. Nephron 22: 239-248, 1978.
70. Nielsen, H. E.: Bone mineral content in renal transplant patients. Clin. Nephrol. 10:196-200, 1978.
71. Lucas, B. St. C., and Castro, J. E.: Calculi in renal transplants. Br. J. Urol. 50, 302-306, 1978.
72. Normann, E., Fryjordet, A., and Halvorsen, S.: Stones in renal transplants. Scand. J. Urol. Nephrol. 14:73-76, 1980.
73. Sakhaee, K., Nicar, M. J., Glass, K., and Pak, C. Y. C.: Post menopausal osteoporosis as a manifestation of renal hypercalciuria with secondary hyperparathyroidism. J. Clin. Endocrinol. Metab. 61:368-373, 1985.
74. Sakhaee, K., Nicar, M. J., Hill, K., and Pak, C. Y. C.: Contrasting effects of potassium citrate and sodium citrate therapies on urinary chemistries and crystallization of stone-forming salts. Kidney Int. 24:348-352, 1983.

75. Preminger, G. M., Sakhaee, K., Skurla, C., and Pak, C. Y. C.: Prevention of recurrent calcium stone formation with potassium citrate therapy in patients with distal renal tubular acidosis. J. Urol. 134:20-23, 1985.
76. Preminger, G. M., Sakhaee, K., and Pak, C. Y. C.: Altered intestinal calcium absorption occurring independently of vitamin D in distal renal tubular acidosis. Metabolism, 1986 (accepted for publication).

9

Gastrointestinal and Liver Complications

DAVID H. VAN THIEL
University of Pittsburgh School of Medicine, Pittsburgh, Pennsylvania

I. STRUCTURE AND FUNCTION OF THE GASTROINTESTINAL TRACT

The gastrointestinal tract is in direct contact with the environment. Thus, like the skin and lungs, it must provide a mechanical barrier to a wide variety of environmental toxins and infectious agents. In contrast to these other two organs, however, the gastrointestinal tract must accomplish this task while allowing the entry of a wide variety of nutrients and essential vitamins, yet limiting the entry of the resident microflora that are present throughout its length. The physiologic, cellular, enzymatic, and humoral mechanisms that allow the survival and proliferation of a unique microflora within the gastrointestinal tract while preventing tissue invasion by these same micro-organisms are shown in Table 1.

The numbers and kinds of bacteria encountered by the host and present within the gastrointestinal tract change markedly as one progresses from the mouth to the anus. So also do the histological and physiologic functions and defenses of the gut.

The oral cavity, particularly the gingival crevices, are heavily colonized with a mixed bacterial flora that on average achieves levels of 10^7-10^8 aerobes and 10^8-10^9 anerobes per milliliter of saliva. The normal ecological balance of this mixed bacterial flora is maintained by several types of interbacterial competitions and inhibitions and the secretion of salivary enzymes and secretory IgA. Many oropharyngeal bacteria and food contaminated by bacteria are swallowed daily; few survive the normal acidity of the stomach. Specifically, most bacteria are destroyed within 15 min exposure to gastric acid (pH 3.5 or less). The

Table 1 Defense Mechanisms of the Gastrointestinal Tract

Defense	Function
Gastric acid	Kills bacteria or limits their replication
Peristalsis	Evacuates infectious agents and their toxic products
Bile	Prevents bacterial proliferation
Secretory glycoproteins and glycolipids	Competes with glycoproteins and glycolipids on bacterial membranes or intrinsic to viral coats that allow for pathogen adherence
Indigenous flora	Produces bacteriotoxins, alters the microenvironment pH, O_2 content, redox state
Local antibody production	Prevents attachment of organisms by agglutinating them

few exceptions are spore-forming bacteria, a few gram-positive streptococci, lactobacilli, and fungi.

Those organisms that are capable of surviving the acidic environment of the stomach are carried by gastric peristalsis into the small bowel where the conditions for their continued survival are considerably more favorable. By the time the ileum is reached, bacteria are present in concentrations of 10^6 organisms per milliliter of luminal content. Across the ileocecal valve, the colon, and particularly the cecum, provide the most favorable environment within the entire gastrointestinal tract for bacterial growth, with both aerobic and anerobic organisms reaching concentrations of 10^{10}-10^{11} bacteria per milliliter of luminal material or gram of feces. The predominant anerobic organisms within the cecum include those of the genus *Bacteroides.* The most common aerobes within the cecum are those of the family Enterobacteriaceae.

Not only do the various components of the gastrointestinal tract differ functionally and environmentally, but they also differ structurally and histologically. As a result of these structural differences, the different component parts of the gastrointestinal tract are also uniquely susceptible to different pathogens [14]. For example, sites such as the mouth, pharynx, esophagus, and anus (and perineum), which have a squamous epithelial surface, are more susceptible to *Candida* infections, and those that have a secretory epithelial surface, like the small bowel, are more susceptible to viral and enteric pathogens that have cell surface ligands (pilae, surface coats, and so on) that interact with various epithelial cell surface glycoproteins that enable localization and infestation of specific pathogens at particular sites.

Returning to Table 1 it can be seen that the various intrinsic defense mechanisms of the gastrointestinal tract actually consist of three main factors. These are factors that (1) inhibit pathogen proliferation, such as gastric acid, bile, and the endogenous flora; (2) those that limit pathogen attachment to gastrointestinal cells, such as secreted and luminally degraded glycoproteins and glycolipids and secretory IgA; and (3) those that enhance evacuation or limit cell surface contact time, such as peristalsis and the factors listed above (those that limit attachment). In addition to agglutinating bacteria, secretory IgA inactivates a variety of bacterial toxins and enzymes that would otherwise damage the mucosa or alter the balance within the endogenous flora.

The process of organ transplantation alters the various intrinsic defense mechanisms in a variety of ways [29,30]. Clearly, the surgical trauma associated with organ transplantation has a direct effect at barrier disruption, particularly if the organ being transplanted is the liver. But even with less gastrointestinally related types of transplantation, the ileus associated with these surgical procedures and the frequent use of decompressing nasogastric tubes and feeding tubes, for example, also disrupt the normal flora, traumatize the mucosa, and allow unusual pathogens to attach, replicate, and/or directly injure mucosal surfaces that otherwise would not be susceptible to such injury. Moreover, the concomitant use of antibiotics and antirejection medicines (steroids) also greatly impairs the natural defense mechanisms of the gastrointestinal tract by altering the rate and type of secretions, such as gastric acid and mucus, bile, and many poorly defined intestinal glycoproteins and glycolipids [14]. Moreover, these same agents also alter the fine balance that exists between the various components of the endogenous flora, leading to alterations within it that allow one or another organism to predominate or new organisms to take hold (staphylococci, *Clostridium difficile,* and others) and induce disease symptoms. In addition, these same agents may affect the replicative function of the mucosa, making it a less adequate defense barrier either altering by its intrinsic structure (biochemically as well as histologically) or its regenerative (repair and/or reserve) capacity.

Finally, these same drugs (steroids and antirejection drugs) can have intrinsic toxicity for the gastrointestinal tract and its appendages. Specifically, the use of steroids predisposes the proximal gastrointestinal tract to acid-peptic disease and occasionally induces pancreatitis. Such drugs as azathioprine have intrinsic hepatotoxicity and in rare cases also can induce pancreatitis.

Not only are the primary or intrinsic defenses of the gastrointestinal tract disturbed as a result of the medicines used to control or prevent rejection, but so also are the secondary defenses, which consist of the phagocytic activity of the polymorphonuclear and mononuclear cells present within the lamina propria.

II. FUNGAL INFECTIONS

The fungal infections of the gastrointestinal tract primarily involve the upper gastrointestinal tract, including the mouth, pharynx, esophagus, and stomach (Table 2). The most common of these infections is that due to *Candida albicans* [25-29]. Such infections usually are local but can become invasive and at times systemic.

Once *Candida* organisms invade the bloodstream, polymorphonuclear cells appear to be the major host defense. Thus control of such infections can be shown to coincide with the ability of the individual to initiate and maintain polymorphonuclear leukocyte (PMN) mobilization. Any delay in leukocyte mobilization, as routinely occurs with steroid therapy, can be followed by the establishment of a systemic fungal infection. About one-third of the *Candida* ingested by polymorphonuclear leukocytes are killed within 1-4 hr of being phagocytized. Such killing appears to be both myeloperoxidase dependent and nonmyeloperoxidase dependent. Polymorphonuclear cells also appear to kill or damage fungi by injuring their hyphal elements, presumably as a consequence of the release of lysosomal enzymes.

Major risk factors for fungal, especially *Candida,* sepsis in transplant patients, in addition to the use of immunosuppressive agents (particularly steroids and others), include the frequent use of antibiotics and the need for hyperalimentation and prolonged venous access.

The most frequent manifestations of candidiasis in transplanted patients are fever and dysphagia. Occasionally mucosal bleeding occurs, and rarely it can be life threatening, although it usually is only mild to moderate in magnitude, albeit chronic. Urine analysis will show *Candida* in at least one-third of cases, and urine cultures have been shown to be positive in 80% of the cases, and urine cultures have been shown to be positive in 80% of the cases ultimately shown to have

Table 2 Gastrointestinal Fungal Infections that Complicate Transplant Procedure and Occur as a Consequence of Immune Suppression

Infection	Predisposing factors	Mechanisms
Candida *Aspergillus*	Steroid therapy and other immunosuppression therapy; abdominal surgery; use of IV catheters	Defective cell-mediated immunity; defective phagocytosis and killing; increased portals of entry
Zygomycosis *Mucor* *Rhizopus*	Acidosis plus above	As above

Candida sepsis. Ocular findings of *Candida* sepsis have been reported and should be sought in all febrile transplant patients in whom a specific focus of infection is not obvious.

Aspergillus organisms are second only to *Candida* in terms of the frequency with which they are the pathogen responsible for a fungal infection of the gastrointestinal tract in patients with organ transplants. Aspergilli have been isolated from the normal gastrointestinal tract and commonly can be found to contaminate certain commercial foods, particularly fresh fruits and vegetables. Both the oral ingestion and the inhalation of organisms are common routes of *Aspergillus* infection in transplanted patients. Any part of the gastrointestinal tract can be involved, but the esophagus and stomach are particularly frequent sites. The typical lesion is an ulcer covered with exudate, which on histological examination is shown to consist of necrotic tissue and fungal hyphae. Bleeding of such lesions is common and can be massive, as the fungus commonly invades and destroys vascular walls.

The antemortum diagnosis of invasive *Aspergillus* infection is difficult as the clinical interpretation of a finding of aspergilli in sputum, urine, and fecal and body fluid cultures is quite difficult.

Zygomycosis is becoming an increasingly common infection in transplant patients. Infections, particularly of the sinuses and gastrointestinal tract, are usual with these organisms. Acidosis due either to diarrhea and/or uremia is a common predisposing factor for such infections. These organisms usually produce focally invasive lesions consisting of ulcers, which can lead to bowel perforation, peritonitis, and intestinal hemorrhage. Because these organisms can tolerate the acidic environment of the stomach, this location is a common site of involvement with these organisms in infected patients.

The definitive diagnosis of zygomycosis requires the demonstration of characteristic hyphae in tissue biopsies. The clinical management of such infections is very difficult and usually requires prolonged courses of amphotericin B.

III. VIRAL INFECTIONS

The common viral infections of the gastrointestinal tract of organ transplant recipients are those due to herpes, cytomegalovirus (CMV), the Epstein-Barr virus (EBV), and adenovirus, as well as the various hepatitis viruses (A, B, non-A, non-B). The easiest way to consider the various viral infections of the gastrointestinal tract and its various appendages (the liver and pancreas) that occur in transplant recipients is to consider them in terms of the specific organs or sites of involvement (Table 3). All these agents can under certain circumstances (immunosuppression) produce a "hepatitis" [1-11]. Cases of herpes, CMV, adenovirus, and even EBV hepatitis in transplant patients tend to be particularly severe. The clinical picture is usually one of chills and fever with rigors and progressive

Table 3 Viral Infections of the Gastrointestinal Tract in Transplant Patients

Mouth and pharynx
Herpes
EBV
Adenoviruses
Esophagus
Herpes
CMV
Stomach: CMV
Small intestine
Adenovirus
Rotavirus
Coxsackievirus
Caliciviruses
Astroviruses
CMV
Colon and rectum
CMV
Herpes
Pancreas
Coxsackievirus
Adenoviruses
Liver
Hepatitis A, B, non-A, non-B
Δ Agent
EBV
Herpesviruses
CMV
Adenovirus

increases in the serum level of the various liver injury tests (AST, ALT, and LDH) and bilirubin. Hepatic enlargement and tenderness are common also and may be the first localizing sign. A current or recent generalized viremia is common in hepatitis involvement with these viruses and should suggest the diagnosis. The prognosis for herpes hepatitis, adenovirus hepatitis, and Δ agent hepatitis (coinfection with hepatitis B) is very poor. The prognosis of EBV, CMV, type A, B, and non-A, non-B hepatitis in transplant patients is less poor as they tend to produce a less severe form of hepatitis in such patients than do the previously discussed viruses. However, type B hepatitis, non-A, non-B hepatitis, and EBV hepatitis can uncommonly produce a form of chronic liver disease in transplanted patients characterized by hepatomegaly, occasional fever, intermittent abdominal pain, and chronic fatigue. Histologically, focal cell necrosis and a diffuse parenchymal mononuclear cell, as well as a portal inflammatory infiltrate, is noted on liver biopsy. Cirrhosis can follow such chronic hepatic infections and frequently does after 5 years or more of continual low-grade but chronic hepatic injury.

Acyclovir is useful in the management of herpes infection of the liver as well as other gastrointestinal organs [12]. No therapy currently exists for the other viruses, with exception of dihydroxymethylpropoxymethylguanine (DHPG), which has been used experimentally in cases of CMV infection of the gastrointestinal tract in the patients with the acquired immune deficiency syndrome (AIDS) [13].

Clinical pancreatic disease occurring in transplant patients and due to viral infections is uncommon but can occur as part of a widespread organ involvement, part of a high-grade or chronic viremia. When it does occur it usually manifests itself as an elevation of the amylase activity and becomes clinically evident following a more severe coexistent clinical hepatitis and may signal the imminent demise of the patient.

CMV infections of the gastrointestinal tract of transplant patients usually manifest themselves as focal areas of erythema, erosions, and ulceration [15-24]. They tend to predominate in the duodenum, terminal ileum, cecum, and rectum, areas where the lymphoid tissue is most abundant. Such lesions can progress to transmural bowel perforations. Thus any localized abdominal pain associated with an ileus or overt peritoneal signs in a transplant patient known to have CMV should suggest the diagnosis of bowel perforation and lead to an aggressive diagnostic evaluation and early surgical closure of any perforation. Occasionally CMV infections or ulcers of the esophagus, small bowel, and colon can be the site of considerable gastrointestinal bleeding.

Those viruses that primarily attack the small intestine usually produce a watery diarrhea that, in a transplant patient, can be quite protracted and lead to dehydration, acid-base abnormalities, and progressive malnutrition and adversely affect the absorption of a variety of medicines including those used to prevent or manage rejection [15,18,20-22,30]. Histologically, the triad of villous atrophy, crypt hyperplasia, and increased numbers of intraepithelial lymphocytes is seen commonly in the jejunum of patients with viral enteritis who have had a prior organ transplant. Similar abnormalities have been reported recently in patients with AIDS [76,77].

Oral, pharyngeal, and esophageal viral infections present as vesicles or shallow ulcers that are frequently surrounded by an erythematous halo and tend to be quite painful and are therefore associated with odynophagia [24].

IV. BACTERIAL INFECTIONS

Clinically important, bacterial infections of the gastrointestinal tract of transplant patients rarely exist in the absence of some local trauma or tissue injury. Those that do occur, however, tend to be characterized by their ability to survive in macrophages and invade the tissues of persons with T-cell deficiency syndromes. Such organisms include those of the *Salmonella* and *Shigella* groups, *Yersinia, Campylobacter,* and *Mycobacterium avium* [31-39]. They all tend to present as diarrheal illnesses that can be associated with either overt or more often occult gastrointestinal bleeding and focal involvement of the colon and/or distal small bowel. Differentiation of *Yersinia, Campylobacter,* and *M. avium* infections from Crohn's disease can be quite difficult and may be impossible in the absence of a biopsy or culture. The recognition of *M. avium* infection as an entity separate from Whipple's disease in a transplant patient can be established by special staining and culture techniques for mycobacteria and should be considered before the diagnosis of Whipple's disease is accepted in such patients [54-58].

It almost goes without saying that *C. difficile* infection should be sought for and eliminated as the cause of any diarrhea in transplant patients, particularly if they have been on antibiotics of any type recently [59,60]. An examination of the stool for *C. difficile* toxin is usually sufficient for a diagnosis. It also should be remembered that the absence of endoscopic proctitis and/or pseudomembranes in the distal colon does not exclude this diagnosis from being present more proximally in the colon.

Nocardia are aerobic gram-positive filamentous bacteria that fragment into bacillary forms that tend to be acid fast. They are native to the soil and are worldwide in distribution. *Nocardia* infections are relatively common in individuals who receive glucocorticoids and are therefore not uncommon in transplant recipients. Typically, such infections begin in the lungs, but metastatic lesions are very common, particularly those involving arterioles. The hepatic artery is a common secondary site of nocardial involvement and such infections frequently result in either focal or diffuse hepatic infarction.

V. NONFUNGAL PARASITIC INFECTIONS

Although any parasitic infection present in a patient prior to organ transplantation can become more evident following the application of immunosuppressive therapy, two such infections (*Cryptosporidium* and *Strongloides sterocoralis*) have been found to be particular problems in such patients, and a third (amebiasis) occasionally can be a major threat to the transplant patient's survival.

Infection with *Cryptosporidium* usually presents as a severe watery diarrhea [40-48]. A specific diagnosis is possible following identification of the parasite in stool using the sucrose flotation method or rectal and/or small intestinal biopsy material using either a modified Ziehl Nielson or auramine staining procedure. Recently, spiramycin has been shown to be the only agent known to be effective in treating this particular enteric parasitic infection [46,47].

Hyperinfection with *S. stercoralis* is usually characterized by profound malabsorption, diarrhea, various electrolyte disturbances, and secondary gram-negative enteric or opportunistic fungal infections that commonly lead to systemic sepsis, coma, and death. Eosinophilia is usually present in such patients and should suggest the possibility of the diagnosis and cause one to examine the stool or duodenal content for the worm [49-53]. Untreated, this particular parasitic infection is universally fatal. Even with appropriate therapy with thiabendazole, the mortality rate approaches 50%.

Chronic quiescent amebiasis of the colon can become activated and a major health problem for transplant patients on immunosuppressive drugs. In such cases, activated disease can progress to form hepatic abscesses and occasionally other metastatic foci of infection, as in the brain, meninges, and skin.

VI. DRUG-RELATED GASTROINTESTINAL INJURIES

Organ transplantation requires that the recipient indefinitely take drugs designed to prevent graft rejection. Many of these agents have actions that are capable of adversely altering gastrointestinal function or gastrointestinal histological integrity. Most antirejection regimens include a glucocorticoid agent known to inhibit phospholipase activity and thereby inhibit prostaglandin synthesis and disturb endogenous "cytoprotective" mechanisms that help to prevent proteolytic and acid-associated mucosal injury and promote healing of such injuries, should they actually occur. Thus acid-peptic disease in all of its forms in the esophagus, stomach, and duodenum are common in transplant patients. In addition to glucocorticoids, a variety of alkalating agents (usually cytoxan) and various antimetabolites (azathioprine, 6-mercaptopurine, and methotrexate) are commonly taken in combination with the glucocorticosteroids to prevent rejection. All these agents are capable of producing intestinal villous atrophy that occasionally can be the cause of clinically important malabsorption (particularly lactose intolerance), and some of them can also initiate hepatic fibrosis, which occasionally progresses to cirrhosis or hepatic veno-occlusive disease [61-63]. Recently, hepatic sinusoidal dilation associated with portal hypertension has also been reported in transplant patients and is believed to be due to the azathioprine used by the patients described [62].

More recently, cyclosporine has been used in combination with glucocorticoids rather than either the alkalating agents or the antimetabolite drugs previously used to prevent and/or treat rejection. It is frequently administered in milk and can result in the clinical expression of occult lactase deficiency in susceptible patients. Cyclosporine can be hepatotoxic and at high doses produces a centrolobular bland necrosis. At the doses used most often clinically, it can produce a cholestasis manifested by an elevated plasma level of bile salts rather than overt hyperbilirubinemia. In particularly severe cases hyperbilirubinemia also occurs.

VII. REJECTION AND GRAFT-VERSUS-HOST REACTIONS

Rejection is manifest only in the transplanted organ. Currently, among the various gastrointestinal organs, only the liver and pancreas are being transplanted, although gut transplants have been performed experimentally and probably will continue to be done sporadically.

Hepatic rejection can be characterized as either acute or chronic in nature. Acute rejection is manifested biochemically by elevations of the serum total bilirubin and aminotransferase levels and clinically by hepatic dysfunction. The biochemical hallmark of chronic hepatic rejection is the finding of a disproportionate elevation of the serum γ-glutamyltranspeptidase level and hyperbilirubinemia. Histologically, acute hepatic rejection consists of a mixed portal inflammatory infiltrate rich in large plasmacytoid lymphocytes, portal and hepatic venous endotheliitis, and a characteristic bile injury. In contrast, chronic rejection is characterized histopathologically by a portal fibrosis, the presence of small or absent portal areas, which demonstrate bile duct paucity, and a subintimal accumulation of macrophages within medium-sized hepatic arteries. Pancreatic rejection is characterized by islet fibrosis and hyalinization, which leads to a progressive loss of functioning islets and functional failure of the endocrine pancreas.

Graft-versus-host disease and gut allograft rejection are quite similar histopathologically and functionally and therefore are nearly identical in their clinical presentation [64-71]. Thus acutely both interstitial and intracellular edema and liquefication and coagulative necrosis of the epithelium leading to a loss of villus height and focal crypt necrosis are common to each histopathologically. Clinically, diarrhea with a massive protein-losing enteropathy is the major symptom of both. Chronic rejection is characterized histologically by villous atrophy, bowel wall thickening with edema, and fibrosis and clinically by malabsorption.

Graft-versus-host disease also involves the liver and produces hepatic changes similar to those of chronic hepatic rejection, such as bile duct paucity, portal fibrosis, and a diffuse portal chronic inflammatory mononuclear infiltrate [67, 71]. Both of these hepatic injuries can progress to produce a picture similar to that of primary biliary cirrhosis and/or chronic active hepatitis with cirrhosis.

Clinically less important, but nonetheless a symptomatic problem for the patient with graft-versus-host disease, is the progressive loss of the lacrimal and salivary glands, with the resultant dry mouth and eyes and an overt sicca (Sjögren's) syndrome.

VIII. GASTROINTESTINAL NEOPLASIA

Cancer development is a constant threat to transplant patients who survive 4 years or more. The gastrointestinal sites of such immunosuppression-related cancers are the mouth, pharynx, and larynx and histocytic lymphoma and lymphoproliferative syndromes that can involve the intestine [72-75]. It is of some interest that each of these tumors has been associated with the Epstein-Barr virus and that the EBV genome has been isolated from the DNA of such tumors, particularly the lymphomas and/or the lymphoproliferative syndromes [73,74]. More important, however, is the clinical observation that some of these "lymphomas" resolve spontaneously if the immunotherapy is stopped or drastically reduced. Such action not uncommonly leads to graft injury or failure due to enhanced rejection and may necessitate retransplantation following resolution of the "tumor."

IX. SUMMARY

As must be evident from the above presentation, organ transplantation has taught us much about the immunologic function of the gut and its appendage organs. It also has taught us much about virology and it has provided unique insights into the important problem of neoplastic transplantation of cells and tissues. It also has produced new diseases (graft-versus-host, rejection, and a large number of opportunistic infections) for us to deal with, manage, and, we hope, prevent. Most importantly, however, it has provided our patients with a chance for a new, more healthy life.

ACKNOWLEDGMENT

This work was supported in part by grants from the NIAAA, #AA04425, and the NIDDK #AM32556 and the Gastroenterological Medical Research Foundation of Southwestern Pennsylvania.

REFERENCES

1. Lee, J. C., and Fortuny, E. I.: Adult herpes simplex hepatitis. Hum. Pathol. 3:277-281, 1972.
2. Briggs, W. A., Lazarus, J. M., Birtch, A. G., Hampers, C. L., Hager, E. B., and Merrill, J. P.: Hepatitis affecting hemodialysis and transplant patients. Arch. Intern. Med. 132:21-28, 1973.
3. Freiberger, Z., Anuras, S., Koff, R. S., and Bonney, W. W.: Chronic active hepatitis without hepatitis B antigenemia in renal transplant recipients. Gastroenterology 66:1187-1194, 1974.
4. Henson, D. E., Grimley, P. M., and Strano, A. J.: Postnatal cytomegalovirus hepatitis. An autopsy and liver biopsy study. Hum. Pathol. 5:93-103, 1974.
5. Mozes, M. F., Ascher, N. L., Balfour, H. H., Simmons, R. L., and Najarian, J. S.: Jaundice after renal allotransplantation. Ann. Surg. 188:783-790, 1978.
6. Ware, A. J., Luby, J. P., Hollinger, B., Eigenbrodt, E. H., Cuthbert, J. A., Atkins, C. R., Shorey, J., Hull, A. R., and Combes, B.: Etiology of liver disease in renal-transplant patients. Ann. Intern. Med. 91:364-371, 1979.
7. Toussaint, C., Dupont, E., Vanherweghem, J. L., Cappel, R., DeRoy, D., Vereerstraeten, P., Kinnaert, P., Thiry, L., and Van Geertruyden, J.: Liver disease in patients undergoing hemodialysis and kidney transplantation. Adv. Nephrol. 8:269-294, 1979.
8. Rustgi, V. K., Hoofnagle, J. H., Gerin, J. L., Gelmann, E. P., Reichert, C. M., Cooper, J. N., and Macher, A. M.: Hepatitis B virus infection in the acquired immunodeficiency syndrome. Ann. Intern. Med. 101:795-797, 1984.
9. Stevens, C. E., Aach, R. D., Hollinger, F. B., Mosley, J. W., Szmuness, W., Kahn, R., Werch, J., and Edwards, V.: Hepatitis B virus antibody in blood donors and the occurrence of non-A, non-B hepatitis in transfusion recipients. Ann. Intern. Med. 101:733-738, 1984.
10. Jones, J. F., Ray, C. G., Minnich, L. L., Hicks, M. J., Kibler, R., and Lucas, D. O.: Evidence for active Epstein-Barr virus infection in patients with persistent, unexplained illnesses: Elevated anti-early antigen antibodies. Ann. Intern. Med. 102:1-7, 1985.
11. Straus, S. E., Tosato, G., Armstrong, G., Lawley, T., Preble, O. T., Henle, W., Davey, R., Pearson, G., Epstein, J., Brus, I., and Blaese, M.: Persisting illness and fatigue in adults with evidence of Epstein-Barr virus infection. Ann. Intern. Med. 102:7-16, 1985.
12. Griffin, P. J. A., Colbert, J. W., Williamson, E. P. M., Fiddian, A. P., Hickmott, E., Sells, R. A., and Salaman, J. R.: Oral acyclovir prophylaxis of herpes infections in renal transplant recipients. Transplant. Proc. XVII:84-85, 1985.
13. van der Waaij, D.: Colonization resistance of the digestive tract: Clinical consequences and implications. J. Antimicrob. Chemother. 10:263-270, 1982.
14. Kotler, D. P., Gaetz, H. P., Lange, M., Klein, E. B., and Holt, P. R.: Enteropathy associated with the acquired immunodeficiency syndrome. Ann. Intern. Med. 101:421-428, 1984.

15. Henson, D.: Cytomegalovirus inclusion bodies in the gastrointestinal tract. Arch. Pathol. 93:477-482, 1972.
16. Rosen, P., Armstrong, D., and Rice, N.: Gastrointestinal cytomegalovirus infection. Arch. Intern. Med. 132:274-276, 1973.
17. Underwood, J. C. E., and Corbett, C. L.: Persistent diarrhoea and hypoalbuminaemia associated with cytomegalovirus enteritis. Br. Med. J. 22:1029-1030, 1978.
18. Peterson, P. K., Balfour, H. H., Marker, S. C., Fryd, D. S., Howard, R. J., and Simmons R. L.: Cytomegalovirus disease in renal allograft recipients: A prospective study of the clinical features, risk factors and impact on renal transplantation. Medicine (Baltimore) 59:283-300, 1980.
19. Knapp, A. B., Horst, D. A., Eliopoulos, G., Gramm, H. F., Gaber, L. W., Falchuk, K. R., Falchuk, Z. M., and Trey, C.: Widespread cytomegalovirus gastroenterocolitis in a pateint with acquired immunodeficiency syndrome. Gastroenterology 85:1399-1402, 1983.
20. Gertler, S. L., Pressman, J., Price, P., Brozinsky, S., and Miyai, K.: Gastrointestinal cytomegalovirus infection in a homosexual man with severe acquired immunodeficiency syndrome. Gastroenterology 85:1403-1406, 1983.
21. Blackman, E., Vimadalal, S. and Nash, G.: Significance of gastrointestinal cytomegalovirus infection in homosexual males. Am. J. Gastroenterol. 79:935-940, 1984.
22. Frank, D., and Raicht, R. F.: Intestinal perforation associated with cytomegalovirus infection in patients with acquired immune deficiency syndrome. Am. J. Gastroenterol. 79:201-205, 1984.
23. Freedman, P. G., Weiner, B. C., and Balthazar, E. J.: Cytomegalovirus esophagogastritis in a patient with acquired immunodeficiency syndrome. Am. J. Gastroenterol. 80:434-437, 1985.
24. Brabander, J. O. W., Blank, F., and Butas, C. A.: Intestinal moniliasis in adults. Can. Med. Assoc. J. 77:478-483, 1957.
25. Eras, P., Goldstein, M. J., and Sherlock, P.: Candida infection of the gastrointestinal tract. Medicine (Baltimore) 51:367-379, 1972.
26. Kane, J. G., Chretien, J. H., and Garagusi, V. F.: Diarrhoea caused by candida. Lancet 1:335-336, 1976.
27. Klein, R., Harris, C. A., Small, C. B., Moll, B., Lesser, M., and Friedland, G. H.: Oral candidiasis in high-risk patients as the initial manifestation of the acquired immunodeficiency syndrome. N. Engl. J. Med. 311:354-358, 1984.
28. Musola, R., Franzin, G., Mora, R., and Manfrini, C.: Prevalence of gastroduodenal lesions in uremic patients undergoing dialysis and after renal transplantation. Gastrointest. Endosc. 30:343-346, 1984.
29. Booth, I. W., Chrystie, I. L., Levinsky, R. J., Marshall, W. C., Pincott, J., and Harries, J. T.: Protracted diarrhoea, immunodeficiency and viruses. Eur. J. Pediatr. 138:271-272, 1982.
30. Yolken, R. H., Bishop, C. A., Townsend, T. R., Bolyard, E. A., Bartlett, J., Santos, G. W., and Saral, R. Infectious gastroenteritis in bone-marrow-trans-recipients. N. Engl. J. Med. 306:1009-1012, 1982.

31. Gillin, J. S., Urmacher, C., West, R., and Shike, M.: Disseminated *Mycobacterium avium*-intracellulare infection in acquired immunodeficiency syndrome mimicking Whipple's disease. Gastroenterology 85:1187-1191, 1983.
32. Malebranche, R., Arnous, E., Guerin, J. M., Pierre, G. D., Laroche, A. C., Pean-Guichard, C., Elie, R., Morisset, P. H., Spira, T., Mandeville, R., Drotman, P., Seemayer, T., and Dupuy, J. M.: Acquired immunodeficiency syndrome with severe gastrointestinal manifestations in Haiti. Lancet 2:873-877, 1983.
33. Pasternak, J., Bolivar, R., Hopfer, R. L., Fainstein, V., Mills, K., Tios, A., Bodey, G. P., Fennell, C. L., Totten, P. A., and Stamm, W. E.: Bacteremia caused by campylobacter-like organisms in two male homosexuals. Ann. Intern. Med. 101:339-341, 1984.
34. Rolston, K. V. I., and Hopfer R. L.: Diarrhea due to *Plesiomonas shigelloides* in cancer patients. J. Clin. Microbiol. 20:597-598, 1984.
35. Smith, P. D., Macher A. J., Bookman, M. A., Boccia, R. V., Steis, R. G., Gill, V., Manischewitz, J., and Gelmann, E. P.: *Salmonella typhimurium* enteritis and bacteremia in the acquired immunodeficiency syndrome. Ann. Intern. Med. 102:207-209, 1985.
36. Dworkin, B., Wormser, G. P., Rosenthal, W. S., Heier, S. K., Braunstein, M., Weiss, L., Jankowski, R., Levy, D., and Weiselberg, S.: Gastrointestinal manifestations of the acquired immunodeficiency syndrome: A review of 22 cases. Am. J. Gastroenterol. in press.
37. Jacobs, J. L., Gold, J. W. M., Murray, H. W., Roberts, R. B., and Armstrong, D.: Salmonella infections in patients with the acquired immunodeficiency syndrome. Ann. Intern. Med. 102:186-188, 1985.
38. Glaser, J. B., Morton-Kute L., Berger, S. R., Weber, J., Siegal, F. P., Lopez, C., Robbins, W., and Landesman, S. H.: Recurrent *Salmonella Typhimurium* bacteremia associated with the acquired immunodeficiency syndrome. Ann. Intern. Med. 102, 1985.
39. Current, W. L., Reese, N. C., Ernst, J. V., Bailey, W. S., Heyman, M. B., and Weinstein, W. M.: Human cryptosporidiosis in immunocompetent and immunodeficient persons. N. Engl. J. Med. 308:1252-1257, 1983.
40. Andreani, T., Modigliani, R., leCharpentier, Y., Galian, A., Brouet, J. C., Liance, M., Lachance, J. R., Messing, B., and Vernisse, B.: Acquired immunodeficiency with intestinal cryptosporidiosis: Possible transmission by Haitian whole blood. Lancet 1, 1983.
41. Miller, R. A., Holmberg, R. E., and Clausen, C. R.: Life-threatening diarrhea caused by *Cryptosporidium* in a child undergoing therapy for acute lymphocytic leukemia. J. Pediatr. 103:256-259, 1983.
42. Payne, P., Lancaster, L. A. Heinzman, M., and McCutchan, J. A.: Identification of cryptosporidium in patients with the acquired immunodeficiency syndrome. N. Engl. J. Med. 309:613-614, 1983.
43. Navin, T. R., and Juranek, D. D.: Cryptosporidiosis: Clinical, epidemiologic, and parasitologic review. Rev. Infect. Dis. 6, 1984.

44. Cohen, J. D., Rhlig, L., Jayich, S. A., Tong, M. J., Lechago, J., and Snape, W. J.: Cryptosporidium in acquired immunodeficiency syndrome. Dig. Dis. Sci. 29:773-777, 1984.
45. Portnory, D., Whiteside, M. E., Buckley, E., and MacLeod, C. L.: Treatment of intestinal cryptosporidiosis with spiramycin. Ann. Intern. Med. 101: 202-204, 1984.
46. Collier, A. C., Miller, R. A., and Meyers, J. D.: Cryptosporidiosis after marrow transplantation: Person-to-person transmission and treatment with spiramycin. Ann. Intern. Med. 101:205-206, 1984.
47. Dobbins, W. O., and Weinstein, W. M.: Electron microscopy of the intestine and rectum in acquired immunodeficiency syndrome. Gastroenterology 68: 738-749, 1985.
48. Lima, J. P., and Delgado, P. G.: Diangosis of strongyloidiasis: Importance of Baermann's method. Am. J. Dig. Dis. 6.899-904, 1961.
49. Cruz, T., Reboucas, G., and Rocha, H.: Fatal strongyloidiasis in patients receiving corticosteroids. N. Engl. J. Med. 275:1093-1096, 1966.
50. Rivera, E., Maldonado, N., Velez-Garcia, E., Grillo, A. J., and Malaret, G.: Hyperinfection syndrome and *Strongyloides stercoralis*. Ann. Intern. Med. 72:199-204, 1970.
51. Purtilo, D. T., Meyers, W. M., and Connor, D. H.: Fatal strongyloidiasis in immunosuppressed patients. Am. J. Med. 56:488-493, 1974.
52. Berry, A. J., Long, E. G., Smith, J. H., Gourley, W. K., and Fine, D. P.: Chronic relapsing colitis due to *Strongyloides stercoralis*. Am. J. Trop. Med. Hyg. 32:1289-1293, 1983.
53. Zakowski, P., Fligiel, S., Berlin, O. G. W., and Johnson, B. L.: Disseminated *Mycobacterium avium*-intracellulare infection in homosexual men dying of acquired immunodeficiency. JAMA 248:2980-2982, 1982.
54. Greene, J. B., Sidhu, G. S., Lewin, S., Levine, J. F., Masur, H., Simberkoff, M. S., Nicholas, P., Good, R. C. Zolla-Pazner, S. B., Pollock, A. A., Tapper, M. L., and Holzman, R. S.: *Mycobacterium avium*-intracellulare: A cause of disseminated life-threatening infection in homosexuals and drug abusers. Ann. Intern. Med. 97:539-546, 1982.
55. Macher, A. M., Kovacs, J. A., Gill, V., Roberts, G. D., Ames, J., Park, C. H., Straus S., Lane, H. C., Parrillo, J. E., Fauci, A. S., and Masur, H.: Bacteremia due to *Mycobacterium avium*-intracellulare in the acquired immunodeficiency syndrome. Ann. Intern. Med. 99:782-785, 1983.
56. Roth, R. I., Owen, R. L., Keren, D. F., and Volberding, P. A.: Intestinal infection with *Mycobacterium avium* in acquired immune deficiency syndrome (AIDS). Histological and clinical comparison of Whipple's disease. Dig. Dis. Sci. 30:497-504, 1985.
57. Wong, B., Edwards, F. F., Fiehn, T. E., Whimbey, E., Donnelly, H., Bernard, E. M., Gold, J. W. M., and Armstrong, D.: Continuous high-grade *Mycobacterium-avium*-intracellulare bacteremia in patients with the acquired immune deficiency syndrome. Am. J. Med. 78:35-40, 1985.

58. Milligan, D. W., and Kelly, J. K.: Pseudomembranous colitis in a leukaemia unit: A report of five fatal cases. J. Clin. Pathol. 32:1237-1243, 1979.
59. Dosik, G. M., Luna, M., Valdivieso, M., McCredie, K. B., Gehan, E. A., Gil-Extremera, B., Smith, T. L., and Bodey, G. P.: Necrotizing colitis in patients with cancer. Am. J. Med. 67:646-656, 1979.
60. McDonald, G. B., Sharma, P., Matthews, D. W., Shulman, H. M., and Thomas, E. D.: Venocclusive disease of the liver after bone marrow transplantation: Diagnosis, incidence, and predisposing factors. Hepatology 4:116-122, 1984.
61. Gerlag, P. G. G., Lobatto, S., Driessen, W. M. M., Deckers, P. F. L., Van Hooff, J. P., Schroder, E., Assmann, K. M., and Van Haelst, U. J. G.: Hepatic sinusoidal dilatation with portal hypertension during azathioprine treatment after kidney transplantation. J. Hepatol. 1:339-348, 1985.
62. McMaster, K. R., and Hennigar, G. R.: Drug-induced granulomatous hepatitis. Lab. Invest. 44:61-73, 1981.
63. Slavin, R. E., and Santos, G. W.: The graft versus host reaction in man after bone marrow transplantation: Pathology, pathogenesis, clinical features, and implication. Clin. Immunol. Immunopathol. 1:472-498, 1973.
64. Berman, M. D., Rabin, L., O'Donnell, J., Gratwohl, A. A., Graw, R. G., Deisseroth, A. B., and Jones, E. A.: The liver in long-term survivors of marrow transplant—chronic graft-versus-host disease. J. Clin. Gastroenterol. 2:53-63, 1980.
65. Sullivan, K. M., Shulman, H. M., Storb, R., Weiden, P. L., Witherspoon, R. P., McDonald, G. B., Schubert, M. M. Atkinson, K., and Thomas, E. D.: Chronic graft-versus-host disease in 52 patients: Adverse natural course and successful treatment with combination immunosuppression. Blood 57:267-276, 1981.
66. Fennell, R. H.: Ductular damage in liver transplant rejection. Its similarity to that of primary biliary cirrhosis and graft-versus-host disease. Pathol. Annu. 16:289-294, 1981.
67. Beschorner, W. E., Tutschka, P. J., and Santos, G. W.: Chronic graft-versus-host disease in the rat radiation chimera. Transplantation 33:393-399, 1982.
68. Beschorner, W. E., Tutschka, P. J., and Santos, G. W.: Sequential morphology of graft-versus-host disease in the rat radiation chimera. Clin. Immunol. Immunopathol. 22.203-224, 1982.
69. Beschorner, W. E., Tutschka, P. J., and Santos, G. W.: Chronic graft-versus-host disease in the rat radiation chimera. Transplantation 35:224-230, 1983.
70. Fennell, R. H., Shikes, R. H., and Vierling, J. M.: Relationship of pretransplant hepatobiliary disease to bile duct damage occurring in the liver allograft. Hepatology 3:84-89, 1983.
71. Geis, W. P., Iwatsuki, S., Molnar, Z., Giacchino, J. L., Kerman, R. H., Ing, T. S., and Hano, J. E.: Pseudolymphoma in renal allograft recipients. Arch. Surg. 113:461-466, 1978.
72. Sullivan, J. L., Medveczky, P., Forman, S. J., Baker, S. M., Monroe, J. E., and Mulder, C.: Epstein-Barr virus induced lymphoproliferation. N. Engl. J. Med. 311:1163-1168, 1984.

73. Hanto, D. W., Frizzera, G., Gajl-Peczaiska, K. J., Balfour, H. H., Simmons, R. L., and Najarian, J. S.: Acyclovir therapy of Epstein-Barr virus-induced posttransplant lymphoproliferative diseases. Transplant. Proc. 18:89-92, 1985.
74. Touraine, J. L., Bosi, E., El Yafi, M. S., Chapuis-Cellier, C., Blanc, N., Dubernard, J. M., Piatti, P. M., Chevalier, M., Pouteil-Noble, C., Lenoir, G., Trepo, C., Gelet, A., Creyssel, R., and Traeger, J.: The infectious lymphoproliferative syndrome in transplant patients under immunosuppressive treatment. Transplant. Proc. 17:96-97, 1985.
75. Reichert, C. M., O'Leary, T. J., Levens, D. L., Simrell, C. R., and Macher, A. M.: Autopsy pathology in the acquired immune deficiency syndrome. Am. J. Pathol. 112:357-382, 1983.
76. Jaffe, H. W., Bregman, D. J., and Selik, R. M.: Acquired immune deficiency syndrome in the United States: The first 1,000 cases. J. Infect. Dis. 148: 339-345, 1983.
77. Welch, K., Finkbeiner, W., Alpers, C. E., Blumenfeld, W., Davis, R. L., Smuckler, E. A., and Beckstead, J. H.: Autopsy findings in the acquired immune deficiency syndrome. JAMA 252:1152-1159, 1984.

the articular end of the bone is involved, joint deformity can ensue and lead to symptomatic secondary osteoarthritis.

Glimcher and Kenzora [3] have pointed out that the pathological findings in posttransplant avascular necrosis differ from the pathological findings in posttraumatic avascular necrosis following hip dislocation or femoral neck fracture. In posttransplantation avascular necrosis of the femoral head, subchondral bone becomes necrotic in the weight-bearing area. A fracture then occurs immediately beneath the articular cortex, rendering this bony platform unstable and permitting collapse of the overlying articular surface. The earliest radiographic finding in renal avascular necrosis is the crescent sign produced by this fracture (Fig. 1a). Andresen and Nielsen [4] found the crescent sign to be the presenting radiographic sign in 21 of 25 necrotic femoral heads. This gross irregularity of the femoral head may then be followed by acetabular degeneration and loss of articular cartilage on both sides of the joint (Fig. 1b). Posttraumatic avascular necrosis presents with woven bone applied to trabeculae of necrotic bone. This produces an early sign of patchy areas of increased bone density. The crescent sign appears later.

B. Etiology

Although loss of nutrition to the osteocyte produces the picture we see of avascular necrosis, its precise cause in the transplant patient remains a matter of considerable debate and study. Almost all workers believe that the steroids used to prevent graft rejection are an important etiologic factor or, at least, a modulating factor [5]. Difference of opinion persists as to the mechanism of steroid action and the relationship of avascular necrosis to total steroid dose. Corticosteroids decrease osteoblastic activity [6,7] and suppress osteoclastic bone resorption [8] while enhancing macrophage-mediated bone resorption [9]. Parathormone activity is inhibited [10], and 1,25-hydroxyl receptors in vitamin D metabolism are stabilized [11]. Corticosteroids alter fat metabolism and may cause marrow fat cell hypertrophy, thus occluding intramedullary circulation. Intestinal calcium absorption is also decreased. Although most workers find no relationship between avascular necrosis and total dose of steroid [12-14], some do believe there is such a relationship, as evidenced by a greater number of treated rejection episodes in those with osteonecrosis compared with those without osteonecrosis [15-17].

Microembolic fat may be an important consideration in avascular necrosis in the alcoholic patient but does not appear to play a part in posttransplant avascular necrosis [18,19]. Uittenbogaart and coworkers [19] found no evidence of fat emboli or of vasculitis in these patients.

Secondary hyperparathyroidism may persist for at least 1 year after transplantation, and some have supported the related osteopenia as a cause [7,20]. On the other hand, most researchers have found no correlation [6,21,22].

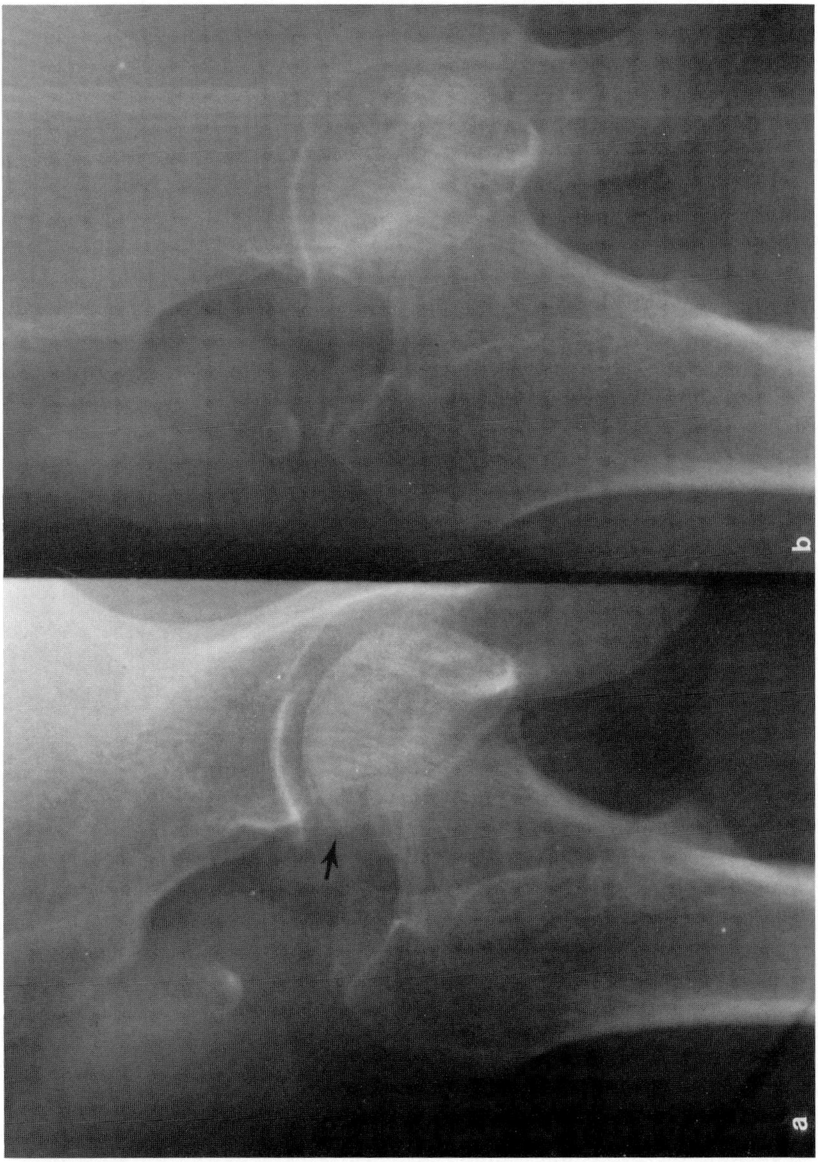

Figure 1 (a) First radiographic appearance of avascular necrosis 6 months after transplantation. The arrow indicates the crescent sign. (b) There is collapse of the femoral head 8 months later.

An attractive hypothesis relates to osteopenia. The patient enters the posttransplant period in a more or less osteopenic state relating to pre-existing renal osteodystrophy [23-26] and length of time on dialysis. Steroids are then given postoperatively, which enhances this osteopenia. Weight-bearing stress now may produce microfractures with little if any healing, leading to avascular necrosis [6]. The question of which comes first, the microfractures or the avascular necrosis, remains [3].

C. Diagnosis

Avascular necrosis usually presents to the orthopedist as involving the femoral head, femoral condyles, humeral head, or talar dome. Almost all appendicular bones have been involved, including metatarsal and metacarpal heads and the tarsal navicular [27]. The condition is most disabling in the weight-bearing joints of the lower extremities. If the patient is on crutches or uses a walker, the upper extremities then must bear weight and a previously asymptomatic humeral head necrosis may become painful.

Diagnosis is rather obvious once radiographic changes appear at a symptomatic joint. Early diagnosis prior to radiographic signs is best made by technetium ^{99}m methylene diaphosphonate bone scan showing increased uptake (Fig. 2). This is nonspecific, but the most common cause of increased local uptake in the posttransplant patient in the femoral head is avascular necrosis. Ficat and Arlet [28] have demonstrated that intramedullary pressure studies and venography along with core biopsy can make the diagnosis and provide treatment as well as decompress the hypertensive femoral head.

In the femoral condyles and talus, avascular necrosis often presents as an extensive osteochondritis dissecans with progressive and severe collapse of the underlying bone (Fig. 3) [29]. These lesions are far more extensive and involve far more bone than the more common, idiopathic osteochondritis dissecans.

D. Treatment

Avascular necrosis of the femoral head is best treated prior to subchondral fracture with its crescent sign and, in fact, prior to any radiographic sign. Core decompression should be considered in symptomatic, bone scan-positive, radiography-negative patients [30]. This procedure will provide the diagnosis and is the most conservative operation to relieve symptoms and yet preserve the femoral head. McBeath and Oeljen [31] reported success with the Phemister bone graft in such cases, but the added morbidity of tibial or fibular bone grafting is not worthwhile. Once radiographic changes present, we employ a period of protected weight bearing and anti-inflammatory medication, since not all patients have progressive symptoms. Andresen and Nielsen [4] found that 26%

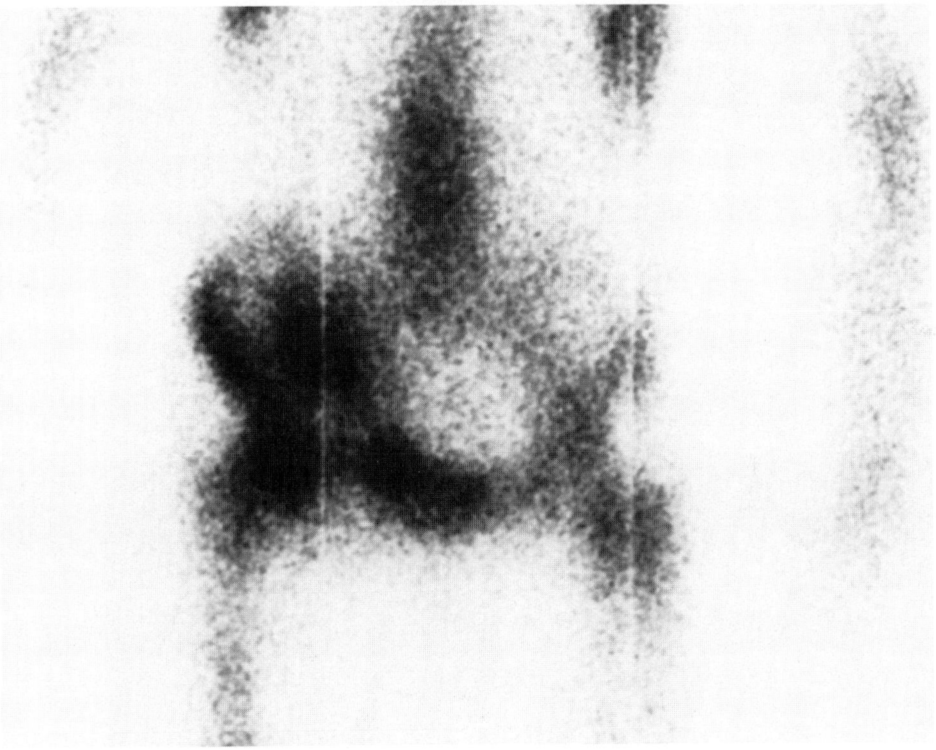

Figure 2 Technetium ^{99}m-methylene diaphosphonte bone scan of the patient in Figure 1 at onset of symptoms.

regressed, 32% progressed, and 42% of these hips remained stable. Thus, the mere fact of diagnosis does not necessarily mean operation. Failure of conservative treatment in the patient with an uninvolved acetabulum (Fig. 1b) is managed with a cemented, bipolar, femoral head endoprosthesis. Cementless fixation [32] is tempting in these relatively young patients, but pre-existing renal osteodystrophy may interfere with bony ingrowth. We have had satisfactory short-term results in two patients.

In more advanced cases, acetabular changes proscribe hemiarthroplasty. The standard total hip arthroplasty with cement provides excellent pain relief and function [5,12-14,19,29,33]. Bradford and coworkers [34] obtained an average Harris hip score of 97 of a possible 100 points in 51 patients. Cementless porous ingrowth fixation can be considered in the young patient. There are several reports of an increased incidence of subluxation and dislocation in these

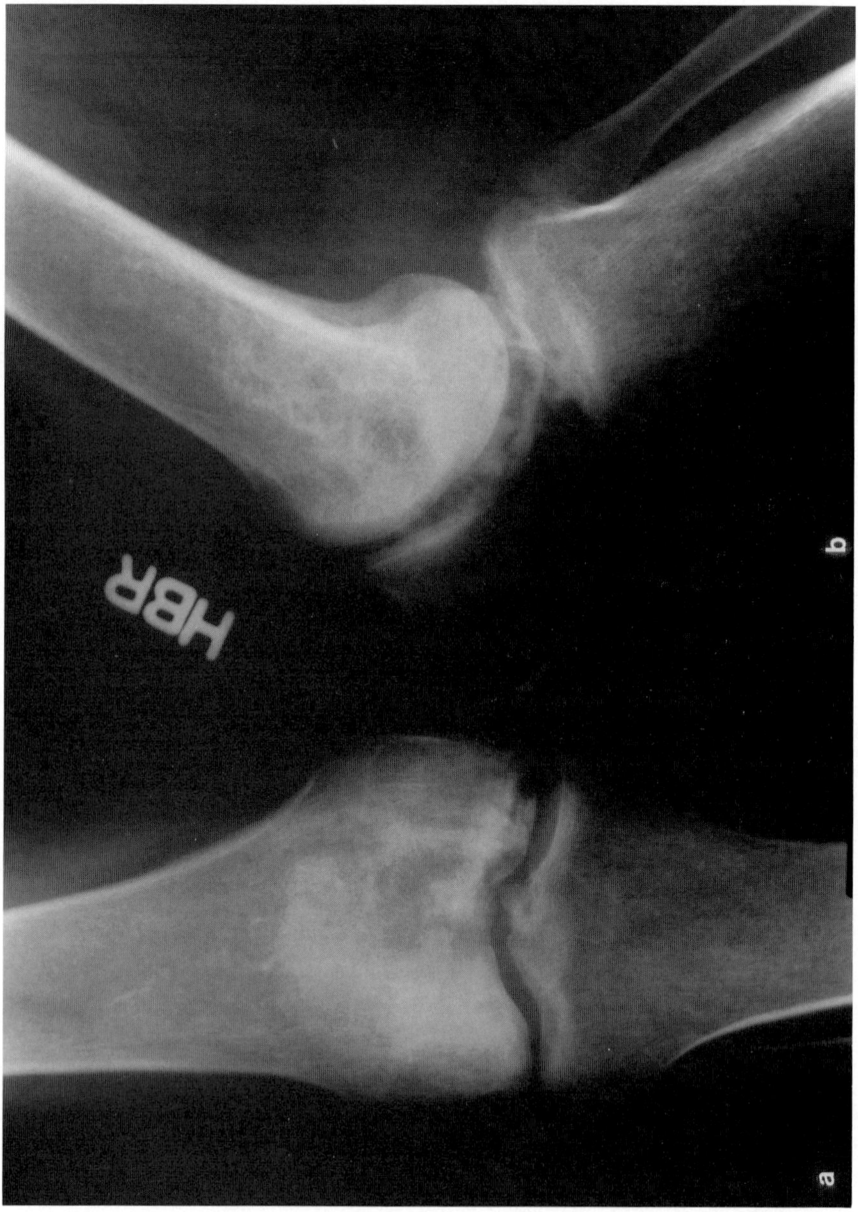

Figure 3 (a) Anteroposterior radiograph of avascular necrosis of medial femoral condyle. (b) Lateral view. Note the similarity to an exaggerated osteochondritis dissecans.

posttransplant patients. Kyd [13] reported a 30% subluxation rate; Bradford et al. [34] noted a 16.2% dislocation rate. This rate is sixfold or more greater than the dislocation rate in the usual total hip arthroplasty. Bradford et al. [34] believe the tissues are more lax in the transplant patient and suggested capsular retention and repair. He states that the posterolateral approach should be avoided in favor of the anterolateral, since more dislocations occur with the posterolateral even in the nontransplant patient.

Avascular necrosis involving the femoral condyles at the knee can usually be managed nonoperatively with rest and anti-inflammatory medication. Our attempts at fixing the separated subchondral bone and articular cartilage to the femoral condyles have failed, because of both the extensive underlying area of necrotic bone and the late extension of the necrosis to previously uninvolved bone. Because of this late extension, medial or lateral hemiarthroplasty may also fail. Total knee arthroplasty is the most reliable procedure in those knees that do require operation.

Osteonecrosis of the humeral head is usually well tolerated. The glenoid is not often involved. Those patients who are symptomatic may benefit from humeral head replacement.

II. STRESS FRACTURES AND NEUROTROPHIC JOINTS

Stress fractures are common and troublesome during the first 4 years after transplantation. Thompson et al. [35] found increasing frequency during the first 2 years, peaking at 4 years and then declining. Of all stress fractures, 69% present in the axial skeleton [33]. Pubic rami fractures are the most common [36,37]. Microfractures of vertebral end plates occur, producing symptomatic radiographic changes [38]. Stress fractures occur most frequently in the diabetic posttransplantation patient. It is also in the diabetic patient that the stress fracture may go on to produce a neurotrophic joint with joint destruction (Fig. 4) [35].

A. Etiology

The chance of sustaining a stress fracture is strongly correlated with bone quality at the time of transplantation [25,36,39]. Renal osteodystrophy continues for at least 1 year following transplantation, and should it persist longer, the frequency of fracture increases. Elmstedt [37] correlated stress fracture in the early posttransplant period with low steroid doses, noting that higher doses protected the patient from the osteoclastic effects of secondary hyperparathyroidism.

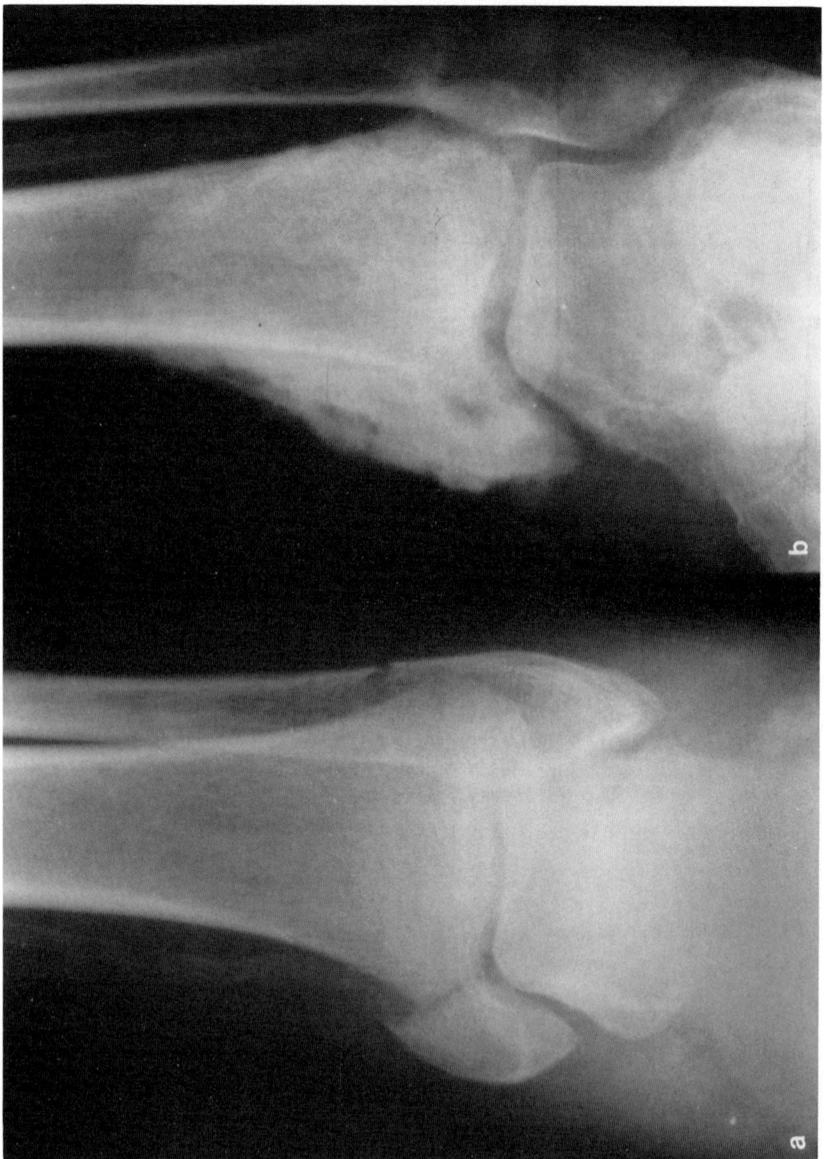

Figure 4 (a) Spontaneous fractures of the medial and lateral malleoli 4 years posttransplantation in a diabetic patient. (b) Final healing with a painless, neurotrophic joint.

B. Treatment

Most of these fractures do not present serious problems. Elmstedt and Svahn [33] reported no pseudarthroses or delayed unions. They did not find avascular necrosis after femoral neck fracture. Our experience with internal fixation of these femoral neck fractures has been poor, with both failure of union and bending of fixative devices (Fig. 5). Thornhill and Creasman (American Academy of Orthopaedic Surgeons, Las Vegas, Nevada, January 24, 1985) reported loss of reduction or nonunion in 11 spontaneously occurring femoral neck fractures treated with internal fixation devices. We suggest femoral head replacement as the initial treatment for these fractures. If internal fixation is elected, close follow-up with consideration of prompt femoral head replacement is indicated should there be delayed union or early loss of fixation. Most other stress fractures will heal with time and immobilization. Standard treatment techniques suffice. A patient presenting with a painful, or even painless, swollen foot with negative radiographs should be treated non-weight bearing or with a walking cast for 2 weeks, at which time repeat films may reveal a stress fracture. A bone scan will demonstrate these fractures within 2-3 days of their occurrence if prompt diagnosis is required.

III. INFECTION

A. Pyogenic Infection

Sepsis is the leading cause of death in renal transplant recipients. The combination of immunosuppressive agents and steroids plays a significant role. Our experience and that of Nicholls et al. [40] indicate that osteomyelitis is extremely unusual. Septic arthritis, however, occurs with some frequency. In addition to the pyogenic infections, fungi, mycobacteria, and viruses can be the infecting agents. Culture media should be selected accordingly. Negative routine cultures do not rule out infection. Synovial fluid analysis can be helpful if attention is directed to cell count, differential white cell analysis, and glucose concentration. A pre-existing joint abnormality produces fertile ground for secondary infection. The previously symptomatic joint that shows some increased swelling and pain may be harboring secondary infection. The signs and symptoms may not be as intense as we are accustomed to seeing in the usual infected joint. A similar phenomenon is seen in the steroid-dependent rheumatoid patient.

B. Tuberculous Infection

Ascher et al. [41] reported three cases of monarticular tuberculosis in 835 transplant patients. Skin tests were not helpful in the face of immunosuppression. He

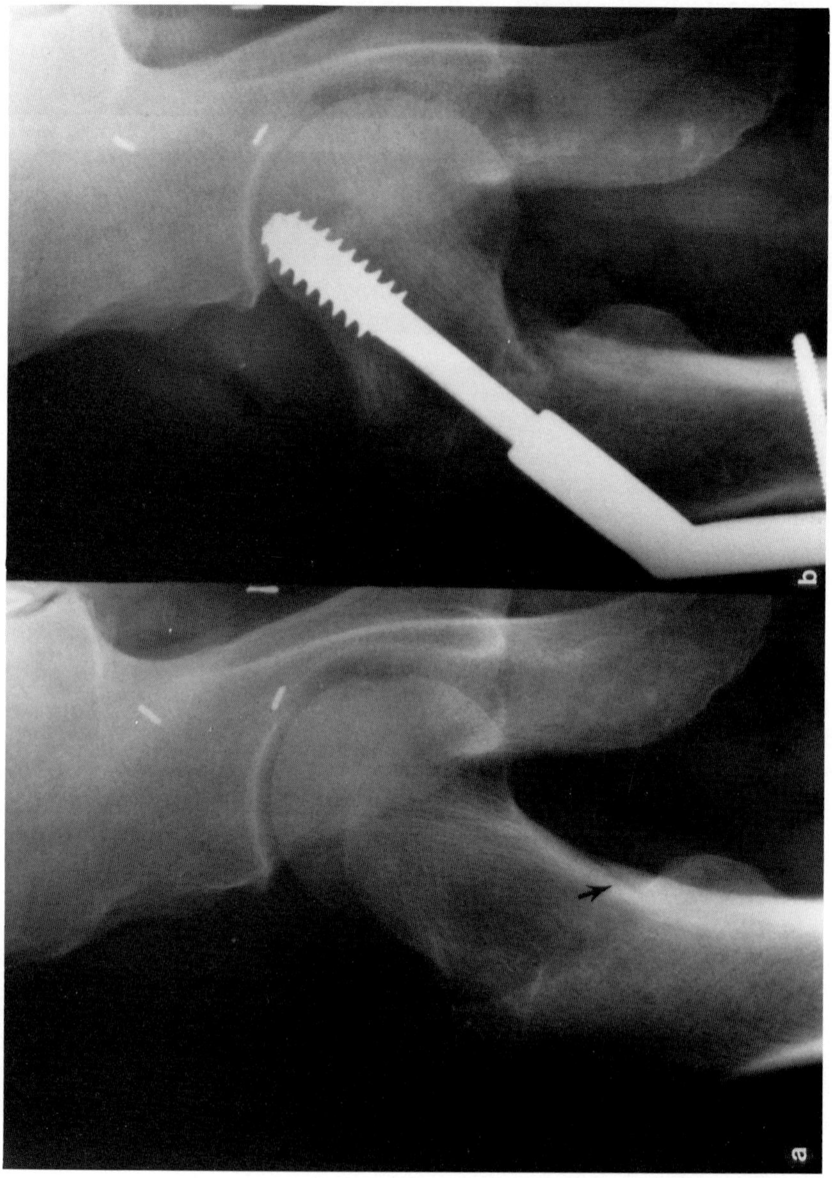

Figure 5 (a) Early femoral neck stress fracture. (b) Failure of fixation with a Richards hip screw. There has been collapse at the fracture site.

found isoniazid a useful antibiotic. Rifampin potentiates hepatic degradation of steroids and therefore should be used with caution.

C. Fungal and Viral Infections

Cryptococcosis [42], *Nocardia* [43], and cytomegalovirus [44] have been reported. *Candida* [45] infection of the hip joint has been successfully treated with 5-flurocytosine and joint resection.

IV. ARTHRALGIA AND EFFUSION

Joint effusions have been common in our postoperative renal transplantation patients. Their condition has persisted for a few months. Complete synovial fluid analysis with culture has revealed a noninflammatory type of fluid. This fluid is normal in all respects, other than the increased quantity. MacFarlane et al. [46] studied 37 patients between 9 days and 3 months posttransplantation. Of these, 11 had joint effusions, of which 2 were painful. Normal joint fluids were found and symptoms persisted from 1 day to 9 months. Bone scans, biopsy specimens, and electron microscopy were normal. They believed that the fluid was a transudate similar to the effusion fluid seen in congestive heart failure and nephrosis and that high-dose steroid therapy might be the cause. Friedman et al. [44] reported a 30% incidence of these effusions in 27 consecutive patients.

Transplant patients can suffer acute arthralgia secondary to steroid withdrawal. Symptoms are usually self-limited. Both Friedman and MacFarlane reported a 16% rate of these painful joints. Joint aspiration for synovial analysis and culture is indicated. Infection must be ruled out. Treatment is rest, mild analgesics, and time, since the condition is self-limited.

V. MALIGNANCY

Immunosuppressive management in the posttransplantation patient increases the risk of malignancy, particularly of bone marrow neoplasms. Various studies indicate a 30-fold increase in malignant lymphoma, especially non-Hodgkin's lymphoma [47,48]. Reiche [49] has published an extensive review of this subject.

REFERENCES

1. Pietrograndi, V., and Mastromarino, R.: Osteopatia da prolungato trattamento cortisonico. Orthop. Traumat. Appar. Mot. 25:791-810, 1957.
2. Starzl, T. E., Marchioro, T. L., Porter, K. A., Moore, C. A., Rifkind, D., and

Waddell, W. R.: Renal homotransplantation: Late function and complications. Ann. Intern. Med. 61:470-497, 1964.
3. Glimcher, M. J., and Kenzora, J.: The biology of osteonecrosis of the human femoral head and its clinical implication. II. Clin. Orthop. 139:283-312, 1979.
4. Andresen, J., and Nielsen, H. E.: Osteonecrosis in renal transplant recipients. Early radiological detection and course. Acta Orthop. Scand. 52:475-479, 1981.
5. Gottlieb, M. N., Stephens, M. K., Lowrie, E. G., Griffiths, H. J., Kenzora, J., Strom, T. B., Lazarus, J. M., Tilney, N. L., and Merill, J. P.: A longitudinal study of bone disease after successful renal transplantation. Nephron 22: 239-248, 1978.
6. Feletti, C., DiFelice, A., Scolari, M. P., and Bonomini, V.: Glucocorticoids and avascular bone necrosis in renal transplantation. Adv. Exp. Med. Biol. 171:361-368, 1984.
7. Slatopolsky, E., and Martin, K.: Glucocorticoids and renal transplant osteonecrosis. Adv. Med. Biol. 171:353-359, 1984.
8. Raisz, L. G., Trummez, C. L., and Wener, J. A.: Effect of glucocorticoids on bone resorption in tissue culture. Endocrinology 90:961-967, 1972.
9. Teitelbaum, S. L., Malone, J. D., and Kahn, A. J.: Glucocorticoid enhancement of bone resorption by rat peritoneal macrophages in vitro. Endocrinology 108:795-799, 1981.
10. Reiss, E., and Canterbury, J. M.: Genesis of hyperparathyroidism. Am. J. Med. 50:679-685, 1971.
11. Manolagas, S. C., and Anderson, D. C.: Glucocorticoids regulate the concentration of 1,25-dihydroxycholecalciferal receptors in bone. Nature 277:314-315, 1979.
12. Hulbert, J., Brockis, J. G., Gilmour, W. N., Golinger, D., House, A. K., and Van Merwyk, A.: Orthopaedic problem of renal transplantation. Aust. N. Z. J. Surg. 49:76-80, 1979.
13. Kyd, R. K.: Bone and joint complications of maintenance haemodialysis and renal transplantation. N.Z. Med. J. 89:4-7, 1979.
14. Susan, L. P., Braun, W. E., Banowsky, L. H., Straffon, R. A., and Bergfeld, V. A.: Avascular necrosis following renal transplantation. Experience with 449 allograft with and without high-dose steroid therapy. Urology 11:225-229, 1978.
15. McGeown, m. G., Douglas, J. F., Brown, W. A., Donaldson, R. A., et al.: Advantages of low-dose steroid from the day after renal transplantation. Transplantation 29:287-289, 1980.
16. Elmstedt, E.: Incidence of skeletal complications in renal graft recipients. Acta Orthop. Scand. 53:853-856, 1982.
17. Dumler, F., Levin, N. W., Szego, G., Vulpetti, A. T., and Preuss, L. E.: Advantage of long-term alternate day steroid therapy in renal transplantation: A controlled study. Proc. Dial. Transplant. Forum 10:215-219, 1980.
18. Cruess, R. L., Blennerhassett, J., MacDonald, F. R., et al.: Aseptic necrosis following renal transplantation. J. Bone Joint Surg. 50A:1577-1589, 1968.

19. Uittenbogaart, C. H., Isaacson, A. S., Stanley, P., et al.: Aseptic necrosis after renal transplantation in children. Am. J. Dis. Child, 132:765-767, 1978.
20. Memmos, D. E., Williams, G. B., Eastwood, J. B., et al.: The role of parathyroidectomy in the management of hyperparathyroidism in patients on maintenance haemodialysis and after renal transplantation. Nephron 30:143-148, 1982.
21. Elmstedt, E.: Avascular bone necrosis in the renal transplant patient. A discriminant analysis of 144 cases. Clin. Orthop. 158:149-157, 1981.
22. Nielsen, H. E., Christensen, N. S., Melsen, F., and Torring, S.: Bone disease, hypophosphatemia and hyperparathyroidism after renal transplantation. Adv. Exp. Med. Biol. 81:603-610, 1977.
23. Ruderman, R. J., Poehling, G. G., Gray, R., et al.: Orthopaedic complications of renal transplantation in children. Transplant. Proc. XI(1):104-106, 1979.
24. Melsen, F., and Nielsen, H. E.: Osteonecrosis following renal allotransplantation. A quantative histological study of iliac bone. Acta Pathol. Microbiol. Scand. [A] 85:99-104, 1977.
25. Andresen, J., and Nielsen, H. E.: Osteonecrosis and spontaneous fractures following renal transplantation. Acta Orthop. Scand. 52:397-404, 1981.
26. Hely, D., Fennell, R. S., III, Petty, W., et al.: Osteonecrosis of the femoral head and condyle in the post transplantation courses of children and adolescents. Int. J. Pediatr. Nephrol. 3:297-303, 1982.
27. Al-Kotoubi, M.: Avascular necrosis of metacarpal head following renal transplantation. Br. J. Radiol. 55:79-80, 1982.
28. Ficat, R. P., and Arlet, J.: *Ischemia and Necrosis of Bone,* Baltimore/London: Williams & Wilkins, 1980.
29. Stern, P. J., and Watts, H. G.: Osteonecrosis in renal transplantation in children. J. Bone Joint Surg. 61A:851-856, 1979.
30. Madsen, S., Olgaard, K., Heerfordt, J., Brix, E., and Vistisen, L.: Scintigraphic skeletal changes in dialysis and kidney transplanted patients. Adv. Exp. Med. Biol. 81:611-619, 1977.
31. McBeath, A. A., and Oeljen, C. G.: Phemister bone graft for osteonecrosis post-renal transplant. Clin. Orthop. 123:164-168, 1977.
32. Maguire, W. B., Muscio, P., and Dodd, P. A.: The results of joint replacement surgery in renal transplant patients. Aust. N.Z. J. Surg. 51:534-537, 1981.
33. Elmstedt, E., and Svahn, T.: Skeletal complications following renal transplantation. Acta Orthop. Scand. 52:279-286, 1981.
34. Bradford, D. S., Szalapski, E. W., Jr., Sutherland, D. E. R., Simmons, R. L., and Najarian, J. S.: Osteonecrosis in the transplant recipient. Surg. Gynecol. Obstet. 159:321-334, 1984.
35. Thompson, R. C., Havel, P., and Goetz, F.: Presumed neurotrophic skeletal disease in diabetic kidney transplant recipients. JAMA 249:1317-1319, 1983.
36. Levine, E., Erken, E. H., Price, H. I., et al.: Osteonecrosis following renal transplantation. AJR 128:985-991, 1977.
37. Elmstedt, E.: Skeletal complications in the renal transplant recipient. A clinical study. Acta Orthop. Scand. (Suppl. 190), 52, 1981.

38. Ansell, G.: Complications of adrenocortical therapy, a radiological survey. J. Fac. Radiol. 9:113-126, 1958.
39. Aird, E. G. A., and Pierides, A. M.: Photon absorptiometry of bone after successful renal transplantation. Br. J. Radiol. 50:350-356, 1977.
40. Nicholls, A., Edward, N., and Catto, G. R. D.: Staphylococcal septicoemia, endocarditis; and osteomyelitis in dialysis and renal transplant patients. Postgrad. Med. J. 56:642-648, 1980.
41. Ascher, N. L., Simmons, R. L., Marker, S., et al.: Tuberculous joint disease in transplant patients. Am. J. Surg. 135:853-856, 1978.
42. Leff, R. D., Smith, E. J., Aldo-Benson, M. A., et al.: Cryptococcal arthritis after renal transplantation. South. Med. J. 74:1290, 1981.
43. Rao, K. V., O'Brien, T. J., and Anderson, R. C.: Septic arthritis due to *Nocardia asteroides* after successful kidney transplantation. Arthritis Rheum. 24:99-101, 1981.
44. Friedman, H. M., Pincus, T., Gibilisco, P., et al.: Acute monoarticular arthritis caused by herpes simplex virus and cytomegalovirus. Am. J. Med. 69:241-247, 1980.
45. Specht, E. E.: *Candida* pyarthrosis of the hip and renal hemotransplantation. Clin. Orthop. 126:176-177, 1977.
46. MacFarlane, J. D., Filo, R. S., and Brandt, K. D.: Joint effusions after kidney transplantation. Arthritis Rheum. 22:164-169, 1979.
47. Hoover, R., and Fraumen, J. R., Jr.: Risk of cancer in renal transplant recipients. Lancet 2:55-57, 1973.
48. Barenfanger, J., Mazur, J. M., Mody, N., et al.: Malignant fibrous histiocytoma of bone in a renal transplant patient. J. Bone Joint Surg. 62A:297-300, 1980.
49. Rieche, K.: Carcinogenicity of antineoplastic agents in man. Cancer Treat. Rev. 11:39-67, 1984.

11
Neurological and Psychiatric Complications

JOHN GILROY
Wayne State University, Detroit, Michigan

The impact of chronic organ failure and the effect of organ transplantation on the individual is that of prolonged stress that has few parallels in medical experience. The process is one of ill health of months' or years' duration superseded by an improvement in well-being accompanied by new stresses and fears. Despite this, many patients survive with relatively few emotional scars and are able to live productive and happy lives—a tribute to the resilience of the human spirit as much as to the skill and sophistication of modern medicine and surgery.

The success of organ transplantation has been followed by the development of new centers for these procedures with the disquieting thought that this mode of surgery may be regarded by many as an innovation that can be incorporated into the activities of any forward-looking surgical department. Such a notion should be viewed with caution, since the best results are only obtained when there is input from psychologists, psychiatrists, social workers, and neurologists in addition to the medical and surgical members of the transplantation unit. This approach allows identification of medical, surgical, ethical, psychological, social, and economic problems, which are an inevitable pressure on the organ recipient, and permits the institution of appropriate treatment without delay.

Problems related to organ transplantation are not confined to the patient. The family is inevitably involved in the process, and the emotional input may have a ripple effect on those close to the patient, who may in turn develop psychoneurotic reactions that require treatment. Consequently, the family must be involved in the process of caring for the patient with the object of producing maximum benefit for all.

The role of the psychiatrist and psychologist may be crucial in many situations following organ transplantation and should be recognized as an integral part of the overall care of the patient.

I. THE PRETRANSPLANTATION STAGE: COPING WITH CHRONIC ILLNESS

Uncomplicated organ failure, that is, chronic congestive heart failure, renal failure with uremia, or aplastic anemia, presents a series of organic and emotional problems. Organic problems, such as anoxia or uremic encephalopathy, and uremic peripheral neuropathy will be discussed later in this chapter. The psychiatric problems are essentially those of any chronic illness plus the problems unique to the failure of a specific organ.

The victim of organ failure feels ill and has lowered energy reserves. He or she has a progressively decreasing ability to cope with everyday tasks and an increasing in dependence on the family for support. Consequently, apprehension about the outcome of the illness, fear of dying, and anger at progressive failure to function independently often lead to depression, chronic anxiety, and hypochrondriasis. Adjustments to chronic organ failure may resemble the emotional stages described by Elizabeth Kubler-Ross in *Death and Dying*—denial, anger, bargaining, depression, and acceptance [15]. The ability to progress through these stages may well depend upon the ability of the transplant team to identify and address the patient's psychological needs.

Additional factors, such as the need for regular hemodialysis, plays a major role in patients with chronic renal failure. The effect of long-term hemodialysis, which has been termed "dialysis stress," is a significant factor in most patients who are awaiting kidney transplantation. These individuals must adjust to dependency on the dialysis machine and accept the need for close physical proximity to the apparatus. Additional problems, such as dietary restrictions, fluid limitations, compliance with a medication schedule, and the continuing patency of access sites, add to the struggle as patients attempt to cope with a complex program of treatment [9].

It is not surprising that the dialysis program dominates the patient's life and that of the family. The latter are subject to their own feelings of anxiety and guilt; their mode of living is inevitably changed to accommodate the demands of chronic illness and regular dialysis. The economic impact is often a concern; the breadwinner may be too fatigued to work, or there may be added expense to the family because of cost of medical care. Consequently, the availability of a donated organ and transplantation surgery may be regarded as a turning point in a slowly deteriorating situation, and the family and patient develop high expectations, such that they may not be prepared for the many new stresses that arise in the postsurgical period [16].

II. THE POSTTRANSPLANTATION STAGE

The immediate period after organ transplantation is spent in an intensive care unit. This is a high-anxiety setting for most patients, even though there is a one nurse to one patient relationship at this stage. It is not unusual for the patient to identify positively with one nurse and to become anxious and demanding at his or her absence during the remaining two shifts of the 24-hr period. The renal transplant recipient is alert postoperatively and frequently experiences a feeling of euphoria as the new organ begins to produce urine. Consequently, delirium and psychotic reactions are unusual in kidney recipients [2] but frequently affect the early postoperative course following cardiac transplantation. Nevertheless, as the donated organ begins to function, there is a feeling of improved health that contributes to both physical and mental well-being. Indeed, to the renal patient who is now free from the debilitating effect of chronic uremia, the constraints of chronic dialysis, and the trauma of bilateral nephrectomies, the transplantation may well promise a return to "normal life."

However, there are emotional restraints following organ transplantation, the first being the fear of organ rejection [4]. To the heart recipient, this is usually equated with death, although successful second heart transplantations have been performed in some cases. The renal patient, on the other hand, faces the prospect of return to chronic dialysis with the concern for shunt care and the burden of dietary restriction once again.

Anxiety over the fate of the graft may be so compelling in some cases that it becomes the prime concern in the patient's existence—the one day at a time syndrome, in which there are limited goals and a poor sense of the continuity of life. In other cases, the recipient develops a feeling of guilt, having received a kidney at someone else's expense.

Given the chronic dependency on dialysis before organ transplantation, it is not unusual to see some reluctance to abandon the dependency role of the sick person after organ transplantation. This may take the form of undue concern about re-entering society or resistance to suggestion that the patient should consider development of plans for gainful employment.

The cushingoid "moon face" resulting from the chronic use of corticosteroids is a cause of depression and withdrawal by some patients, particularly adolescents and young women who naturally believe that the appearance hinders social relations available prior to organ transplantation. This is usually compensated by the improvement in well-being probably accentuated by the use of corticosteroids, and almost all patients prefer existence with a transplant to the life of chronic dialysis. This is borne out by the fact that a high proportion of patients with a successful kidney transplant return to employment within 6 months after surgery, many to full employment, which they maintain despite the burden of frequent medical checks and the side effects of medication.

A. Sexual Function

A significant number of both men and women develop sexual dysfunction in the presence of chronic organ failure [17]. Although transplantation improves function in some cases, impotence remains a major problem in men after kidney transplantation.

Common causes of sexual dysfunction are as follows:

1. Reduction of libido in an individual with a chronic disease.
2. Reduction of libido because of concomitant emotional problems, particularly depression.
3. Impotence associated with the use of antihypertensive drugs, tricyclic antidepressants, or benzodiazepines.
4. Women who receive a kidney transplant from a male donor feel less feminine.
5. Men who receive a kidney from a female donor feel less masculine.
6. Impotence may be due to reduced blood flow through the hypogastric arteries to the internal pudendal arteries supplying the corpora cavernosa in the male. This results from an end-to-end anastomosis between the allograft artery and the recipient's hypogastric artery and is likely to occur after a second allograft. There is, in fact, a cessation of flow through both hypogastric arteries under these circumstances. This means that the second allograft should be performed with an end-to-end anastomosis between the common or external iliac arteries and the allograft artery, sparing the remaining hypogastric artery.
7. The presence of impotence secondary to an associated disease, such as diabetes mellitus.

Male patients who do well after organ transplantation but who continue to complain of impotence may benefit from implantation of a penile prosthesis.

B. Psychological Assessment

The impact of organ failure, the chronic illness, pretransplantation therapy, and the effect of transplantation all effect the emotional life of the patient. In addition, many patients develop organic changes because of chronic organ failure. It is important to document both emotional and organic factors by psychological testing before and after transplantation, since clinical assessment is often inaccurate and follow-up treatment may be modified in response to the psychological report. Once psychological testing has been scheduled, initial reaction by the patient is one of suspicion, fear, anxiety, and anger [8]. There is resistance to the idea that either emotional or organic deterioration may be present, which can be documented with some degree of accuracy by psychological testing. The patient's physician and the psychologist should be aware of this reaction and help the patient adopt a realistic approach to testing. This requires a positive attitude—it is important to have a record of intellectual functioning, cognitive function, and emotional stability before surgery. This will benefit the patient, and follow-up testing will provide a measure of improvement that is expected to occur after transplantation. The emphasis on the positive that is not unrealistic goes a long way in gaining patient confidence and cooperation during the performance of the psychological test battery.

Personality testing and the emotional profile of the patient identify ego resources and the strength of coping mechanisms, and an accurate assessment of anxiety, depression, hypochondriasis, and hysteria is essential for the planning of appropriate support therapy. Intellectual evaluation, particularly with the WAIS, often demonstrates an overall decline in estimated premorbid levels due to impaired visual motor coordination, a restricted ability to learn new material, impaired attention and retention, poor judgment, and loss of abstraction. Such findings, which indicate an encephalopathy, may well be reversed when the metabolic and/or electrolyte abnormalities are corrected posttransplantation. In any case, the results of psychological testing have implications during convalescence and recovery in understanding the patient's attitude towards his illness, the transplantation process, the family, and future employment. The results also permit a realistic approach to employment—has the patient ego strength and the intelligence to resume a previously held position, or should there be an attempt to retrain him or her in a more modest occupation?

C. Effect on the Living Donor

The motives of the living related donor are usually altruistic rather than a search for kudos. Undue family pressure is unusual, and the family seems to regard the related donor as a hero or a fool. Pressures on the donor to resist donation are usually exerted by the spouse, who perceives donation as a threat to health through loss of an organ and by exposure to the hazards of a major surgical procedure. This may lead to family conflict. On the other hand, a reluctant donor may enlist the aid of a spouse to justify a refusal to donate an organ. Again, this has the potential of increasing family conflict, particularly if members have already assumed that the organ donation will be made. It is clear that the physician should avoid exerting pressure on the potential donor since this may initiate or enhance family dissension.

The donor tends to withdraw emotionally as the operative date approaches, and the loss of part of his body is becoming a reality [1]. This tends to clear rapidly in the postsurgical period, and there is usually a feeling of satisfaction after the related donor has given an organ to a near relative. However, this feeling may give way to anxiety and fear of ill health, particularly when the donor is ignored in the general euphoria following a successful transplantation. In general, the donor feels particularly close to the recipient after transplantation and has an ongoing concern about the viability of the donated organ [12]. In most cases, this is a healthy and enduring relationship for both donor and recipient.

D. Rehabilitation

The success of organ transplantation and subsequent rehabilitation require that the recipient give up some pretransplantation dependency. This is usually accomplished when the fear of rejection diminishes. For the heart recipient, this means less fear of death, and the kidney recipient has less apprehension about rejection and return to dialysis.

There is a marked diminution in physical complaints after kidney transplantation and a decrease in psychiatric complaints, with two-thirds of the transplantation patients free from psychiatric symptoms 1 year after surgery. Transplantation patients enter a more normal family relationship, and resumption of sexual activity is very common. The quality of life improves after successful transplantation, particularly for those who resume full-time employment, and there is an increasing ability to enjoy family life.

Nevertheless, depression is not uncommon in the immediate posttransplantation period, particularly in those patients who had unduly high expectation preoperatively. It may be that close medical supervision, regular blood tests, and long-term use of corticosteroids and immunosuppressive drugs perpetuate the dependent state, and hope for independence seems to be illusionary.

Depression is more likely to occur in those who have had one or more episodes of organ rejection, and suicide attempts are particularly common in the adolescent who lacks hope and fears that he or she has no future [19].

E. Physical Enjoyment of Life

Although depression is common in the posttransplantation period, it is offset in many cases by the feeling of well-being that accompanies a successful operation. The patient does in fact enjoy better health, and with it, a freedom from the constant preoccupation with the problems of a chronic organ failure. It is true that there are new problems, owing to the administration of corticosteroids and immunosuppressive drugs and the fear of organ rejection, but the specter of death from organ failure and the necessity for regular dialysis in patients with chronic renal failure becomes less compelling. Patients find that they have time to enjoy their family, and their initial cautious approach to the future becomes more optimistic with the passage of time. Most patients do well in the posttransplantation period, and at least two-thirds have a good response to rehabilitation [7].

F. Attitude Toward Treatment

Following transplantation, the fear of progressive ill health and dying is replaced by fear of organ rejection. In the case of the renal recipient, this means a return to regular dialysis and resumption of the life lead in the pretransplantation period. Other organ recipients once again face the prospect of dying. This may lead to depression or chronic anxiety in the postsurgical period, which may be partially alleviated by the increased feeling of well-being as the donated organ improves bodily function. This feeling may be enhanced by corticosteroids [13] to the extent that the patient and family develop unduly high expectations in the post-operative period. On the other hand, corticosteroids can lead to psychosis, depression, and even suicide unless the physician is alert to these complications.

Noncompliance with drug therapy in the posttransplantation period has been recorded [3]. This is the result of undue concern over the cushingnoid appearance and is likely to occur in the self-conscious adolescent recipient. Cases of noncompliance have also been recorded in which the individual has used this act as a manipulative measure, which has resulted in organ rejection in some cases.

G. Problems of the Diabetic Patient

The expectations of the diabetic patient who is considered a candidate for transplantation—that is, renal transplantation—differ from those of the nondiabetic patient. The diabetic individual is faced with continuing deterioration because of vascular disease, retinopathy, and neuropathy despite successful transplantation, and awareness of the seriousness of these complications is an added stress. The initial improvement in well-being is common to both diabetic and nondiabetic individuals after renal transplantation, but the diabetic patient must still cope with a progressively debilitating illness. Indeed, many diabetic individuals have already experienced multiple medical problems, such as visual impairment [21], hypertension, congestive heart failure, ischemic lesions of the lower limbs, peripheral neuropathy, and autonomic neuropathy prior to transplantation [18]. Consequently, renal transplantation is not the final barrier the diabetic patient must overcome. Unlike the nondiabetic, the diabetic individual faces a continuing downhill course, even though aware that there is good evidence that diabetic patients with end-stage renal disease have higher survival rates following transplantation than their counterparts receiving hemodialysis.

It is not surprising that the initial well-being experienced by the diabetic patient following renal transplantation is soon followed by depression in some patients and that it is prudent to evaluate all diabetic individuals who have evidence of severe complications of diabetes prior to surgery and to offer supportive psychotherapy to those with psychiatric problems. Use of antidepressants may be beneficial in some cases. Amitriptyline is useful in that it may not only alleviate depression but also abolish the pain and discomfort of diabetic neuropathy. The therapeutic dosage of amitriptyline may be lower than expected because of impairment of excretion, and monitoring of serum levels is advised.

III. NEUROLOGICAL COMPLICATIONS

The association of neurological and systemic disease is widely recognized to constitute a considerable percentage of neurological practice. There is increasing recognition of the neurological complications of organ transplantation because of the longest survival of patients with chronic disease in both the pre- and posttransplantation period and because of the use of corticosteroids and immunosuppressive agents. Consequently, a number of neurological problems may be encountered in transplantation patients, many of which respond to appropriate therapy.

A. Central Nervous System Infections

Infection is common in organ transplant patients with impaired host resistance, but the infectious process often follows a unique course that makes identification and management a difficult process [24].

1. The list of potential microbial invaders is large, including pathogens commonly affecting the normal host as well as agents affecting predominantly the compromised host.
2. Infection with more than one agent, or sequential infection, is not uncommon.
3. Multiple organ systems may be simultaneously involved.
4. The manifestations of infection may be masked because of the host's diminished inflammatory response.
5. Meaningful survival is dependent on rapid diagnosis and initiation of effective therapy.

Central nervous system (CNS) infection is a major problem in the immunosuppressed individual, second in frequency only to infection of the lung as a cause of morbidity and mortality [28]. Central nervous system infection is usually associated with renal transplantation, Hodgkin's disease, non-Hodgkin's lymphoma, chronic lymphatic leukemia, and chronic corticosteroid therapy. Clinical presentation is manifested by fever and headache, but signs of meningitis are infrequent, and in many cases, there is no evidence for CNS infection. There may be some alteration of consciousness in patients with aspergillosis brain abscesses and bacterial meningitis, but cryptococcal infections and *Listeria monocytogenes* infections can exist without obtundation or stupor. Focal neurological signs and seizures are usually indicative of aspergillosis brain abscess or progressive multifocal leukoencephalopathy.

There are two distinct periods of transplantation immunodepression. The first, a period of granulocytopenia, is present during the first 4 weeks after transplantation. This is the period when gram-negative sepsis, viral infections, particularly due to herpes simplex virus (HSV), and fungal infections are the major problem. The second period of impaired immunity is a cell-mediated and humoral immunity deficit, which persists for up to 1 year, when viral infections, particularly cytomegalovirus (CMV), interstitial pneumonia, and protozoan infections are encountered.

The main fungal infection aspergillosis is often an overwhelming systemic infection with terminal CNS involvement. It produces a diffuse necrotizing meningoencephalitis although the infection may be localized occasionally to one lobe of the brain with poorly defined abscess formation.

The onset of symptoms occurs shortly after transplantation, when the patient presents with disorientation and confusion progressing to terminal coma. Computed tomography (CT scan) may show areas of irregular contrast-enhanced lesions. The cerebrospinal fluid (CSF) is normal in about 50% of cases, and the diagnosis is established by needle biopsy. Many cases are not suspected until autopsy examination. Both intravenous and intrathecal amphotericin B are recommended for proven cases [5].

Cryptococcosis (torulosis) is another infection produced by a fungus in immunosuppressed individuals, particularly those on long-term steroid therapy [26]. The infection is systemic, but the main impact is on the central nervous system with the development of chronic meningitis and meningoencephalitis. The symptoms are fever and headache, often of many months' duration; focal neurological signs are rare. The diagnosis is established by CSF examination that shows a high opening pressure, less than 20 monocytes mm^{-3}, a low or normal glucose content, slight to moderate elevation in protein content, the presence of cryptococci on smear, and high titers of cryptococcal antigen in the CSF and serum. Amphotericin B intravenously of several months' duration produces remission in the majority of cases, but relapse is common, and patients often receive repeated courses of the drug in an attempt to control the infection.

Mucormycosis due to infection by fungi of the family Mucoraceae usually occurs in diabetic patients and is also encountered following renal transplantation, again particularly in diabetics or in those who are receiving high doses of corticosteroids. The infection usually begins in the palate or nasal sinuses and spreads through the paranasal sinuses into the orbit and then into the brain [20]. Orbital involvement results in involvement of the optic third, fourth, and sixth nerves; spread to the brain is followed by cavernous sinus thrombosis or thrombosis of one or both internal carotid arteries. The clinical picture is that of a blind proptotic eye draining necrotic pus. There is ptosis, pupillary dilatation, and complete ophthalmoplegia. Involvement of the brain results in obtundation stupor and focal neurological signs. The diagnosis is established by biopsy and the demonstration of Mucoraceae. Treatment consists of amphotericin B in high doses (1.0 mg/kg per day) and surgical excision of infected tissue. Since this is a highly mutilating procedure, early diagnosis is critical.

Herpes simplex viral encephalitis usually presents as a subacute encephalitis without CSF pleocytosis, in contrast to the fulminating encephalitis with predominantly temporal lobe involvement seen in the nonimmunosuppressed individual [18]. The diagnosis depends upon suspicion that the HSV encephalitis may be present in an immunosuppressed individual in the presence of an encephalopathy that cannot be explained by metabolic abnormalities. Treatment with cytosine arabinoside or acyclovir is successful in patients who have not deteriorated to the point of coma.

Systemic cytomegalovirus infections are common in immunosuppressed individuals, and between 70 and 90% of renal transplant recipients who survive for more than 2 weeks after surgery may show virological or immunological evidence of CMV infection [6]. Transplant patients with disseminated CMV infection may occasionally develop encephalitis. The clinical findings are nonspecific, and the cerebrospinal fluid is often normal. When recognized, treatment with cytosine arabinoside may be effective in some cases. Since the diagnosis is difficult, it is quite possible that CMV encephalitis is more common than previously recorded in immunosuppressed individuals.

The protozoa *Toxoplasmosis gondii* has been reported as a cause of encephalitis in immunosuppressed patients after organ transplantation. The infection occurs in patients with a high level of immunosuppression and presents with diffuse muscle pain, myoclonus, seizures, and focal neurological abnormalities. The cerebrospinal fluid may be normal or show a mild to moderate mononuclear pleocytosis with elevated protein and normal glucose levels. The diagnosis is established by the demonstration of a positive Sabin-Feldman dye test or indirect fluorescent antibody titer of 16,000 or higher in the presence of an IgM-IFA titer of 160 or more. Therapy with sulfadiazine and pyrimethamine has been successful in some cases [10].

Listeria monocytogenes meningitis occurs early or late in the immunosuppressive process and is one of the commonest bacterial infections encountered in immunocompromised patients. Most present with fever, headache, and signs of meningeal involvement, and neurological deficits are often absent. Diagnosis is established by lumbar puncture, the CSF showing increased pressure, polymorphonuclear pleocytosis, increased protein, and low glucose content. CSF and blood cultures are often positive for *Listeria.*

Treatment consists of high doses of penicillin G (12-24 million units/day) for 6 weeks or ampicillin (12 g/day) alone or in combination with gentamicin chloramphenicol or oxacillin for 4-6 weeks. A relapse rate of 35% has been reported in patients who are treated for less than 3 weeks [25].

Other bacterial infections can cause meningitis in immunosuppressed individ uals. The organisms encountered include *Hemophilus influenzae, Streptococcus pneumoniae, Pseudomonas aeruginosa, Escherichia coli,* and *Staphylococcus epidermidis.* Infection may be associated with septicemia or local infection of paranasal sinuses. Symptoms include fever, rigors, headache, and obtundation, but signs of meningeal irritation are often absent. The diagnosis is established by lumbar puncture. Treatment consists of administration of high doses of the appropriate antibiotic.

B. Brain Abscess

The occurrence of single or multiple abscesses in the brain and other organs is not uncommon in the immunosuppressed individual who develops septicemia due to infection by bacterial or fungi in the posttransplantation period [22]. Disseminated aspergillosis can produce multiple abscesses in the brain that frequently remain undetected in the presence of overwhelming infection [27]. Epidural or intracerebral abscess formation can occur in individuals who have chronic paranasal sinus infection by bacteria, such as *S. epidermidis* or *P. aeruginosa* [10]. Such cases present with fever, headache, lethargy, and meningism. Examination may reveal papilledema, but focal neurological abnormalities are often mild and late in appearance. The cerebrospinal fluid may show the presence of concomitant meningitis; there may be x-ray evidence of paranasal sinusitis or osteomyelitis. Brain abscess produces a characteristic appearance by CT scanning, with a homogenous zone of decreased density and an oval rim of increased density demonstrated after injection of contrast material. There may be considerable surrounding edema [28].

C. Cerebrovascular Disease

Most immunosuppressed individuals develop some degree of thrombocytopenia in the period following organ transplantation. This is often associated with bleeding at various sites in the body, yet intracerebral and subdural hemorrhage is relatively uncommon. There is an increased incidence of nonbacterial thrombotic endocarditis (NBTE) in organ transplant individuals and a significant increase in cerebral infarction due to embolism [14]. Consequently, a stroke following organ transplantation is likely to be an ischemic infarction in a patient with NBTE. There is a lesser risk of multiple hemorrhagic infarction in immunosuppressed individuals who develop septicemia, acute bacterial endocarditis, and septic embolism.

D. Progressive Multifocal Leukoencephalopathy

Progressive multifocal leukoencephalopathy is a predominantly white matter disease of the central nervous system due to papovaviral infection in patients with suppression of a cell-mediated immune response. The condition can occur in the presence of chronic neoplastic disease or acquired autoimmune deficiency syndrome or in individuals who are immunosuppressed after organ transplantation. The presenting symptoms are usually a progressive impairment of cognition and memory, but some cases present with focal features, such as visual loss, dysphagia, or hemiparesis [10]. The course is one of steady progression and decreasing mentation, visual impairment, cranial nerve palsies, and motor and cerebellar dysfunction. Occasionally the deficits are localized to the brain stem or cerebellum. The outcome is usually fatal due to overwhelming infection, but arrest and survival has been reported. Electroencephalography may show loss of α rhythm with a background θ activity and slowing in the δ range. Computed tomography of the brain shows one or more areas of decreased attenuation in the white matter corresponding to the site of focal δ activity in the EEG. The diagnosis can be established by a brain biopsy of one of the abnormal areas. Electron microscopy demonstrates the presence of intranuclear occlusions compatible with papovavirus and is diagnostic.

There have been some reports of successful treatment of progressive multifocal leukoencephalopathy with cytosine arabinoside hydrochloride.

E. Hypertensive Encephalopathy

Severe elevation of blood pressure in patients with ischemic renal disease may result in encephalopathy. The essential changes consist of intense vasospasm, cerebral edema, and increased intracranial pressure. Patients present with increasing headache, drowsiness, seizures, papilledema, and focal neurological deficits due to microinfarction and petechial hemorrhages.

Hypertensive encephalopathy is a neurological emergency requiring immediate treatment. The blood pressure should be lowered by

1. Diazoxide (Hyperstat), 300 mg IV bolus, or
2. Nitropresside (Nipride), 3.0 mg/kg per minute IV (not more than 200 mg/min IV)

Nitropresside (Nipride) should be prepared by dissolving 50 mg of the drug in 500 mL of 5% dextrose solution. Infusion of 3.0 mg/kg per minute IV should be associated with continuing monitoring of blood pressure, and the flow rate should be adjusted to maintain diastolic pressure at a desired normal level.

F. Anoxic Encephalopathy

Mild occult anoxic encephalopathy is not unusual in patients with congestive heart failure or repeated episodes of hypertensive encephalopathy. The condition is manifested by slowing of response, impaired judgment, lack of insight, and some memory failure. This may be compounded by multiple infarcts, which may occur in hypertensive encephalopathy.

Although it is to be expected this process would be less likely to occur following organ transplantation, patients are particularly susceptible to further damage should there be prolonged hypotensive episodes during the transplantation process. Consequently, any tendency to hypotension or cardiac dysrhythmia with reduced cardiac output should be promptly corrected by the transplantation team as soon as it develops.

It is not uncommon to see a brightening of mentation following organ transplantation, which is probably due to improvement in brain circulation and oxygenation. This means that the anoxic changes suffered during the pretransplantation period were a reversible phenomenon, which is not unusual in such cases.

G. Metabolic Encephalopathy

Metabolic acidosis is not unusual in renal failure, and although usually seen in the pretransplantation period may occur following transplantation and organ rejection. The condition is characterized by increasing drowsiness leading to stupor and coma and Kussmaul breathing. The diagnosis can be established by demonstration of a pH less than 7.3; P_{CO_2} less than 35, and bicarbonate less than 10 mEq/L.

Other encephalopathies may be encountered with hypernatremia due to dehydration or inappropriate use of intravenous fluids. In these cases, patients show alteration of the levels of consciousness associated with tremulousness and convulsions leading to coma. Hyponatremia, on the other hand, is a well-recognized complication of dialysis and is associated with alteration in the levels of consciousness leading to coma. Hypokalemia, a condition that is not usual in patients receiving corticosteroids, is associated with alterations in the level of consciousness, profound weakness, and cardiac dysrhythmias.

The treatment in each case is correction of the cause when possible. Hyponatremia requires water restriction rather than attempting to increase the sodium content by infusion, which may lead to further neuronal damage due to rapid changes in intracellular osmolality.

H. Toxic Encephalopathy

Immediate and delayed neurotoxicity has been reported in patients with aplastic anemia and hematologic malignancies who underwent marrow transplantation after preparation with mechlorethamine [23]. Early signs of toxicity consisted of confusion, disorientation, headache, hallucinations, and seizures. The acute symptoms subside in less than 2 weeks but may be followed by personality changes, confusion, seizures, and dementia some months later. The brain shows neuronal degeneration, increased vascularity, gliosis, and perivascular fibrosis.

The possibility that neurotoxicity from immunosuppression could occur in other types of organ transplantation should be borne in mind.

I. Uremic Encephalopathy

Patients with chronic renal disease often show episodes of confusion associated with apathy, fatigue, and irritability. This may be followed by stupor associated with hallucinations and myoclonic jerks when the patient is aroused. If untreated, the patient may develop convulsions. It should be noted that uremic encephalopathy can occur with only moderate elevation in blood urea nitrogen and creatinine levels and is probably multifactorial in etiology. There is often a gratifying improvement in the patient's condition following renal transplantation.

J. Uremic Neuropathy

Some degree of peripheral neuropathy is not an uncommon complication of chronic renal failure, and in some cases the condition can be disabling. The initial symptoms are those of progressive sensory loss involving the lower extremities more than the upper extremities and extending from the distal regions toward the more proximal areas of the limbs. Many patients experience vague discomfort associated with this neuropathy and have the disturbing complication of "restless legs syndrome," particularly in bed at night. In others, there is frank pain, which can be disabling and lead to depression. In patients receiving dialysis, the symptoms of peripheral neuropathy may fluctuate, showing improvement after the completion of a dialysis session.

Motor involvement is less frequently encountered than sensory changes in uremic neuropathy; however, motor involvement can be severe in some cases who present with bilateral foot drop and even paraparesis.

The onset of uremic neuropathy is an indication for dialysis or renal transplantation. Symptoms of pain and the restless leg syndrome can be controlled with the use of amitriptyline (Elavil), beginning with 25 mg at night and increasing slowly up to 150 mg/day, if necessary. A slow increase in this medication will avoid side effects, such as drowsiness. It should be noted that some patients are extraordinarily susceptible to amitriptyline, presumably due to reduction of excretion of metabolites through damaged kidneys.

IV. ENCEPHALOPATHY

A. Dialysis Encephalopathy

This condition is probably due to rapid changes in water content of neurons following dialysis. In many ways it is similar to water intoxication. Patients complain of headache, nausea, weakness, and agitation, which may continue into drowsiness and convulsions. The symptoms usually appear 3-4 hr after dialysis and may last for several hours. In some cases, a longer period of dialysis produces less rapid changes in the water content of the brain and is sufficient to avoid these symptoms.

B. Dialysis Dementia

This is an unusual complication in patients who are receiving dialysis and can occur either pre- or posttransplantation and presents with a characteristic impairment of speech that resembles a motor dysphasia but is, in fact, an apraxia of speech. This initial symptom is followed by a progressive decline in intellectual functioning, the appearance of myoclonic jerks, which may be focal or generalized, and focal or generalized seuzures. The symptoms occur intermittently at first but gradually become established, and the condition is steadily progressive over the next year to 18 months. The average survival has been reported as 6 months once the symptoms appear.

The cause of dialysis encephalopathy is uncertain at this time, but it has been speculated that it is the result of an accumulation of aluminum in cerebral neurons. The source of the aluminum is in the dialyzate or from the administration of aluminum gels during treatment.

C. Wernicke's Encephalopathy

There is an increased risk of developing Wernicke's encephalopathy following kidney transplantation with the use of corticosteroids and immunosuppressant drugs.

The basic problem is a deficiency of thiamine, and the pathological changes consist of demyelination and loss of neurons in the perivascular regions of the thalamus and hypothalamus and the periaqueductal regions of the midbrain and the floor of the fourth ventricle. In addition, there are similar lesions in the mamillary bodies and the anterior part of the cerebellum, particularly in the vermis.

The initial symptoms are usually those of an ocular disturbance with a combination of gaze palsies and involvement of individual oculomotor nerves. There may be paralysis of gaze in any direction, but it is commoner in horizontal and upward gaze. There is often a combination of gaze palsy with bilateral involvement of the sixth nerve with bilateral lateral rectus palsy. In some cases, there may be complete ophthalmoplegia.

Cerebellar ataxia produces a wide-based gait and bilateral intention tremor of lesser degree.

Most patients show some evidence of an acute dementia, with poor attention span, impaired judgment, impaired insight, poor retention and recall, and marked impairment of recent memory.

Laboratory abnormalities include a mild to moderate elevation of CSF protein, elevation of blood pyruvate level, and marked reduction of erythrocyte transketolase levels. The EEG is often diffusely abnormal.

There is a prompt response to the administration of thiamine, and the patient should be given 50-100 mg intravenously followed by 50 mg intramuscularly every day until able to take an adequate diet with vitamin supplement.

D. Brain Lymphoma

The risk of developing lymphoma after kidney transplantation is about 35 times higher than normal. Almost all tumors are reticulum cell sarcoma, and the excess risk appears within a year of transplantation and remains at the same level for 5 years or more. More than 50% of posttransplantation lymphomas occur in the brain [11].

Symptoms usually encountered include headache, intellectual dulling, drowsiness, and neck stiffness followed by focal signs of cerebral, cerebellar, brainstem, or cranial nerve involvement. Computed tomography of the brain may be positive for a single or multiple areas of density associated with edema. The spinal fluid is abnormal in most cases, with a pleocytosis, elevated protein content, and normal glucose content [20].

REFERENCES

1. Abram, H. S., and Buchanan, D. C.: The gift of life: A review of the psychological aspects of kidney transplantation. Int. J. Psychiatry Med. 7:153-164, 1977.
2. Abram, H. S.: The psychiatrist, the treatment of chronic renal failure, and the prolongation of life. III. Am. J. Psychiatry. 128:84-89, 1972.
3. Armstrong, S. H., and Weiner, M. F.: Noncompliance with post-transplant immunosuppression. Int. J. Psychiatry Med. 11:89-95, 1981.
4. Beard, B. H.: The quality of life before and after renal transplantation. Dis. Nerv. Syst. 32:24-31, 1971.
5. Britt, R. H., Enzmann, D. R., and Remington, J. S.: Intracranial infection in cardiac transplant recipients. Ann. Neurol. 9:107-119, 1981.
6. Dorfman, L. J.: Cytomegalovirus encephalitis in adults. Neurology (NY) 23: 136-144, 1973.
7. George, C. R. P., Tiller, D. J., et al.: Life with a transplanted kidney. Med. J. Aust. 1:461-466, 1970.
8. Greenberg, R. P., Davis, G., and Massey, R.: The psychological evaluation of patients for a kidney transplant and hemodialysis program. Am. J. Psychiatry 130:274-277, 1973.
9. Gulledge, A. D., Buszta, C., and Montague, D. K.: Psychosocial aspects of renal transplantation. Urol. Clin. North Am. 10:327-333, 1983.

10. Hooper, D. C., Pruitt, A. A., and Rubin, R. H.: Central nervous system infection in the chronically immunosuppressed. Medicine (Baltimore) 61:166-188, 1982.
11. Hoover, R., and Fraumeni, J., Jr.: Risk of cancer in renal transplant recipients. Lancet 2:55-57, 1973.
12. Kamstra-Hennen, L., Beebe, J., et al.: Ethical evaluation of related donation: The donor after five years. Transplant. Proc. 12:60-61, 1981.
13. Kaplan De-Nour, A., and Shanan, J.: Quality of life on dialysis in transplanted patients. Nephron 25:117-120, 1980.
14. Kooiker, J. C., Maclean, J. M., and Sumi, S. M.: Cerebral embolism, marantic endocarditis and cancer. Arch. Neurol. 33:260-264, 1976.
15. Kubler-Ross, E.: Death and Dying, New York: Macmillan, 1979.
16. Lefebure, P., Crombez, J. C., and LeBeuf, J.: Psychological dimension and psychopathological potential of acquiring a kidney. Can. Psychiatr. Assoc. J. 18:495-500, 1973.
17. Levy, N. B., and Wynbrandt, G. D.: The quality of life on maintenance hemodialysis. Lancet 1:1328-1330, 1975.
18. Peterson, L. G., and Perl, M.: Diabetic patients and the impact of renal transplantation. Psychomat. 23:173-185, 1982.
19. Poznanski, E. O., Miller, E., et al.: Quality of life for long-term survivors of end-state renal disease. JAMA 239:2343-2347, 1978.
20. Schober, R., and Herman, M. M.: Neuropathology of cardiac transplantation. Lancet 1:962-967, 1973.
21. Simmons, R. G., Kamstra-Hennen, L., and Thompson, C. R.: Psychosocial adjustment five to nine years post transplant. Transplant. Proc. 13:40-43, 1981.
22. Solberg, C. O., Meuwissen, H. J., et al.: Infectious complications in bone marrow transplant patients. Br. Med. J. 1:18-23, 1971.
23. Sullivan, K. M., Storb, R., et al.: Immediate and delayed neurotoxicity after mechlorethamine preparation for bone marrow transplantation. Ann. Intern. Med. 97:182-189, 1982.
24. Turcotte, J. C.: Infection and renal transplantation. Surg. Clin. North Am. 52:1501-1512, 1972.
25. Watson, G. W., Fuller, T. J., et al.: *Listeria* cerebritis—relapse of infection in renal transplant patients. Arch. Intern. Med. 138:83-87, 1978.
26. Wilson, T. S., Fleming W. A., et al.: Cryptococcal meningitis associated with steroid therapy. J. Clin. Pathol. 23:657-663, 1970.
27. Young, R. C., Bennett, J. E., et al.: Aspergillosis. The spectrum of the disease in 98 patients. Medicine (Baltimore) 49:147-173, 1970.
28. Zimmerman, R. A., Bilancuk, L. T., et al.: Evolution of cerebral abscess: Correlation of clinical features with computed tomography. Neurology 27:14-19, 1977.

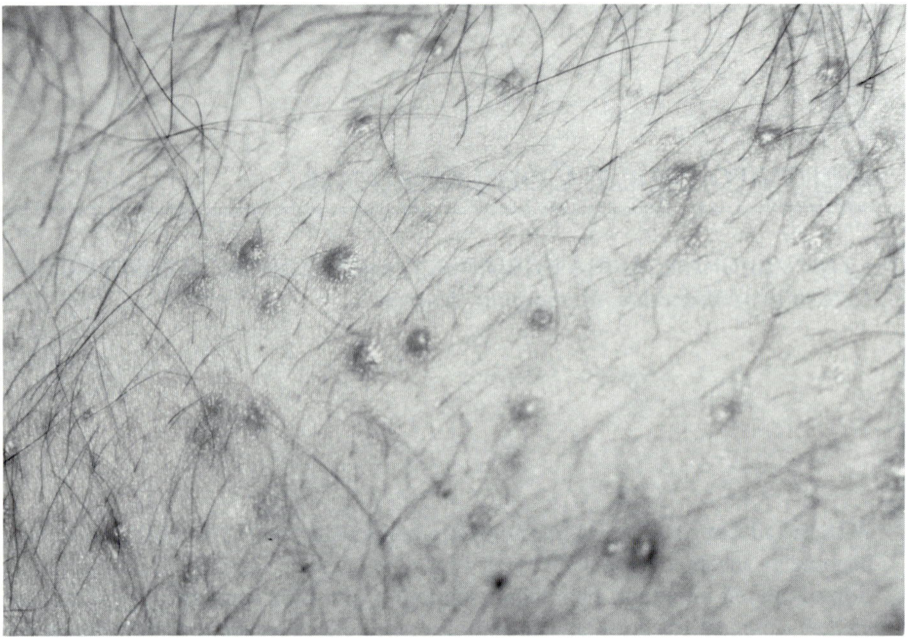

Figure 1 Steroid acne.

diminished scar formation. This atrophic dermis also provides less support to a more fragile cutaneous vasculature, allowing the formation of petechiae and ecchymoses with minimal trauma.

Broad, violaceous striae usually are seen on the abdomen, buttocks, and thighs [7]. As the steroid level is lowered the color fades, but the atrophy tends to remain. This cutaneous lesion is another manifestation of the loss of dermal connective tissue integrity.

Follicular hyperkeratosis is commonly seen with glucocorticoid administration. It is characterized by dilatation of follicles by keratotic plugs. The alteration in the follicular walls probably also plays a role in steroid-induced acne [7]. Steroid acne is manifest by small, closed comedones in a uniform stage of development (Fig. 1). Absent is the open comedo or "blackhead" of regular acne. The distribution is predominantly over the forehead, cheeks, chin, and chest. The time of onset is generally 2-3 weeks after the initiation of high-dose steroids. As the steroid dose is lowered, the acne lesions tend to regress but may persist in up to one-third of the patients [1].

Alteration of fat distribution is another cutaneous complication of corticosteroid therapy. This is clinically seen as increased deposition of fat in the supraclavicular and suprasternal areas, the back of the neck (buffalo hump), the cheeks (moon facies), and the abdomen. The truncal obesity may be accompanied by a decrease in subcutaneous fat of the extremities and a flattening and narrowing of the buttocks. Other cutaneous features seen in patients receiving oral glucocorticoids include alopecia, increased hair growth of the fine vellus type, telangiectasias, and erythema of sun-exposed areas.

Wolfson et al. describes an entity they have termed transplant elbow, which may also be attributed to exogenous steroid administration. "Transplant elbow" is the name given to the phenomenon of recurrent cellulitis in and around the elbow [8]. It is characterized by marked cutaneous atrophy, decreased skin tensile strength, and increased susceptibility to trauma associated with steroid-induced proximal myopathy of the legs. Transplant elbow then results from repetitive trauma when patients push off with their elbows when arising from a sitting position.

II. CANCER AND TRANSPLANTATION

The development of de novo malignant neoplasms is an acknowledged complication of immunosuppression and organ transplantation [1,2,9-17]. The University of Colorado Medical Center and Denver Veterans Administration Hospital series of 678 recipients showed an incidence of 5.9% [13] and an Australian series of 1884 patients a 7% incidence of the development of de novo malignancies [18]. Penn calculated this incidence to be approximately 100 times greater than that in individuals in the general population in the same age range [13,19]. The average time to diagnosis of malignancy from transplantation is 37 months [13], with an increasing incidence of cancer as the transplant interval increases [1,18,20]. The vast majority of these neoplasms are lymphomas and epidermoid carcinomas [13,21].

The most common malignancies are those of the skin. Cancer of the skin and lower lip occurred in 41% of the patients who developed neoplasms in the series by Penn [13], with the overall incidence of cutaneous cancer approximating 3.5% [1].

In the general population, basal cell carcinomas outnumber squamous cell carcinomas; the opposite is true in renal transplant recipients [20,22]. In the transplant population, cutaneous squamous cell carcinoma occurs 36.4 times more frequently than expected, with the overall risk of skin cancer 7.1 times more than expected [21]. The mean interval from transplantation to the time of diagnosis of the first cutaneous carcinoma ranges from 34 to 43.4 months [1,21,22]. Most of the skin carcinomas described have been on sun-exposed areas, such as the face, lower lip, neck, forearms, and hands [1,22,23]. These lesions are seen at a younger age in transplant patients and tend to increase in incidence with time from the date of transplantation [1,20,21]. Squamous cell carcinoma in particular may present with multiple lesions and be more aggressive and prone to recurrence and metastases [1,9,20,21,23].

A full range of premalignant and malignant cutaneous lesions may be seen in the transplant population. These include actinic keratoses, keratoacanthomas, Bowen's disease, and malignant melanoma, as well as squamous and basal cell carcinomas (Fig. 2a-f). Actinic keratoses are the most frequently seen precancerous lesion [2] (Fig. 2a). They tend to be multiple, occur on sun-exposed forearms and hands, and present at a younger age compared with the normal population [2]. In the general population, approximately 20% of actinic keratoses evolve into squamous cell carcinoma [24]. In the immunosuppressed patient, cutaneous actinic keratoses evolve more rapidly into squamous cell carcinoma [2,23].

A keratoacanthoma is defined as a benign epithelial tumor that tends to regress spontaneously (Fig. 2b). In transplant recipients, although this lesion may present with a typical appearance, it may behave atypically, occurring more frequently, persisting longer, and recurring after local excision [23].

Cutaneous malignant melanoma is stated to occur approximately five times more than expected in transplant recipients [9,25] (Fig. 2d). Greene et al. suggest that cutaneous malignant melanomas in renal transplant patients evolve from precursor nevi in the immunosuppressed host who is unable to mount a tumor-specific cellular immune response [25]. Recipients with dysplastic nevi show only a 22-month interval from transplantation to melanoma diagnosis compared with 40 months for all recipients who develop melanoma. This observation suggests that dysplastic nevi should be considered markers for an increased melanoma risk.

Multiple factors probably play a role in the increased risk of cutaneous neoplasms. The observation that most skin cancers arise on sun-exposed skin [22, 23], combined with the observation that the frequency of cutaneous malignancy increases with the transplant interval as well as the extent of sun exposure [22, 26], points to ultraviolet (UV) light as a possible cofactor in skin carcinogenesis [27]. In support of this hypothesis is the observation that although the incidence of skin cancer is increased 4- to 7-fold in areas of low sun exposure, such as the United Kingdom and Minnesota, it is increased almost 21-fold in the high sun-exposure area of Queensland, Australia [10,21,22].

Viruses may also play a role in the development of malignant neoplasms in the immunosuppressed transplant population. Transplant patients are known to have an increased incidence of warts [27]. However, it has not been until recently that human papillomavirus type 5 has been identified in skin cancers of a renal allograft recipient, pointing to a possible role for papillomaviruses in the pathogenesis of skin cancers [28].

A complex interplay of numerous factors is probably responsible for the in-

Figure 2a Actinic keratoses.

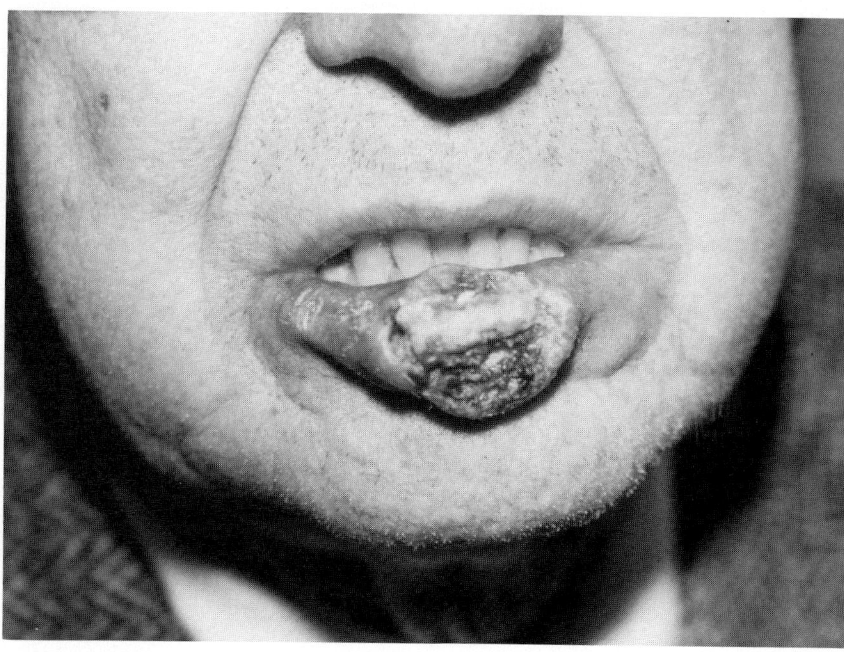

Figure 2b Keratoacanthoma.

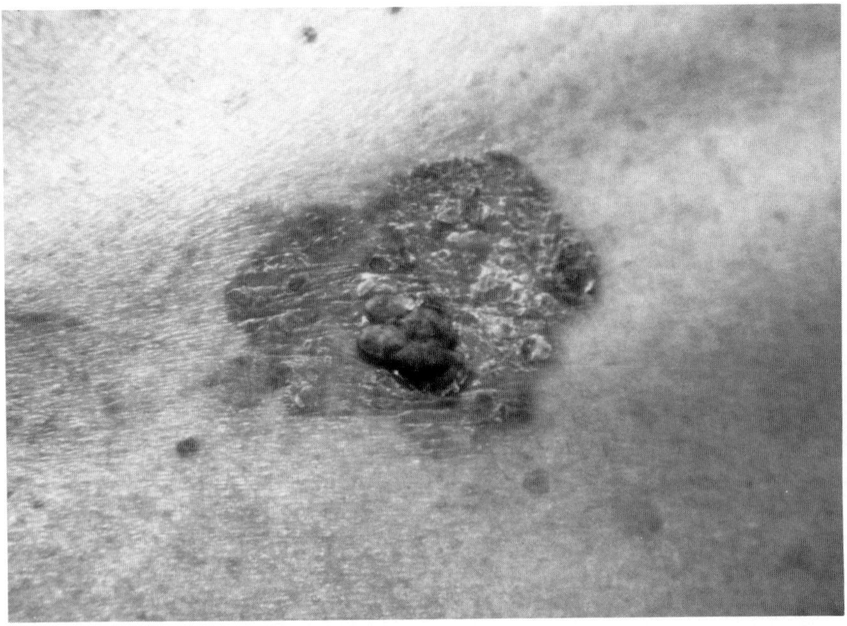

Figure 2c Bowen's disease (squamous cell carcinoma in situ).

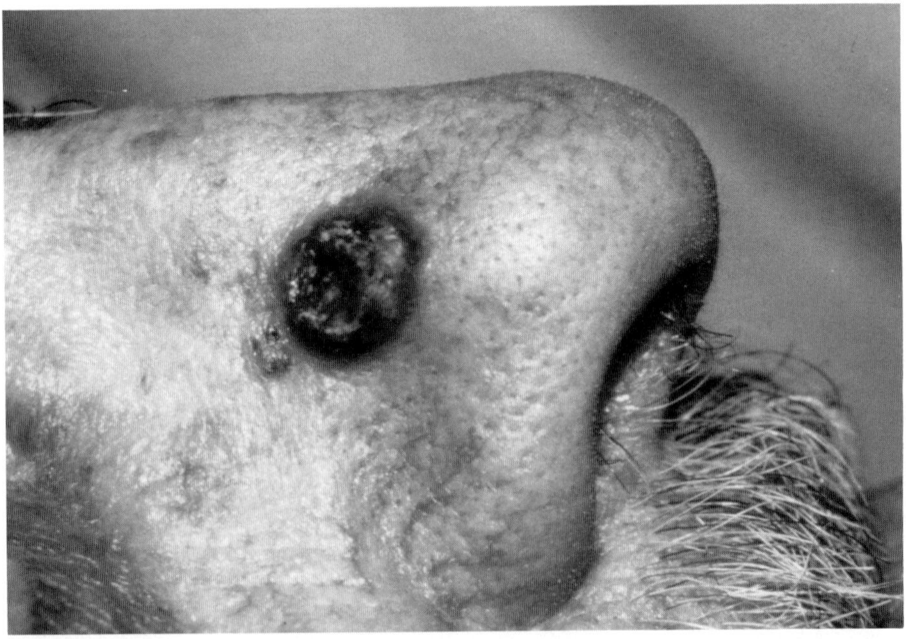

Figure 2d Malignant melanoma.

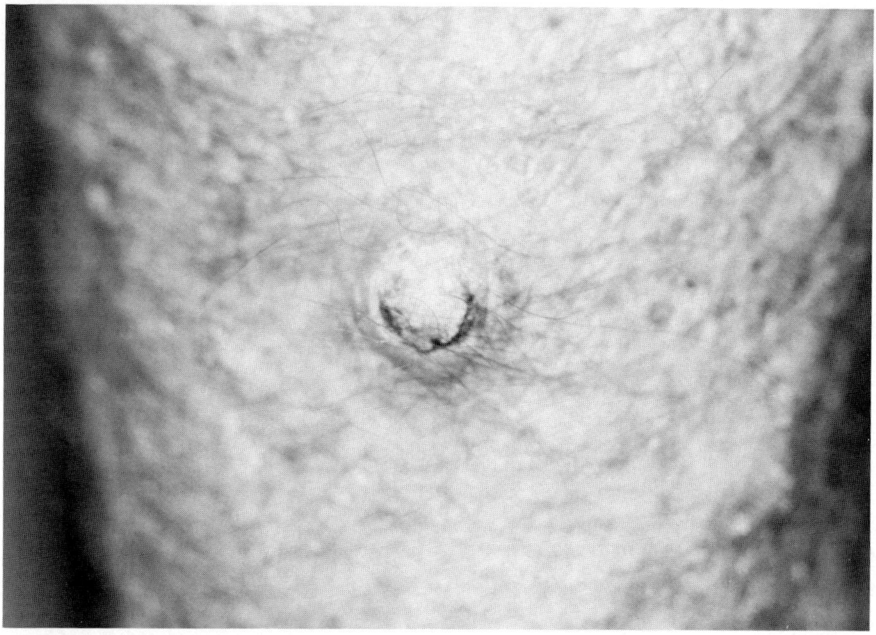

Figure 2e Squamous cell carcinoma.

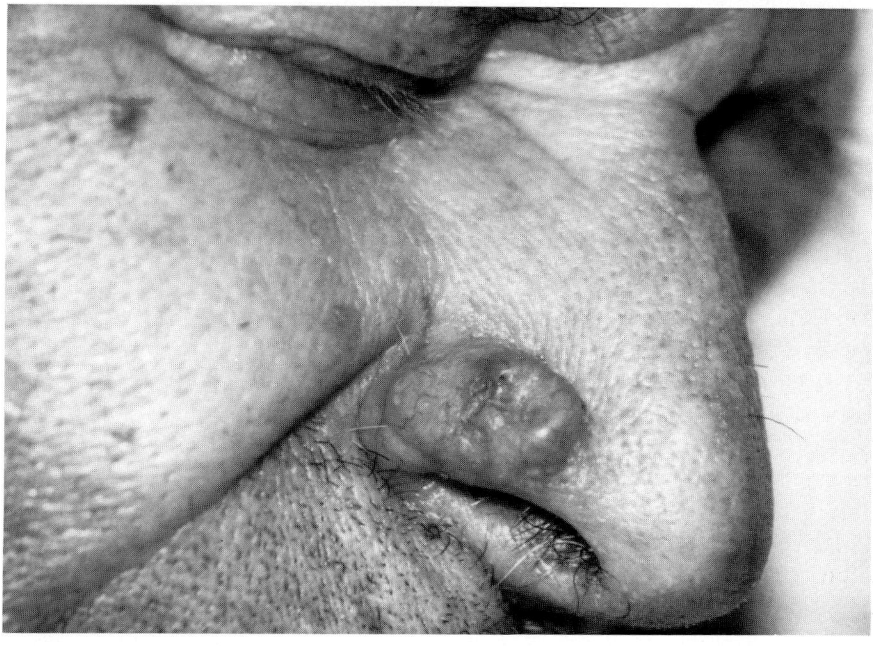

Figure 2f Basel cell carcinoma.

creased development of malignancies in immunocompromised transplant recipients. These factors include (1) the use of immunosuppressive drugs, (2) alteration of immunologic surveillance, (3) potentiation of oncogenic viruses, (4) sustained antigenic stimulation, (5) solar irradiation, (6) chronic uremia, and (7) genetic factors [13,17,20,23]. Interestingly, associated with the occurrence of skin cancers is a decrease in graft rejection [11]. This has been interpreted as follows: the host's depressed immune surveillance system fails to reject the graft and the neoplastic cells such that the renal transplant recipient with the longer graft survival is at greatest risk of cutaneous malignancy [26].

Although skin cancers represent the majority of de novo malignant neoplasms, deaths from skin cancer represent 1-2% of deaths in renal transplant recipients [13, 22]. Despite the fact that cutaneous cancers tend to be multiple, more aggressive. and prone to recurrence, local therapy produces good results [13]. Therefore, the incidence of cutaneous malignancy does not pose a contraindication to the continued clinical use of transplantation [22], nor do most patients with skin cancer necessarily require changes in their immunosuppressive therapy [13]. The exception to this would be the patient with an invasive primary cutaneous malignant melanoma [25]. In this case, sacrifice of the graft may avoid the development of melanoma metastases [25].

The high incidence of skin cancer in transplant patients warrants frequent examination of the skin, biopsy of suspicious lesions, and early treatment of any precancerous or cancerous lesions. Immunosuppressed patients whose nevi meet the criteria for dysplastic nevi may merit an aggressive biopsy policy [25]. All transplant recipients should be counseled to avoid unnecessary sun exposure and to regularly use sun screens.

III. CUTANEOUS MANIFESTATIONS OF INFECTION

The prolonged use of systemic steroids and other immunosuppressive agents in the transplant population alters the host's defense mechanisms, predisposing this population to infectious complications. Several papers have emphasized the frequency of skin infections [1,2,8,29]. The percentage of renal transplant recipients with skin infections has been estimated to be as high as 74-100% [2,29]. The challenge to the dermatologist and transplant surgeon is to determine which of the vast array of potential pathogens is the source of the infection and to appreciate the diversity of the clinical manifestations of cutaneous infections in the posttransplant population.

The incidence of herpes simplex virus (HSV) infection is between 35 and 52% in the renal transplant population [1,30]. The most common clinical presentation is the presence of orofacial lesions [1,2,30]. The lesions tend to be multifocal, hemorrhagic, and persistent [2]. Intraoral lesions may also occur but are less common [1]. Herpetic lesions may be the classic "dewdrops on a rose petal" or may present in an atypical manner, as in the case Haboubi reported; his patient presented with only transcient vesicles on the lingula [31]. Reactivation of varicella zoster virus is also common in transplant recipients. Koranda reported a 13% incidence in 200 patients [1]. These lesions also appear as grouped vesicles on an erythematous base. They usually present in a unilateral dermatomal pattern, are inclined to be hemorrhagic [2], but do not manifest a tendency for dissemination [1,2,8,32].

Viral infections in the first year posttransplantation are almost exclusively due to the herpesviruses [2]. Later, cutaneous viral infections with any one of the types of DNA human papilloma virus or warts are seen [2,8,32]. In the transplant population, the development of warts is most commonly seen 8 months following transplantation [1]. The incidence of infected patients increases with the transplant interval [1,32], with 42% of the patients manifesting warts more than 1 year after transplantation [32] and up to 1% having extensive disease [1]. Clinically, the warts are characterized as multiple in number, more resistant to therapy, and occurring mostly on the hands, but also frequently on the arms, legs, and feet (Fig. 3) [1,2,8,26,32]. Wolfson et al. proposed that the incidence and severity of

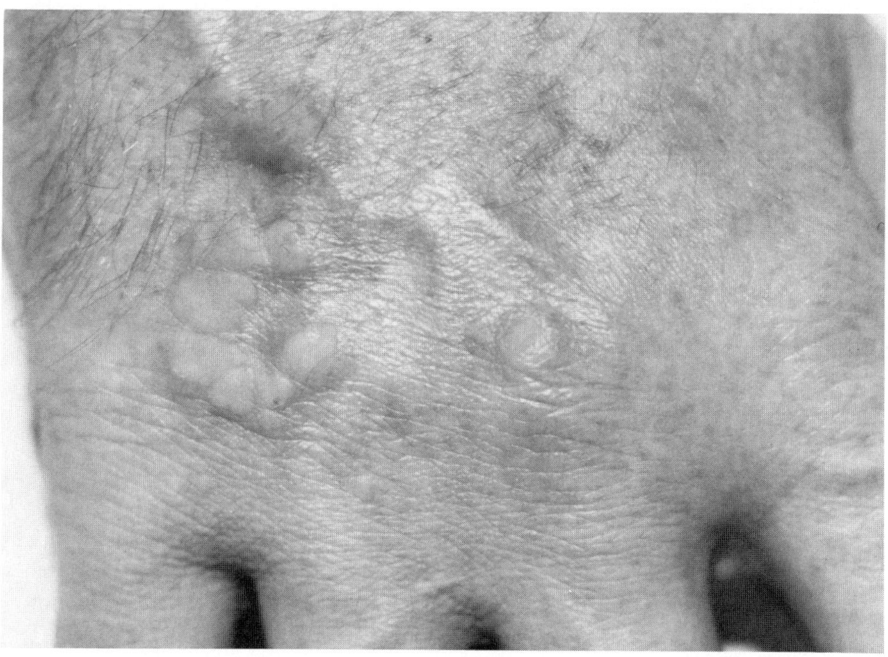

Figure 3 Warts.

papillomavirus-induced skin disease in the transplant population are directly related to immunosuppression [8]. Supporting this hypothesis is the case of one patient whose confluent warts completely resolved with the cessation of steroid therapy [8]. Also of concern to the transplant patient is the potential for malignant transformation in warts, especially those present in sun-exposed areas [26]. DNA human papillomavirus type 5 has been found in both benign warts and skin cancers of a renal allograft recipient [28]. This finding may be coincidental, but it also suggests a role for papillomaviruses in the pathogenesis of skin cancers [28].

Typical types of cutaneous infections, such as cellulitis, secondary to gram-positive organisms, appear to be increased in incidence and severity in the immunocompromised host [8]. With immunosuppression the possibility of unusual infections also has to be considered [8].

Depression of cell-mediated immunity is most important in the development of both typical and atypical mycobacterial infections [33]. In a large survey of renal allograft recipients at the University of Minnesota from 1968 to 1980, the incidence of mycobacterial infections was found to be 0.65% (7 of 1069), with atypical mycobacterial infections accounting for 42.8% of the total [33]. Both these figures exceeded the incidence in the normal population during the same time frame, in whom the expected incidence of *M. tuberculosis* infection was 6.1 per 100,000 and atypical mycobacterial infections were less than 5% of the total [33]. Irrespective of the causative species of *Mycobacterium,* the initial extrapulmonary presentations mimicked acute pyogenic bacterial infections of a joint or the subcutaneous tissue. The high frequency of joint infection and skin involvement, including subcutaneous nodules, abscesses, ulcers, and cellulitis, was at least partially attributed to the increased incidence of atypical myocbacterial infections. Atypical mycobacteria that are reported to infect the renal transplant population include *M. kansasii, M. chelonei, M. haemophilum, M. fortuitum* subspecies *abscessus,* and *M. marinum* [1,8,33-37]. Resistance to conventional therapy is more common in nontuberculous mycobacterial infections [38,39], making it advisable to treat with multidrug regimens for prolonged periods of time in transplant recipients [8,33].

Cutaneous superficial fungal infections also appear to increase in incidence and severity with an increasing interval from transplantation [2]. Tinea versicolor is a common, benign, noninflammatory superficial fungal infection of the skin caused by *Pityrosporon orbiculare* [40,41]. Lesions are characterized by numerous white to fawn-colored to brown scaling macules scattered over the upper trunk that commonly extend to the proximal portions of the extremities and lower abdomen [40,41]. Koranda et al. found an 18% incidence of tinea versicolor in immunosuppressed renal transplant recipients compared with an incidence of 0.5% in normal persons in a temperate climate [1,42]. The distribution of tinea versicolor in the transplant population typically includes the neck, trunk shoulders, and arms [1,2], with a tendency for extensive involve-

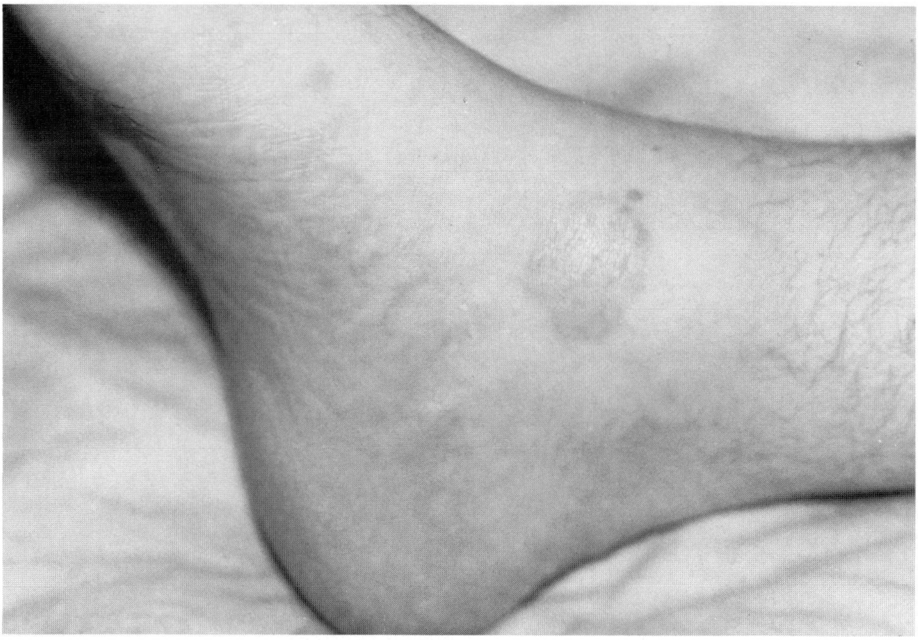

Figure 4 Tinea pedis.

ment [2] and, occasionally, an unusual presentation affecting only the flexural areas [2,41].

Koranda et al. also recovered pathogenic dermatophytes from clinically normal feet in 12% of renal transplant patients [1] (Fig. 4). This contrasts with the 6.8% incidence Davis et al. found in 152 clinically normal, healthy military recruits [1,43]. Other dermatophyte infections Koranda noted were onychomycosis (5%) and tinea corporis (2%) (Fig. 5). In immunocompromised individuals, superficial dermatophyte infections show a high degree of resistance to standard therapy, accompanied by frequent recurrence [8].

Serious mycotic infections may also develop in transplant recipients, in whom immunosuppression enhances infections, determines new manifestations, and allows ubiquitous organisms to become opportunistic pathogens [44]. A complete presentation of deep fungal infections is beyond the scope of this chapter; however, the following infections will be addressed: histoplasmosis and cryptococcosis as disseminated infections metastatic to the skin and dermal alternariasis and *Acremonium falciforme* mycetoma as recently reported primary skin fungal infections.

The frequency of dissemination of histoplasmosis is increased in immunosup-

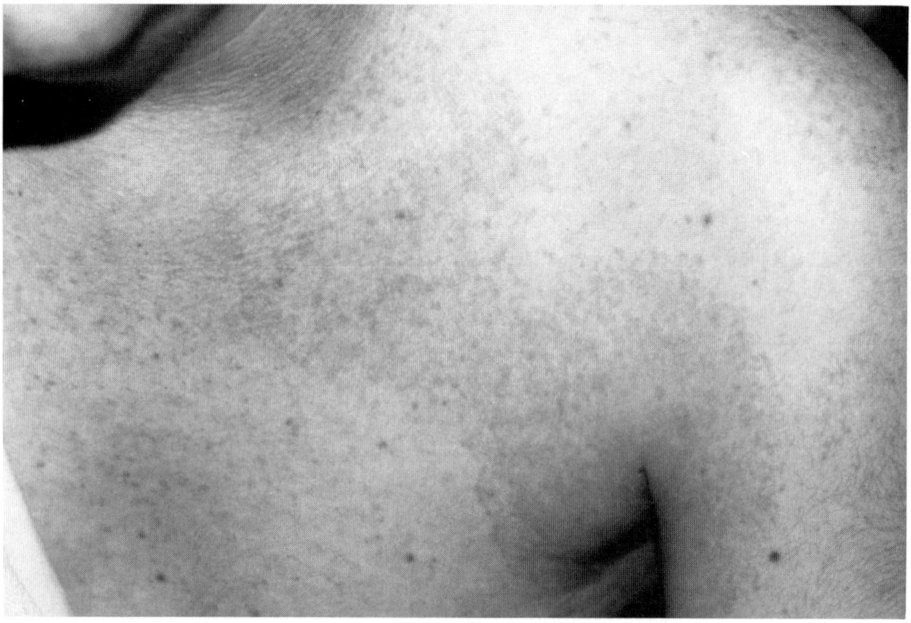

Figure 5 Tinea corporis.

pressed hosts [45], with a tendency toward more frequent cutaneous involvement [46]. When their case was added to those previously reported in the literature, Farr et al. noted a 47% incidence of cutaneous manifestations in renal transplant recipients with disseminated histoplasmosis [47]. Classically, the cutaneous lesions of histoplasmosis have been described as papules, plaques, purpura, and ulcers [48]. Of significance is the addition of cellulitis to the list of cutaneous presentations [46,47,49,50], emphasizing the need for early aspiration and biopsy of cellulitic lesions for diagnosis in transplant recipients, and possibly warranting the initiation of antifungal therapy [47,51].

Cutaneous involvement occurs in 10-15% of patients with disseminated cryptococcosis [7,52,53]. Classic dermatologic manifestations include papules, nodules, ulcers, acneiform pustules, granulomas, and purple plaques [7]. Most recently, acute cryptococcal cellulitis has been reported to occur almost exclusively in patients undergoing long-term immunosuppressive therapy [54-57]. Infection of the central nervous system (CNS) with *Cryptococcus neoformans* is life threatening. Since approximately 20% of patients with cryptococcal meningitis have skin lesions preceding CNS involvement [58], the need for early diagnosis, including aspiration and biopsy of cellulitis and possible therapy with an antifungal agent, is again emphasized [56,57].

Relatively new to the growing list of infections in the transplant patient is dermal alternariasis. This infection initially presents as flesh-colored papules and nodules that subsequently centrifugally spread and end up appearing as lesions with eroded, crusted borders around atrophic central areas [44]. Lesions are located randomly but have a preference for the extremities. The causative organism, *Alternaria tenuis,* has a widespread distribution in the environment, exemplifying a ubiquitous organism that becomes a pathogen.

Acremonium species are saprophytes, ubiquitous to the soil. These organisms have now also entered the league of pathogens that may infect the renal transplant patient. Primary fungal infection of the skin with *Acremonium falciforme* is characterized by induration and draining sinuses, usually on an extremity [59]. Other organisms responsible for cutaneous infections in the immunocompromised host include *Aspergillus* species, *Mucoraceae, Candida* species, *Coccidioides immitus, Blastomyces dermatitides, Paecilomyces* species, *Nocardia* species, and *Prototheca* (Fig. 6) [8,60].

Transplant recipients are not only susceptible to the usual infectious organisms, but by virtue of their immunosuppression become vulnerable to a vast number of pathogens with an unlimited array of manifestations. Therefore, when unusual

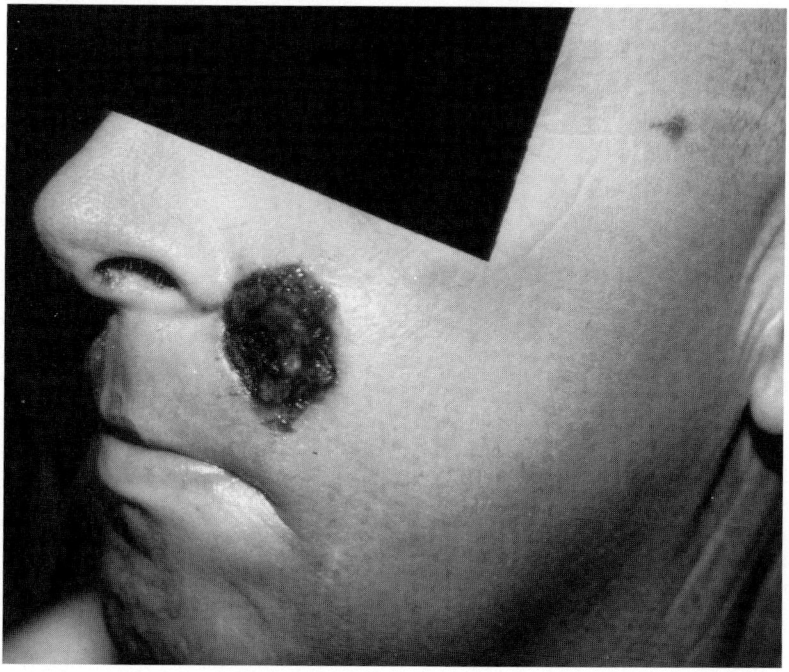

Figure 6 Disseminated aspergillosis.

skin lesions occur or when cutaneous lesions of unclear etiology persist, rapid and varied methods of organism identification are recommended [8,44,60]. In the patient with cellulitis, the rapid procedure of injecting normal saline into the cellulitic lesion, followed by aspiration of fluid and microscopic examination of the material, is recommended [51]. Biopsy material should always be obtained from any suspicious lesion for histological examination and culture [8]. Special stains for fungus, bacteria, and mycobacteria should also be done. Sections of the specimen should also be cultured for the following: aerobic and anerobic bacteria, fungus at 25 and 37°C, mycobacteria, and, if indicated, viruses. Touch preparations and/or ground tissue may be stained with Gram, acid-fast, modified acid-fast, and direct fungal stains. Tzanck preparations may also be done on lesions suspicious for a herpes virus infection. This armamentarium of diagnostic techniques assists the transplant physician in the assessment of cutaneous disease and allows use of the skin as an "early warning system" of serious infection [8].

IV. CONCLUSION

Transplant recipients receiving immunosuppressive therapy may manifest the entire spectrum of common dermatologic diseases, as well as unusual cutaneous complications unique to their immunocompromised state. Some of these cutaneous complications are potentially fatal, making the need for close dermatologic surveillance mandatory.

REFERENCES

1. Koranda, F. C., Dehmel, E. M., Kahn, G., and Penn, I.: Cutaneous complications in immunosuppressed renal homograft recipients. JAMA 229:419-424, 1974.
2. Bencini, P. L., Montagnino, G., DeVecchi, A., Tarantino, A., Crosti, C., Caputo, R., and Ponticelli, C.: Cutaneous manifestations in renal transplant recipients. Nephron 34:79-83, 1983.
3. Fisher, L. B., and Maibach, H. I.: Effect of corticosteroids on human epidermal mitotic activity. Arch. Dermatol. 103:39-44, 1971.
4. Sugimoto, M., and Endo, H.: Effect of hydrocortisone on keratinization of chick embryonic skin cultured in chemically defined medium. Nature 222: 1270-1272, 1969.
5. Laurence, E. B., and Christophers, E.: Selective action of hydrocortisone on postmitotic epidermal cells in vivo. J. Invest. Dermatol. 66:222-229, 1976.
6. Dorfman, A., and Schiller, S.: Effects of hormones on the metabolism of acid mucopolysaccharide of connective tissue. Recent Prog. Horm. Res. 14:427-456, 1958.

7. Fitzpatrick, T. B., Eisen, A. Z., Wolff, K., Freedberg, I. M., and Austen, K. F.: Dermatology in General Medicine, New York: McGraw-Hill, 1979.
8. Wolfson, J. S., Sober, A. J., and Rubin, R. H.: Dermatologic manifestations of infections in immunocompromised patients. Medicine (Baltimore) 64: 115-133, 1985.
9. Sheil, A. G. R.: Cancer in organ transplant recipients: Parts of an induced immune deficiency syndrome. Br. Med. J. 288:659-661, 1984.
10. Penn, I.: Depressed immunity and the development of cancer. Clin. Exp. Immunol. 46:459-474, 1981.
11. Disler, P. B., MacPhail, A. P., Meyers, A. M., and Myburgh, J. A.: Neoplasia after successful renal transplantation. Nephron 29:119-123, 1981.
12. Kinlen. L. J., Sheil, A. G. R., Peto, J., and Doll, R.: Collaborative United Kingdom-Australasian study of cancer in patients treated with immunosuppressive drugs. Br. Med. J. 2:1461-1466, 1979.
13. Penn, I.: Development of cancer in transplantation patients. Adv. Surg. 12: 155-191, 1978.
14. Penn, I.: Development of cancer as a complication of clinical transplantation. Transplant. Proc. 9:1121-1127, 1977.
15. Hoover, R., Fraumen, J. F., Jr.: Risk of cancer in renal transplant recipients. Lancet 2:55-57, 1973.
16. Penn, I., and Starzl, T. E.: A summary of the status of de novo cancer in transplant recipients. Transplant. Proc. 4:719-732, 1972.
17. Penn, I., and Starzl, T. E.: Malignant tumors arising de novo in immunosuppressed organ transplant recipients. Transplantation 14:407-417, 1972.
18. Sheil, A. G. R.: Cancer in renal allograft recipients in Australia and New Zealand. Transplant. Proc. 9:1133-1136, 1977.
19. Penn, I.: Malignant Tumors in Organ Transplant Recipients. New York: Springer-Verlag, 1970.
20. Marshall, V.: Premalignant and malignant skin tumors in immunosuppressed patients. Transplantation 17:272-275, 1974.
21. Hoxtell, E. O., Mandel, J. S., Murray, S. S., Schuman, L. M., and Goltz, R. W.: Incidence of skin carcinoma after renal transplantation. Arch. Dermatol. 113:436-538, 1977.
22. Hardie, I. R., Strong, R. W., Hartley, L. C. J., Woodruff, P. W. H., and Clunie, G. J. A.: Skin cancer in Caucasian renal allograft recipients living in a subtropical climate. Surgery 87:177-183, 1980.
23. Walder, B. K., Robertson, M. R., and Jeremy, D.: Skin cancer and immunosuppression. Lancet 2:1282-1283, 1971.
24. Montgomery, H., and Dorffel, J.: Verruca senilis and keratoma senile. Arch. Derm. Symph. 166:286-298, 1932.
25. Greene, M. H., Young, T. I., Clark, W. H., Jr.: Malignant melanoma in renal transplant recipients. Lancet 1:1196-1199, 1981.
26. Boyle, J., Briggs, J. C., Mackie, R. M., Junor, B. J. R., and Aitchison, T. C.: Cancer, warts and sunshine in renal transplant patients. Lancet 1:702-705, 1984.

Table 1 De Novo Cancers in Organ Allograft Recipients

Type of neoplasm	No. patients[a]
Cancers of skin and lips	914
Lymphomas	325
Carcinomas of uterus	156
Cervix	140
Body	16
Carcinomas of the lung	106
Carcinomas of colon and rectum	87
Kaposi's sarcomas	85
Carcinomas of breast	74
Carcinomas of the vulva, perineum, penis, or scrotum	65
Carcinomas of the kidney	65
Host kidney	59
Allograft kidney	6
Leukemias	59
Carcinomas of the head and neck (excluding thyroid parathyroid and eye)	58
Metastatic carcinomas (primary site unknown)	57
Carcinomas of urinary bladder	43
Carcinomas of liver and bile ducts	38
Carcinomas of thyroid	33
Soft tissue sarcomas	31
Cancers of stomach	29
Ovarian cancers	23
Testicular carcinomas	23
Carcinomas of prostate gland	23
Cancers of the pancreas	20
Brain neoplasms (excluding lymphomas)	14
Miscellaneous neoplasms	33
Total	2361

[a]There were 2211 patients, of whom 143 (6.5%) had more than one type of tumor involving different organ systems. Of these patients, 7 each had three separate types of neoplasia.

carcinoma of the uterine cervix, are not increased in incidence in transplant recipients [1-9]. Instead, the CTTR data show that certain neoplasms occur with remarkable frequency (Table 1). Skin and lip cancers are the most common tumors [7]. Their incidence varies with the amount of exposure to sunshine. In areas with limited exposure, there is a 4- to 7-fold increase, but in regions with plentiful exposure there is an almost 21-fold increase above the already high incidence seen in the local control population [1,2,7]. A study of 934 renal transplant recipients from a single Swedish center shows that lip cancers are increased 29-fold in incidence compared with controls [11]. Two epidemiological studies indicate that the incidence of non-Hodgkin's lymphomas is 28- to 49-fold above that encountered in age-matched controls. In situ carcinomas of the uterine cervix have a 14-fold increase over controls [12]. Nonmelanoma skin cancers and in situ carcinomas of the uterine cervix are usually excluded from cancer statistics. If we omit them from the CTTR data, then several other neoplasms show a substantial increase in incidence. Kaposi's sarcoma (KS) then makes up 5.2% of malignancies in the CTTR, in comparison with its incidence in the general population in the United States (before the AIDS epidemic started), where it comprised only 0.02-0.07% of all tumors [3,8]. The high incidence of KS in this worldwide collection of patients is comparable to that seen in areas of the world where it occurs with greatest frequency, namely, in the rain forest area of Africa, where it makes up 3-9% of all cancers [13]. These observations are in keeping with findings of a 400- to 500-fold increase in the incidence of KS in renal transplant recipients compared with a control population of the same ethnic origin [14]. Carcinomas of the vulva and perineum comprise 4.0% of tumors in the CTTR, a much higher figure than in the general population [1-3]. This finding is consonant with a 100-fold increase in the incidence of carcinomas of the vulva and anus in renal transplant patients compared with controls [11]. Transplant patients also are prone to small increases in the incidence of leukemia, carcinomas of the kidney, and carcinomas of the liver and biliary passages [15].

C. Time of Appearance of Neoplasms

As the length of follow-up of organ transplant recipients has increased, it has become evident that certain tumors become manifest at fairly distinct periods after transplantation [1-5,7-9]. In contrast with other known oncogenic stimuli in humans, which often take 15-20 years or more before they cause obvious malignancies, cancers appear a relatively short time after transplantation [1-9,15,16]. KS is the first to appear at an average of 23 (range 2½-225½) months after transplantation [3,8]. Lymphomas appear at an average of 36 (range, 1-154) months after transplantation. Other neoplasms (excluding carcinomas of the vulva and perineum) appear at an average of 61 (range, 1-221½) months following transplantation. Carcinomas of the vulva and perineum appear at the longest interval after transplantation, at an average of 89 (range, 9-215) months.

The incidence of malignancies rises as the length of follow-up after transplantation increases [1-5]. Of 418 renal transplant patients who survived at least 1 year, 26% had cancers; at 10 years, 14 of 30 survivors (47%) were so affected [17]. Similarly, in 124 cardiac transplant recipients the actuarial risk of developing cancer was 2.7 ± 1.9% at 1 year and 25.6 ± 11.0% at 5 years [18]. These statistics underline the need to follow transplant patients indefinitely [1-9].

D. Age and Sex of Patients

The malignancies occurred in a relative young group of patients whose average age at the time of transplantation was 40 years (range, 7 months to 72 years) [1-9]. Of these patients, 49% were under the age of 40 years at the time of transplantation; 64% were male and 36% female, in keeping with the 2:1 ratio of male to female patients who undergo renal transplantation.

E. Malignancies of the Skin and Lips

The most commonly encountered tumors were those of the skin and lips [1-9, 19]. They made up 914 of 2361 (39%) cancers in the CTTR (Table 1). Their incidence increased with the duration of follow-up after transplantation. In an Australian study, skin cancers occurred in 8% of patients who survived 1 year or more after transplantation, but they affected 17% of those who lived 4 years or longer [20]. In addition, premalignant keratoses occurred in 28% of the 4-year survivors.

The skin cancers seen in transplant patients show some unusual features when compared with their counterparts in the general population [1-9,19,20]. Basal cell carcinomas outnumber squamous cell carcinomas in the general population, but the opposite is true in transplant patients in whom squamous cell carcinomas comprised 53% and basal cell carcinomas 28% (Table 2). Another 13% of patients have both types of neoplasm. Another difference is the youth of the transplant patients, whose average age was 30 years younger than those with similar malignancies in the general population [7,21]. In addition, the incidence of multiple skin cancers, which were present in at least 392 of 914 patients (43%), is remarkably high and is comparable to that seen only in areas of plentiful sun exposure [7]. Several individuals each had more than 50 skin cancers. Malignant melanomas comprised 5% of the skin cancers in this series, in contrast to an incidence of 2.7% in the general population of the United States [22].

Most skin cancers were of low-grade malignancy, but a number were very aggressive [1-3,7]. Lymph node metastases were present in 70 patients (8%), 58 of whom had squamous cell carcinomas, 10 of whom had malignant melanomas, and 2 of whom had Merkel's cell tumors. Of the squamous cell carcinomas with lymph

Table 2 Carcinomas of the Skin and Lips

Type of malignancy	No. patients	
Squamous cell carcinomas	478	
Basal cell carcinomas	254	
Squamous and basal cell carcinomas	118	
Malignant melanoma	46	(16)[a]
Unclassified	11	
Merkel's cell carcinoma	4	(1)
Malignant sweat gland carcinoma	2	
Intracystic subaceous gland carcinoma	1	(2)
Total	914	

[a]Numbers in parentheses are patients who also had squamous or basal cell carcinomas.

node metastases, 39 involved the skin, 11 affected the lips, and 8 were cases with skin and lip involvement. The metastases probably arose from the skin lesions in 4 patients in the last group. In 2 they arose from the lip lesions, and in 2 the origin was unclear. Metastases caused the deaths of 59 patients with skin cancer (6%), 38 with squamous cell carcinomas, 19 with malignant melanomas, 1 with basal cell carcinoma, and 1 with Merkel's cell tumor. Of the fatalities caused by squamous cell carcinomas, 29 were caused by lesions arising in the skin, 3 by lesions from the lips, and 6 by lesions involving the lips and skin, with the skin lesions apparently responsible for fatal metastases in 3 patients and the lip lesions in 2, and in 1 it was not clear which lesions caused the lethal outcome. Not included in the above figures are 7 patients, all with squamous cell carcinomas, who are alive with pulmonary, cerebral, hepatic, and osseous metastases and 2 patients who died of complications of chemotherapy given for treatment of an advanced squamous cell carcinoma and a Merkel's cell tumor, respectively. All these findings are in keeping with a more than 10-fold increased mortality from squamous cell carcinomas of the skin observed in Australian renal transplant recipients [12]. The behavior of skin tumors in the present series is in marked contrast with that seen in the general population, in whom they cause only 1-2% of all cancer deaths, the great majority of which are from malignant melanomas [23].

Organ transplant recipients must be taught about prevention of skin cancer [1,2,7]. As exposure to sunlight is a major etiologic factor, patients should be warned to avoid prolonged exposure. If their occupations or hobbies do not permit this, they should wear wide-brimmed hats, sunvisors, and protective clothing and shield the skin with effective sunscreen preparations.

Hyperkeratoses and warts are common in transplant patients and usually present in areas exposed to sunlight. Some lesions may be indistinguishable clinically from skin cancers [1,2,7,19]. In such instances one should biopsy any suspicious areas. Lip carcinomas also may create diagnostic problems as often they are atypical and appear as superficial ulcers without an indurated base and rolled everted edge [1,2,7]. Occasionally, two superficial lip cancers may be present simultaneously. One should biopsy all lip ulcers that persist for more than a month, except during the early posttransplant period, where herpetic ulcers are encountered frequently.

Treatment of skin and lip cancers includes surgical excision, cryosurgery, and radiotherapy [1,2,7]. Topical applications of 5-fluorouracil or other chemotherapeutic agents are useful for extensive areas of Bowen's disease or multiple superficial carcinomas [1,2,7]. In the general population, some patients with multiple skin tumors have been treated satisfactorily with topical immunotherapeutic agents, such as DNCB, BCG, or PPD. However, transplant physicians are reluctant to employ these immunopotentiating agents in immunosuppressed patients for fear of causing serious adverse effects.

F. Lymphomas

Lymphomas in transplant patients show several unusual features, in contrast to their behavior in the general population [1-6,8,9,15]. They comprise 3-4% of all neoplasms in the community at large [23], but make up 325 of 2361 cancers (14%) in the CTTR. If we exclude nonmelanoma skin malignancies and in situ carcinomas of the uterine cervix, the incidence is 20%.

One would prefer to classify lymphomas according to the cell of origin, such as T cell, B cell, or null cell. However, many lymphomas in the present series were reported before immunologic methods of identifying lymphocyte markers became available [1-6,8,9]. Of cases studied, 42 lymphomas and 7 lymphoproliferations, which were suspected to be lymphomas, were of B-cell origin (Table 3). In several other lymphomas the cells did not demonstrate cellular immunoglobulin and could not be characterized further. Thus far, 4 T-cell neoplasms have been reported, including 1 case of mycosis fungoides. There has been 1 case of null cell lymphoma.

An unusual feature of the lymphomas is the rarity of Hodgkin's disease [1-6, 8,9]. There were only 12 cases among 325 patients (4%) with lymphomas. This is much lower than its incidence in the general population, in whom it makes up 18% of all lymphomas. If we exclude the 12 patients with Hodgkin's disease and another 10 with myelomas (plasma cell lymphomas), we are left with 302 patients with non-Hodgkin's lymphomas (NHL). In several respects these

Table 3 Lymphomas in Organ Transplant Recipients

Type of lymphoma	No. patients
Reticulum cell sarcomas[a]	182[b]
Unclassified lymphomas	47
B-cell lymphomas	42
Lymphosarcomas	13[b]
Hodgkin's disease	12
Plasma cell lymphomas	10
B-cell hyperplasias (lymphomas ?)	7
Lymphoreticular malignancies	4
T-cell lymphomas (1 case of mycosis fungoides)	4
Burkitt's lymphoma	1
Histiocytic medullary reticulosis	1
True histiocytic lymphoma	1
Null cell lymphoma	1
Total	325

[a]Also classified as histiocytic lymphoma, microglioma, immunoblastic sarcoma, reticulosarcoma, and large cell lymphoma.
[b]A reticulum cell sarcoma in 1 patient underwent spontaneous regression, and 2 years later he developed a lymphocytic lymphoma.

lymphomas were markedly different from those seen in the general population [1-3,9]. Extranodal involvement was reported in from 24 to 48% of NHL patients in the general population [24,25]. In the present series, the distribution of NHL was unknown in 2 patients and extranodal disease occurred in 227 (76%) of the remaining 300 patients. Most of the 73 patients with nodal involvement had widespread disease involving mainly the liver, lungs, spleen, bone marrow, renal allograft, and brain. In the 227 recipients with extranodal disease, a single organ was affected in 152 (67%). The organ most frequently involved was the central nervous system (CNS), which was affected in 85 of 152 patients (56%). Overall, 110 of the 300 patients (37%) had CNS involvement. Patients with meningeal involvement were not included in these statistics. Lesions of the CNS almost always involved the brain but rarely affected the spinal cord. The brain lesions frequently had a multicentric distribution. The remarkably high incidence of brain involvement contrasts with a 1% incidence of focal cerebral involvement by NHL in a series of 1039 patients in the general population (meningeal involvement occurred in 3.7%) [26]. A possible explanation for the frequency of brain involvement is that it has poor immunologic reactions so that lymphoma cells that arise in the brain itself or are carried there from other areas grow more readily in this relatively immunologically privileged site than in other regions [1-3,5,9].

The physician should consider the possibility of a CNS lymphoma whenever a transplant patient develops neurological symptoms [1-6,9]. A thorough work-up is necessary and may include examination of the cerebrospinal fluid, computed axial tomography, electroencephalography, radionuclide brain scan. cerebral angiography, and nuclear magnetic resonance. These tests help to exclude the more common causes of neurological symptoms in transplant patients, such as hypertensive encephalopathy, meningitis, brain abscess, or intracranial bleeding.

The gastrointestinal tract is frequently involved by NHL in transplant patients. A quite common presentation is acute perforation of an intestinal lymphoma with resultant peritonitis.

A remarkable finding in the 302 recipients with NHL was the frequency of lymphomatous involvement of the allograft, which occurred in 43 recipients (14%); 38 renal, 2 cardiac, 2 pancreatic, and 1 hepatic [1-3,9]. Another unusual feature was that NHL presented in the soft tissues at the sites of injection of antilymphocyte or antithymocyte globulin in at least 4 patients.

The mortality of lymphomas in renal transplant recipients is 48-fold greater than that observed in age-matched controls in the general population [12].

Disagreements have appeared in the literature about whether lymphomas are monoclonal or polyclonal in origin [27-29]. (At least some of the differences may be due to different methods used to determine clonality.) In addition, questions have been raised about whether some posttransplant lymphomas may be nonneoplastic virally induced lymphoproliferations rather than true lymphomas. Some authors describe a spectrum of lesions ranging from benign polyclonal B-cell lymphoproliferations, on the one hand, to frank malignant monoclonal B-cell lymphomas, on the other, with an intermediate phase in which a polyclonal B-cell proliferation undergoes a clonal cytogenetic alteration leading to malignant transformation [27]. Arguments about clonality are not merely intellectual exercises but may have therapeutic implications [27-29]. Hanto et al. [27] believed that at least some polyclonal lesions are caused by the Epstein-Barr virus and treated these with the antiviral agent acyclovir. They obtained remissions in 4 patients with polyclonal lesions so treated, but monoclonal lesions did not respond to acyclovir and were treated by surgery, radiotherapy, or chemotherapy. In addition, immunosuppression was reduced or discontinued in a few patients. Of their 19 patients, 5 survived without recurrence of the tumors. Cleary et al. [28] emphasized the need to establish monoclonality because such lesions required antineoplastic therapy (radiation and chemotherapy), perhaps with reduction in immunosuppressive therapy. However, they did not describe the results obtained following treatment of their 10 patients. In contrast, Starzl et al [29] found that the majority of their patients had complete remissions after reduction or cessation of immunosuppressive therapy and that several seemingly monoclonal lesions regressed as readily as did polyclonal lymphomas. They did not recommend the use of acyclovir, radiotherapy, or chemotherapy. Following treatment, 11 of their 17 patients were alive and free of malignancy. Several deaths in their series occurred in patients who were not appropriately treated because of failure to make a timely diagnosis. The conflicting opinions expressed above indicate the need for additional studies of larger numbers of patients to determine the importance of clonality and the appropriate forms of treatment of various lymphomas.

G. Kaposi's Sarcoma (KS)

There were 85 patients with this disorder, 59 males and 26 females. The 2:1 ratio of males to females is the same as that seen in transplant patients with other neoplasms but is much less than the 9:1 to 15:1 ratio seen with KS in the general population [8]. KS was most common in transplant patients who were Jewish, black, or of Mediterranean ancestry [8]. Of the 85 patients 7 (8%) had other cancers, an incidence similar to that seen in the general population [30]. Of the 85 patients, 59 (69%) had "benign" KS involving the skin, conjunctiva, or oropharyngolaryngeal mucosa, and 26 (31%) had the "malignant" variety with involvement of the internal organs. Following treatment, complete remissions occurred in 32 of the 59 patients (54%) with benign disease. Of these 32 remissions, 6 (19%) occurred when the *only* treatment was a drastic reduction of immunosuppressive therapy [1-3,8]. The other 26 remissions followed surgery, radiotherapy, or chemotherapy. In the malignant group, 4 of the 26 patients (15%) had complete remissions after chemotherapy or radiotherapy together with alteration of immunosuppressive therapy. Of the 50 patients with nonvisceral KS, 20 died, usually of causes unrelated to the KS, whereas 19 of the 26 patients with visceral KS are dead, the major cause being the malignancy.

The physician should suspect KS whenever a transplant patient develops reddish blue macules or plaques in the skin or oropharyngeal mucosa or has apparently infected granulomas that fail to heal. If the diagnosis is confirmed, a comprehensive workup is needed to determine whether there is involvement of the internal viscera [1-3,8]. Upper and lower gastrointestinal endoscopy and computed axial tomography are particularly valuable studies.

H. Carcinomas of the Uterus

Carcinomas of the cervix occurred in 140 of the 787 women in this series (18%) [1-5]. In situ lesions made up at least 80% of the cases. These tumors are probably more common than is realized. It is, therefore, advisable that all post-adolescent female patients have pelvic examinations and cervical smears done on a regular basis [1-5].

Carcinomas of the body of the uterus are uncommon. Perhaps this is because most transplant patients are young whereas these neoplasms occur mainly in postmenopausal women [1-5].

I. Carcinomas of the Vulva and Perineum

Carcinomas of the vulva, perineum, scrotum, penis, perianal skin, and anus occurred in 65 patients, 49 female and 16 male [1-3]. In contrast with patients who have similar lesions in the general population, the patients were surprisingly young. The average age of the females at the time of transplantation was 30 (range, 15-55) years and of the males 39 (range, 25-60) years. In females there was sometimes a "field effect" with involvement by cancer of the vulva and vagina and/or the cervix of the uterus. Some patients gave a history of condyloma acuminatum or herpes genitalis, suggesting that oncogenic viruses may play an etiologic role in these immunosuppressed patients [1-3].

Small lesions were treated by local excision. More extensive cancers required radical operations, such as total vulvectomy and inguinal node dissection or abdominoperineal resection [1-3].

J. Treatment of De Novo Cancers

In addition to conventional therapy of the cancers, we must consider the value of reduction or cessation of immunosuppressive therapy [1-9]. As mentioned above, several inadvertently transplanted cancers regressed when immunosuppressive therapy was discontinued and the tumor-bearing kidney was removed. Does such treatment help patients who develop de novo tumors? As mentioned above, six cases of KS and several lymphomas regressed following drastic reduction of immunosuppressive therapy [3,8,29]. Thus far, the CTTR has rarely received reports of regression of epithelial tumors with such treatment. Nevertheless, one may try to reduce the immunosuppression in patients with highly malignant, extensive, or advanced malignancies in the hope that the immune system may recover and help to eliminate the cancer. However, such treatment has the inherent risk that the allograft may undergo rejection. This may mean a return to dialysis therapy in renal transplant recipients, but in cardiac or hepatic transplant patients the outcome may be fatal.

In those patients who require cytotoxic therapy for the treatment of widespread malignancies, we must remember that most agents depress the bone marrow [1-2,9]. It is therefore prudent to stop or reduce azathioprine dosage during such therapy to avoid severe bone marrow toxicity. As most chemotherapeutic agents have immunosuppressive side effects, satisfactory allograft function may persist for prolonged periods. Treatment with prednisone may be continued as it is an important constituent of many cancer chemotherapeutic regimens [1,2,9].

K. Etiology of De Novo Cancers

This is discussed in detail elsewhere [2-5,9]. The tumors probably originate as a result of a complex interplay of multiple factors, including depression of immunity, liberation or activation of oncogenic viruses, oncogenic or co-oncogenic effects of the immunosuppressive agents or other treatments administered to the patient, and variations in individual susceptibility to carcinogenic stimuli.

IV. SUMMARY

Although the overall risk of transplant patients developing cancer is small, all of them should be followed indefinitely. Female patients require regular pelvic examinations and cervical smears in order to detect lesions early. Any untoward symptoms should be thoroughly investigated, keeping in mind the most common cancers: carcinomas of the skin and lips, lymphomas, Kaposi's sarcomas, in situ carcinomas of the uterine cervix, and carcinomas of the vulva and perineum. As other lesions in transplant patients frequently mimic cancer, any suspicious areas should be biopsied, if they are accessible.

It may be possible to prevent the development of some malignancies. Donors with cancer should not be used with the exceptions mentioned above. Administration of hepatitis B vaccine to dialysis patients may prevent the development of hepatitis and hepatocellular neoplasms. Avoidance of sunshine exposure, wearing of protective clothing, and the use of sunscreens may prevent skin tumors.

In addition to conventional cancer treatment, drastic reduction of immunosuppression may be worthwhile, particularly in patients with Kaposi's sarcoma and lymphomas. Sometimes the risk of reducing immunosuppressive therapy, as in heart or liver transplant patients, may outweigh the danger of treating a particular neoplasm by conventional means only.

ACKNOWLEDGMENT

The author wishes to thank his many colleagues throughout the world who have generously contributed data concerning their patients to the CTTR.

REFERENCES

1. Penn, I.: The price of immunotherapy. Curr. Probl. Surg. 18(11):682-751, 1981.

2. Penn, I.: The occurrence of cancer in immune deficiencies. Curr. Probl. Cancer 6(10):1-64, 1982.
3. Penn, I.: The occurrence of malignant tumors in immunosuppressed states. In: Klein, E., ed., Acquired Immunodeficiency Syndrome, Basel: Karger, Progress in Allergy Series, Vol. 37, 1986, pp. 259-300.
4. Penn, I.: Chemical immunosuppression and human cancer. Cancer 34: 1474-1480, 1974.
5. Penn, I.: Tumors arising in organ transplant recipients. In: Klein, G., and Weinhouse, S., eds., Advances in Cancer Research, Vol. 28, New York: Academic Press, 1978, pp. 31-61.
6. Penn, I., Hammond, W., Brettschneider, L., and Starzl, T. E.: Malignant lymphomas in transplantation patients. Transplant Proc. 1:106-112, 1969.
7. Penn, I.: Immunosuppression and skin cancer. Clin. Plast. Surg. 7:361-368, 1980.
8. Penn, I.: Kaposi's sarcoma in immunosuppressed patients. J. Clin. Lab. Immunol. 12:1-10, 1983.
9. Penn, I.: Allograft transplant cancer registry. In: Purtilo, D. T., ed., Immune Deficiency and Cancer: Epstein-Barr Virus and Lymphoproliferative Malignancies, New York: Plenum, 1984, pp. 281-308.
10. Weintraub, I., and Warnke, R. A.: Lymphoma in cardiac allograft recipients. Clinical and histological features and immunological phenotype. Transplantation 33:347-351, 1982.
11. Blohme, I., and Brynger, H.: Malignant disease in renal transplant patients. Transplantation 39:23-25, 1985.
12. Porreco, R., Penn, I., Droegemueller, W., Greer, B., and Makowski, E.: Gynecologic malignancies in immunosuppressed organ homograft recipients. Obstet. Gynecol. 45:359-364, 1975.
13. Templeton, A. C.: Kaposi's sarcoma. In: Andrade, R., Gumport, S. L., Popkin, G. L., and Rees, T. D., eds., Cancer of the Skin. Biology-Diagnosis-Management. Philadelphia: W. B. Saunders Co., 1976, pp. 1183-1225.
14. Harwood, A. R., Osaba, D., Hofstader, S. L., Goldstein, M. B., Cardella, C. J., Holecek, M. J., Kunynetz, R., and Giammarco, R. A.: Kaposi's sarcoma in recipients of renal transplants. Am. J. Med. 67:759-765, 1979.
15. Kinlen, L.: Immunosuppressive therapy and cancer. Cancer Surveys 1:565-583, 1982.
16. Kinlen, L. J., Sheil, A. G. R., Peto, J., and Doll, R.: Collaborative United Kingdom-Australasian study of cancer in patients treated with immunosuppressive drugs. Br. Med. J. 2:1461-1466, 1979.
17. Sheil, A. G. R., Mahony, J. F., Horvath, J. S., Johnson, J. R., Tiller, D. J., Stewart, J. H., and May, J.: Cancer following successful cadaveric renal transplantation. Transplant Proc. 13:733-735, 1981.
18. Krikorian, J. G., Anderson, J. L., Bieber, C. P., Penn, I., and Stinson, E. B.: Malignant neoplams following cardiac transplantation. JAMA 240:639-643, 1978.

19. Koranda, F. C., Dehmel, E. M., Kahn, G., and Penn, I.: Cutaneous complications in immunosuppressed renal homograft recipients. JAMA 229:419-424, 1974.
20. Marshall, V.: Premalignant and malignant skin tumors in immunosuppressed patients. Transplantation 17:272-275, 1974.
21. Mullen, D. L., Silberberg, S. G., Penn, I., and Hammond, W. S.: Squamous cell carcinomas of the skin and lip in renal homograft recipients. Cancer 37:729-734, 1976.
22. Sober, A. J.: Diagnosis and management of skin cancer. Cancer 51:2448-2452, 1983.
23. Silverberg, E.: Cancer statistics, 1984. CA 34:7-23, 1984.
24. Freeman, C., Berg, J. W., and Cutler, S. J.: Occurrence and prognosis of extranodal lymphomas. Cancer 29:252-260, 1972.
25. Reddy, S., Pellettiere, E., Saxena, V., and Hendrickson, F. R.: Extranodal non-Hodgkin's lymphoma. Cancer 46:1925-1931, 1980.
26. Herman, T. S., Hammond, N., Jones, S. E., Butler, J. J., Byrne, G. E., Jr., and McKelvey, E. M.: Involvement of the central nervous system by non-Hodgkin's lymphoma. The Southwest Oncology Group experience. Cancer 43:390-397, 1979.
27. Hanto, D. W., Gajl-Peczalska, K. J., Frizzera, G., Arthur, D. C., Balfour, H. H., Jr., McClain, K., Simmons, R. L., and Najarian, J. S.: Epstein-Barr virus (EBV) induced polyclonal B-cell lymphoproliferative diseases occurring after renal transplantation. Clinical, pathologic, and virologic findings and implications for therapy. Ann. Surg. 193:356-369, 1983.
28. Cleary, M. L., Warnke, R., and Sklar, J.: Monoclonality of lymphoproliferative lesions in cardiac-transplant recipients. Clonal analysis based on immunoglobulin-gene rearrangements. N. Engl. J. Med. 310:477-482, 1984.
29. Starzl, R. E., Nalesnik, M. A., Porter, K. A., Ho, M., Iwatsuki, S., Griffith, B. P., Rosenthal, J. T., Hakala, T. R., Shaw, B. W., Jr., Hardesty, R. L., Atchison, R. W., Jaffe, R., and Bahnson, H. T.: Reversibility of lymphomas and lymphoproliferative lesions developing under cyclosporine-steroid therapy. Lancet 1:583-587, 1984.
30. Safai, B., Mike, V., Giraldo, G., Beth, E., and Good, R. A.: Association of Kaposi's sarcoma with second primary malignancies. Possible etiopathogenic implications. Cancer 45:1472-1479.

14

Maternal and Fetal Complications

ROBERT A. WELCH, MARK I. EVANS, and ROBERT J. SOKOL
Wayne State University/Hutzel Hospital, Detroit, Michigan

I. INTRODUCTION

Over 1000 pregnancies have been reported worldwide in kidney transplant patients since the original report by Murray et al. in 1963 of the successful cesarean delivery of a renal transplant recipient [1]. Additional pregnancies have been reported after liver [2] and bone marrow transplants [3]. As the number of transplant procedures continues to grow, the likelihood increases that a physician will encounter the transplant recipient who needs counseling regarding reproduction. This chapter reviews the information accumulated over the past two decades concerning the effects of transplantation on the reproductive process and the resulting offspring. After briefly reviewing reproductive results reported in liver and bone marrow transplantation, a detailed assessment of pregnancy risk in renal transplantation is presented.

II. LIVER TRANSPLANT RECIPIENTS

Pregnancies in liver transplant recipients were recently reported in two patients by Penn and Makowski [4]. One patient became pregnant at 17 and again at 40.5 months after transplantation and the second at 42 months after this precedure. The first patient carried her two pregnancies until full term; the second elected for a therapeutic abortion because parenthood was not desired. These patients were continued on immunosuppressive medications similar to the regimen for renal transplant recipients (see below) throughout pregnancy. No untoward effects were encountered in this very limited experience. No male liver transplant recipients have fathered children.

B. Male Kidney Transplant Recipients

As mentioned above, a major problem confronting the male renal transplant recipient is sexual dysfunction. This is seen in between 22 and 43% of patients despite restoration of satisfactory kidney function [33-35]. Largely of historical interest, inadvertent sterilization by division of the spermatic cord during the transplant process was a primary reason for sterilization during earlier kidney transplant procedures. Since survival has become a reality in these patients, every effort is being made to preserve the spermatic cord [36]. Penn et al. reported that despite occasional problems with sexual dysfunction, including loss of libido and impotence, 50 males in their series were responsible for 67 pregnancies [37].

A major concern is the possibility for abnormal sperm formation secondary to immunosuppressive medications required to inhibit allograft rejection. Rosenkrantz et al. have shown some teratogenic effects of azathioprine in animal models [38]. This agent induces chromosomal aberrations, and it is theoretically possible that sperm could be affected. However, from the combined experience of several centers [37,39-41], it appears that the rate of congenital anomalies associated with azathioprine is small and no specific abnormalities have been found.

C. Female Kidney Transplant Recipients

After kidney transplant, menstruation reappears on the average within 6 months [37]. Improved libido results from the restoration of better renal function, menstruation, and ovulation. Some patients have the mistaken impression that they are incapable of having children even after kidney transplant and fail to take contraceptive precautions. Therefore, it is imperative that potential transplant candidates be thoroughly counseled regarding reproductive function prior to the transplant operation. Should pregnancy not be desired following resolution of renal failure, sterilization should be offered and performed at the time of the kidney transplant.

In those patients who wish to become pregnant, the following recommendations are suggested regarding the appropriate interval between transplant and pregnancy [42,43]:

1. Adequate, stable graft function for 18 months after transplantation
2. Good general health for 18 months after transplantation
3. No significant hypertension
4. No significant proteinuria
5. No evidence of pelvicalyceal dilatation on a recent intravenous pyelogram (IVP)

6. Serum creatinine less than 2 mg/dL
7. Stable low dosage of immunosuppressive drugs (e.g., prednisone, 15 mg/day or less; azathioprine, 3 mg/kg per day or less)

D. Early Pregnancy Outcome

In a review of over 700 gestations reported by Davison and Lindheimer [42], the mean time from renal transplantation to pregnancy was 43 months with a range of 6 weeks to 13 years following transplantation. Of these pregnancies, 8% occurred in women who had received cadaver kidneys. If a pregnancy continued past the first trimester, the likelihood of successful outcome was 80-90%. The majority of pregnancies in transplant recipients have apparently successful outcomes. However, gestation and delivery are not necessarily free of complications.

During the first trimester of pregnancy, approximately 42% of all conceptions end in either therapeutic or spontaneous abortion [42]. Reasons given for ending pregnancy with therapeutic abortion include unplanned pregnancy, psychosocial problems, uncertainty about long-term maternal prognosis, unstable renal function before pregnancy, deteriorating renal function, and/or severe hypertension in pregnancy and hereditary renal disease. About 13% of the first trimester abortions occur spontaneously.

It has been hypothesized [44] that a slightly higher risk of ectopic pregnancy exists in transplant patients because of pelvic adhesions due to previous urologic surgery, peritoneal dialysis, inflammatory disease, or overzealous use of intrauterine contraceptive devices. Approximately 0.5% of all conceptions that occurred in renal transplant patients were probably ectopic pregnancies. Because of the irregular menstrual bleeding and amenorrhea associated with deteriorating renal function, as well as an intrauterine pregnancy, the diagnosis of ectopic pregnancy may be difficult in this patient population. As stated by Davison and Lindheimer [42], "the main clinical pitfall is erroneously attributing genuine gynecological pathology to the transplant because of its location near the pelvis."

E. Kidney Function in Normal Pregnancy

Plasma volume in pregnancy normally rises by 30-45% during the second trimester and is sustained until term [45]. Gradual accumulative retention of 500-900 mm of sodium and 6-8 L of water occurs, and the added salt and water are distributed between the maternal extracellular fluid and the fetoplacental unit. Even though there is an increase in the extracellular fluid volume, blood pressure falls because of a decrease in peripheral vascular resistance thought to be secondary to progesterone.

The normal kidney in pregnancy responds to these changes in extracellular fluid volume by increasing the glomerular filtration rate (GFR) to a level about 30-50% above control by week 12 of gestation [46]. Renal plasma flow changes in a similar manner. The kidney sustains this elevation of GFR until after delivery, and then the GFR rapidly falls to nongravid levels [47,48].

Because of the increased renal plasma flow, GFR, and dilutional effects of pregnancy, BUN and serum creatinine are reduced below nonpregnant values [49]. In addition to changes in the renal handling of sodium and increased GFR, plasma osmolality regularly falls to about 270 mOsm/L in normal pregnancies [50]. Secondary to progesterone-induced respiratory alkalosis, plasma bicarbonate also falls during pregnancy from about 26-28 mm/L to approximately 20 mm/L. The daily excretion of urinary protein, however, is not increased in normal pregnancy, and therefore, rates above 200 mg in a 24-hr period should be regarded as abnormal [46].

F. Allograft Function in Pregnancy

In monitoring the kidney transplant patient, it has been shown that, for the most part, renal function behaves similarly to that in the normal pregnancy [51]. Among renal transplant patients, a transient reduction in GFR may occur in the third trimester. Proteinuria has been seen near term in about 40% of patients but usually disappears postpartum. It may be related to underlying kidney disease or subclinical allograft rejection [52]. However, this phenomenon has also been noted infrequently in normal pregnancies [41,53].

Compromised renal function prior to conception correlates with a greater possibility that permanent renal impairment will result [54,55]. Warren et al. [56] have noted hyperkalemic acidosis in two transplant recipients, associated with a decline in renal function during pregnancy. Following delivery of normal term infants, however, renal function improved and the hyperkalemic acidosis resolved. They concluded that these changes were benign when unaccompanied by other evidence of graft deterioration.

Coulam et al. [57] reported that a 75-year-old kidney was transplanted into a 36-year-old patient with adequate function during a subsequent pregnancy. They concluded that the age of the donor kidney apparently was not a factor in the kidney's ability to respond to the physiologic stresses of pregnancy. In the absence of severe maternal disease, the hazards of pregnancy appear to be no greater in the renal transplant recipient than those faced by the nonpregnant renal transplant recipient.

G. Allograft Rejection During Pregnancy

Allograft rejection occurring during pregnancy does not appear to be increased or decreased compared with risks during the same time interval in a nonpregnant renal allograft recipient [58]. Even though this rejection rate is similar to that in the nonpregnant transplant patient, it might be considered unusually high because of the privileged immunologic state of pregnancy, which should benefit the transplant recipient. There have been reports of reduction or cessation of immunosuppressive therapy during pregnancy without rejection episodes [55, 59,60].

The first signs of the acute rejection phenomenon include fever, oliguria, and elevated serum creatinine and blood urea nitrogen. In the nonpregnant patient, percutaneous biopsy of the renal allograft is safe, and histological study of this biopsy is the best way to confirm the clinical diagnosis of acute rejection [61]. In pregnancy, however, the increased vascularity of tissue biases the procedure of choice to an open biopsy. The rejection phenomenon may be minimized during pregnancy by continuation of immunosuppressive therapy at maintenance levels, along with stress doses of corticosteroids during the puerperium [61,62]. Failing these efforts, deterioration of graft function and rejection are considered sufficient reasons to terminate the pregnancy [62]. Serious rejection is reported in 9% of women whose pregnancies are carried into the third trimester [63].

H. Prenatal Complications

1. Pregnancy-Induced Hypertension

In three reports, the rate of pregnancy-induced hypertension (i.e., preeclampsia) was between 27 and 30% in renal transplant recipients [52,62]. However, the basis for the diagnosis of preeclampsia in these studies was on clinical grounds only. Preeclampsia is generally seen in 5% of the normal pregnant population [64]. Biopsy studies in nontransplant female patients with renal parenchymal disease have shown that the clinical diagnosis of superimposed preeclampsia can be wrong in approximately 50% of cases [65]. A report exists [66] in which a primigravida transplant recipient developed severe preeclampsia that rapidly progressed to eclampsia. Although many of the hypertensive syndromes of any etiology occurring in renal transplant recipients may be severe, this is the only case of eclampsia that, to our knowledge, has been reported in this patient population.

Among the most difficult challenges facing the clinicians caring for the transplant recipient is differentiating the patient who is preeclamptic from the patient with continued underlying renal disease. Serum uric acid level and urine protein excretion are not useful markers for either the onset or severity of preeclampsia in transplant recipients. It has also been suggested that both these indices may be substantially above the norm at any stage of gestation in otherwise uncomplicated pregnancies of renal transplant recipients [67].

2. Risk of Infection

The risk of infection presents another concern in the pregnant transplant recipient. Sciarra et al. [55] indicate that these patients should be carefully monitored for this possibility throughout pregnancy, particularly with regard to urinary tract infection. They suggest that prophylactic antibiotics be given before any surgical procedure, since overwhelming infection is a leading cause of death in these patients. Infections frequently seen with chronically immunosuppressed patients include *Pneumocystic carinii,* cytomegalovirus, and fungal organisms, as well as some of the more common bacterial agents [68,69]. Sciarra et al. indicate that bacterial and viral infections occur in virtually all of these patients during pregnancy or in the puerperium. Waltzer et al. cited infection rates as high as 60% [43]. Nonetheless, Penn et al. found no increase in the rate of infection in transplant patients during pregnancy [62], and Rifle and Traeger support this conclusion regarding urinary tract infections [53]. Meier and Makowski state that, "despite the conflicting opinions, careful observation for infectious complications and aggressive antibiotic therapy are indicated in these patients" [58].

In the immunosuppressed condition, chronic viral infections and the viral carrier state are an additional risk to the pregnant transplant patient and her offspring, as well as those caring for her. Schooley et al. monitored renal transplant recipients for development of herpes virus infections and found 35 primary or reactivation infections in 28 patients during the first 3 months after transplantation [69]. This would represent a significant risk for the pregnant graft recipient and her offspring. At least one case of congenital cytomegalovirus infection has been reported in the offspring of a renal transplant patient [70]. The exact rate of hepatitis B surface antigenemia in the renal transplant recipient is unclear but is very high, since 50% of dialysis patients are hepatitis B surface antigen positive [71]. As a result of their immunosuppressed state, these patients are frequently chronic carriers and present an infectious risk to both the health care provider and the newborn [72]. Evaluation for hepatitis B antigen and antibody in the serum should be performed. The possibility of future hepatic dysfunction and, perhaps, even hepatic malignancy must be considered [71].

I. Management of the Antepartum Course

Penn et al., indicate that pregnant transplant recipients should be followed in a high-risk obstetric clinic by a team including an obstetrician, a transplant nephrologist, a geneticist, a neonatologist, and appropriate psychosocial support personnel [37]. Visits are biweekly until 28 weeks and then weekly thereafter [58]. Since pregnancy cannot be allowed to interfere with the integrity of the renal allograft, immunosuppressive agents are continued at prepregnancy levels [37]. Blood pressure and weight are screened at each visit, and Meier and Makowski [58] reccommend that the patient be seen by both the obstetrician and transplant nephrologist at each visit.

Evaluation of renal function, including blood urea nitrogen, creatinine, and electrolytes, should be performed frequently. Creatinine clearance and protein excretion should be determined with 24-hr urine samples. Urinalysis should be performed at every visit and followed up with culture if the urinalysis is suspicious for infection. Anemia should be evaluated and treated. Serum calcium and phosphate levels should be evaluated at least every trimester, and early signs of hyperparathyroidism fully investigated [58]. Hemolytic disease of the newborn is a potential complication since these patients have commonly received multiple blood transfusions while on dialysis. These patients should be screened for regular and irregular blood antibodies each trimester. Glucose metabolism may be altered because of chronic steroid therapy in transplant recipients. They should receive a 50-g oral glucose load followed by a 1-hr random blood sugar (plasma value $>$ 135 mg/dL considered abnormal) at the initial visit, and at 28-30 weeks' gestational age. A 3-hr glucose tolerance test may be necessary to fully determine their ability to metabolize glucose.

J. Antenatal Fetal Surveillance

Coulam et al. [57] have shown that ordinary hormone excretion tests (24-hr urine estriol) and probably plasma hormone levels (estriol and human placental lactogen) are of no value in these pregnancies. We recommend weekly nonstress tests (NST) beginning at 28 weeks' gestational age, backed up by contraction stress tests (CST) for nonreactive NST. In addition, serial ultrasound studies to follow fetal growth are a useful adjunct to care. If intrauterine growth retardation is suspected, the antenatal testing sequence (NST and/or CST) should be performed every 3-5 days with early delivery for signs of compromised fetal well-being. Evans and coworkers recommended that if evidence of severe intrauterine growth retardation exists, the possibility of congenital cytomegalovirus infection should be ruled out [70].

K. Intrapartum Complications

1. Premature Delivery

The overall preterm delivery rate in renal transplant recipients is approximately 50% [67]. Rudolph and coworkers have postulated that the long-term steroid therapy given to these patients may weaken connective tissues and contribute to an increased rate of premature rupture of membranes [63]. Some transplant patients may go into premature labor because of poor renal function [73]. Although spontaneous premature rupture of membranes and premature labor are frequent in renal transplant recipients, many preterm deliveries are performed upon medical and/or obstetric indications as well.

2. Premature Rupture of Membranes

The issue of management of premature or prolonged rupture of membranes in these patients is conflicting. It has been recommended that cervical culture for β-hemolytic streptococci and other pathogens should be obtained and labor induced [58]. However, this aggressive approach may partially contribute to the high rate of respiratory distress syndrome in these neonates.

L. Management of Delivery

During the intrapartum period, meticulous attention should be paid to aseptic technique. Stress doses of corticosteroids (hydrocortisone, 100 mg IV piggyback every 6 hr), should be administered during labor and for the first 24-hr postpartum. Meier and Makowski recommend the liberal use of prophylactic antibiotics for all surgical procedures related to the peripartum period, including episiotomy [58].

Since the transplanted kidney is generally placed high in the false pelvis, it should not represent an impediment to vaginal delivery. Not only does the transplant not produce mechanical dystocia during labor, it apparently is not damaged during vaginal delivery [67]. Although cesarean section may be necessary for purely obstetric reasons, it is apparent that the rate of 25% or more in these patients reflects fear of the unknown rather than a belief that vaginal delivery will damage the mother and/or the child [67].

There is some evidence that pelvic osteodystrophy may be responsible for pelvic contractures in those patients with previous chronic renal failure (and dialysis) or in relation to prolonged steroid therapy, particularly before puberty [67]. Ideally, this problem may be recognized before attempted vaginal delivery. Sciarra et al. recommended performing simultaneous intravenous pyelogram (IVP), and x-ray pelvimetry at approximately 36 weeks' gestation should doubts concerning kidney compression or the adequacy of the maternal pelvis arise [55]. However, we are not aware of any studies that support this recommendation and would suggest the more standard procedure of awaiting labor to test the pelvis. Should cesarean section ultimately become necessary for delivery, in order to avoid the renal allograft and because of difficulty in exposing the lower uterine segment because of previous pelvic infections or urologic complications, a classic incision may become necessary [58]. Regardless of the route of delivery, management of labor should include close fetal surveillance with electronic fetal monitoring and fetal scalp blood gases when indicated.

M. Postpartum Care

Use of stress dose steroids and antibiotic prophylaxis have already been noted. Several additional questions arise concerning the postpartum period in the kidney transplant recipient. Among these are providing the patient with information regarding breast-feeding, contraception, and pelvic cancer screening.

The available data on breast-feeding in these patients is limited. Briggs et al. have analyzed infants with continued exposure to prednisone and cyclosporine through breast milk and have noted no short-term effects [74]. There is no information currently available about continued exposure of the infant to azathioprine. The decision regarding breast-feeding is parental at this time; however, it must be based on the knowledge that continued exposure of the infant to potent immunosuppressive drugs or metabolites will occur.

For patients who request permanent sterilization, postpartum sterilization by bilateral tubal ligation is the preferred method [58]. Other forms of contraception available to the patient, should she elect to maintain her fertility, would include low-dose oral contraceptive pills (OCP), barrier methods, and the intrauterine device. OCP provide maximum protection against pregnancy but could be associated with an increased risk for thromboembolic complications. It appears that the intrauterine device (IUD) may be a poor choice in these patients because of their chronically immunosuppressed state and the risk of overwhelming sepsis secondary to the presence of an IUD [75]. We believe that use of a barrier method supported by voluntary interruption of pregnancy, if acceptable to the patient in failures, represents the safest method for contraception.

Iatrogenic immunosuppression of patients increases their risk for pelvic malignancy. A 13-fold increase in the rate of squamous cell carcinoma of the cervix has been reported [26,76,77] and is consistent with theories of a viral etiology of cervical cancer. Pelvic examination every 6 months in the nonpregnant patient is recommended, including a Papanicolaou smear and colposcopic examination for the presence of cervical lesions if the smear is abnormal. We would also recommend this for the pregnant transplant recipient, including colposcopically directed cervical biopsy during pregnancy if a suspicious lesion is seen.

N. The Offspring

Parents may be reassured that the likelihood of carrying a normal newborn is high. There are no good data suggesting increased cytogenetic abnormalities in the fetus, and genetic amniocentesis is not indicated solely because of transplantation. The major problem is preterm delivery, occurring in 50% of infants, and approximately 20% of these are noted to be small for gestational age (SGA). This high percentage of SGA babies indicates that the risk for intrauterine growth retardation is significant and close fetal surveillance of additional importance. Scott has suggested the possibility that nonspecific depression of the immune system by immunosuppressive agents like azathioprine could result in intrauterine growth retardation [78]. However, these effects could also be explained by the direct cytotoxic action of azathioprine on the intrauterine contents.

Some problems that have been seen in these offspring suspected to result from chronic immunosuppression include thymic atrophy, transient leukopenia and thrombocytopenia, adrenal insufficiency, reduced blood levels of IgG and IgM, chromosome abberations in lymphocytes, hypoglycemia, and hypocalcemia [55, 79-83]. Penn et al. reported that respiratory distress syndrome occurred in 9% of the newborns in their study, 5% had adrenocorticol insufficiency, and 5% developed septicemia [79].

Reimers and Sluss have suggested that fetuses of mice given mercaptopurine during pregnancy may have reproductive problems at maturation [84]. These exposed offspring were either sterile or had decreased litter size and greater frequency of fetal wastage than in control animals. Whether a similar problem will evolve in humans at present remains unknown. Long-term follow-up will be required for offspring of transplant patients.

Borrell and coworkers initially discovered the antilymphocytic properties of cyclosporin A [85]. This drug is thought to have selective action against the T cells involved in allograft rejection. Graft rejection is inhibited by administering this drug in high doses to the renal transplant patient [86]. It is nephrotoxic at these high dosages, and the consequences for the recipient patient are unknown. Likewise, the amount that crosses the placenta and might affect the offspring's kidneys has not been determined. Lewis et al. have reported a case of pregnancy following transplant in which cyclosporine was used as an immunosuppressent. At this point, the results appear encouraging [87]. Cyclosporine was found in the fetal cord blood at the time of delivery, but no medication was found in the amniotic fluid. It was also found in maternal breast milk 4 days postpartum. Further studies are needed before a determination can be made as to whether breast feeding is safe for the offspring of these patients.

V. CONCLUSION

As transplant technology continues to progress, it is apparent that the transplant team will be frequently confronted with patients asking for advice concerning their future reproductive capacity. At present, the weight of evidence suggests that if the recipient of a renal transplant has had the return of normal renal function for a period of approximately 2 years without complications, pregnancy may be considered. Likewise, hepatic and bone marrow transplant patients have this option. Although further studies are needed on the possibility of long-term teratogenic effects of chemotherapeutic agents used to induce immunosuppression in these patients, currently there is no indication that the offspring of these individuals suffer from teratogenic side effects. The transplant recipient is encouraged to seek the early advice of a member of the transplant team, a nephrologist, her obstetrician, and a psychologist-psychiatrist before attempting pregnancy or at least early in pregnancy.

Although we are unaware of any current reports in the literature, we expect that patients who undergo transplant of other organs and subsequently become pregnant will be reported. It is also anticipated that pregnancies may someday be reported in patients with artificial transplant organs.

REFERENCES

1. Murray, J. E., Reid, D. E., Harrison, J. H., et al.: Successful pregnancies after human renal transplantation. N. Engl. J. Med. 269:341, 1963.
2. Walcott, W. O., Derick, D. E., Jolley, J. J., and Snyder, D. L.: Successful pregnancy in a liver transplantation. Am. J. Obstet. Gynecol. 132:340, 1978.
3. Jacobs, P., and Dubovsky, D. W.: Bone marrow transplantation followed by normal pregnancy. Am. J. Hematol. 11:209, 1981.
4. Penn, I., and Makowski, E. L.: Parenthood in kidney and liver transplant recipients. Transplant. Proc. 13:36, 1981.
5. Moe, P. S., Lethinen, M., Wegelius, R., Friman, S., Krueger, A., and Berg, A.: Progeny of survivors of acute lymphocytic leukaemia. Acta Paediatr. Scand. 68:301, 1979.
6. McKeen, E. A., Muldihill, J. J., Rosner, F., and Zarrabi, M. H.: Pregnancy outcomes in Hodgkin's disease. Lancet 2:590, 1979.
7. Camitta, B. M., et al.: Severe aplastic anemia: A prospective study of the effect of early marrow transplantation on acute mortality. Blood 48:63, 1976.
8. Thomas, E. D., et al.: Marrow transplantation for patients with acute lymphoblastic leukemia in remission. Blood 54:468, 1979.
9. Thomas, E. D., et al.: Marrow transplantation for acute nonlymphoblastic leukemia in first remission. N. Engl. J. Med. 301:597, 1979.
10. Speiser, B., Rubin, P., and Casarett, G.: Aspermia following lower truncal irradiation in Hodgkin's disease. Cancer 32:592, 1973.
11. Sherins, R. H., and DeBita, V. T.: Effective drug treatment for lymphoma on male reproductive capacity. Ann. Intern. Med. 79:216, 1973.
12. Asbjornsen, G., Molne, K., Klepp, O., and Aakbaag, A.: Testicular function after combination chemotherapy for Hodgkin's disease. Scand. J. Haematol. 16:66, 1876.
13. Thomas, P. R. M., Winstanly, O., Peckham, M. J., Austin, D. E., Murray, M. A. F., and Jacobs, H. S.: Reproductive and endocrine function in patients with Hodgkin's disease: Effects of oophoropexy and irradiation. Br. J. Cancer 33:226, 1976.
14. Rostom, A. Y., and White, W. F.: Hodgkin's disease, chemotherapy, and fertility. Lancet 1:555, 1979.
15. Hager, B., Thomas, E., and Ferrebee, J. W.: Fertility of dogs after recovery from "lethal" exposure to radiation. Radiobiol. Radiother. (Berl.) 3:1, 1962.
16. Deeg, H. J., Kennedy, M. S., Sanders, J. E., Thomas, E. D., and Storb, R.: Successful pregnancy after marrow transplantation for severe aplastic anemia and immunosuppression with cyclosporine. JAMA 250:647, 1983.

56. Warren, S. E., Mitas, J. A., and Evertson, L. R.: Pregnancy after renal transplantation: Reversible acidosis in renal dysfunction. South. Med. J. 74: 1139, 1981.
57. Coulam, C. D., Zincke, A., and Sterioff, S.: Relationship between donor age and outcome of pregnancy in renal allograft population. Transplantation 33: 97, 1982.
58. Meier, P. R., and Makowski, E. L.: Pregnancy and the patient with a renal transplant. Clin. Obstet. Gynecol. 27:902, 1984.
59. Kaupman, J. J., Digman, W., Goodwin, W. E., Martin, D. T., Goldman, R., and Maxwell, M. H.: Successful normal childbirth after kidney homotransplantation. JAMA 200:162, 1967.
60. Davison, J. M., Dellagrammatikas, H., and Parkin, J. M.: Fetal haematopoiesis and azathioprine therapy in pregnant patients with renal transplants. Clin. Exp. Hypertens. Bi 209, 1982.
61. Stuart, F. P.: Selection, preparation, and management of kidney transplant recipients. Med. Clin. North Am. 62:1381, 1978.
62. Penn, I., Makowski, E. L., and Harris, P.: Parenthood following renal transplantation. Kidney Int. 18:221, 1980.
63. Rudolph, J. E., Shwihizir, R. T., and Barius, S. A.: Pregnancy in renal transplant patients: A review. Transplantation 27:26, 1979.
64. Pritchard, J. A., MacDonald, P. C., and Gant, M. F.: Williams Obstetrics, 17th Ed. East Norwalk, CN: Appleton-Century-Crofts, 1985, p. 539.
65. Katz, A. I., Davison, J. M., Hayslett, J. P., Sing-Son, E., and Lindheimer, M. D.: Pregnancy in women with kidney disease. Kidney Int. 18:192, 1980.
66. Williams, P. F., and Jelen, J.: Eclampsia in a patient who had a renal transplant. Br. Med. J. 2:972, 1979.
67. Davison, J. M.: Pregnancy in renal transplant recipients: Clinical perspectives. Contrib. Nephrol. 37:170, 1984.
68. Washer, G. F., Schroter, G. P. S., and Starzl, G. E.: Causes of death after kidney transplantation. JAMA 250:49, 1983.
69. Schooley, R. T., et al.: Association of herpes virus infections with T-lymphocyte-subset alterations, glomerulopathy and opportunistic infections after renal transplantation. N. Engl. J. Med. 308:307, 1983.
70. Evans, T. J., McCollum, J. P. K., and Valdemarsson, II: Congential cytomegalovirus infection after maternal renal transplantation. Lancet 1:1359, 1975.
71. Chan, M. K., and Moorehead, J. F.: Hepatitis B and the dialysis in renal transplantation units. Nephron 27:229, 1981.
72. Schweitzer, I. L., Dunn, A. E., Peters, R. L., and Spear, R. L.: Viral hepatitis B in neonates and infants. Am. J. Med. 55:762, 1973.
73. Felding, C. F.: Obstetric aspects in women with histories of renal disease. Acta Obstet. Gynecol. Scand. 48:2, 1969.
74. Briggs, G. C., et al.: Drugs in Pregnancy and Lactation, Baltimore: Williams and Wilkins, 1983.
75. Ferner, J., et al.: Intrauterine contraceptive devices in renal transplant patients. J. Reprod. Med. 26:99, 1981.

76. Penn, I.: Malignancies associated with immunosuppressive or cytotoxic therapy. Surgery 83:492, 1978.
77. Porreco, R., Penn, I., Droegemueller, W., Greer, B., and Makowski, E. L.: Gynecologic malignancies in immunosuppressed organ homograft recipients. Obstet. Gynecol. 45:359, 1975.
78. Scott, J. R.: Fetal growth retardation associated with maternal administration of immunosuppressive drugs. Am. J. Obstet. Gynecol. 128:441, 1971.
79. Penn, I., Makowski, E. L., and Harris, R.: Parenthood following renal transplantation. Kidney Int. 18:221, 1980.
80. Leb, D. E., Weisskopf, B., and Kanovitz, B. S.: Chromosome abberations in the child of a kidney transplant recipient. Arch. Intern. Med. 128:441, 1971.
81. Lower, G. D., Stevens, L. E., Najarian, J. S., and Reemtsma, K.: Problems from immunosuppression during pregnancy. Am. J. Obstet. Gynecol. 111: 1120, 1971.
82. Price, H. V., Salaman, J. R., Laurence, K. M., and Langmain, H.: Immunosuppressive drugs and the fetus. Transplantation 21:294, 1976.
83. Korsch, B. M., Klein, J. D., Negrete, D. F., Henderson, D. J., and Fine, R. M.: Physical and psychological follow-up on offspring of renal allograft recipients. Pediatrics 65:275, 1980.
84. Reimers, T. J., and Sluss, D. M.: 6-Mercaptopurine treatment of pregnant mice: Effects on second and thrid generations. Science 201:65, 1978.
85. Borel, J. F., Feurer, C., Gubler, H. U., et al.: Biological effects of cyclosporine A: A new antilymphocytic agent. Agents Actions 6:468, 1976.
86. Merion, R. M., White, D. J., Thiru, S., et al.: Cyclosporine: 5 years experience in cadaveric renal transplantation. N. Engl. J. Med. 310:148, 1984.
87. Lewis, G. J., et al.: Successful pregnancy in a renal transplant recipient taking cyclosporin A. Br. Med. J. 286:603, 1983.

15

Complications of Pancreatic Transplantation

VIJAY K. MITTAL and LUIS H. TOLEDO-PEREYRA
Mount Carmel Mercy Hospital, Detroit, Michigan

I. INTRODUCTION

Pancreatic transplantation was introduced clinically in 1966 [1]. The aim of this procedure was to achieve a more satisfactory control of carbohydrate metabolism, restore normal glucose homeostasis, and possibly prevent or halt the secondary complications of juvenile diabetes mellitus [2].

Early results of pancreatic transplantation were discouraging because of a high frequency of technical complications and high morbidity and mortality. However, recently the results have improved, mainly by new advances in surgical techniques [3-7]. This chapter will focus on the postoperative complications of pancreatic transplantation. Although rejection has been considered a frequent cause of failure, technical problems related to handling of the pancreatic duct and activation of pancreatic enzymes have accounted for many of the complications.

The complications of pancreatic transplantation can be divided into two major areas: (1) complications in the living related donors secondary to harvesting of the segmental pancreatic graft, and (2) complications in the recipient.

Potential complications that might be encountered in living related donors, from whom a segmental pancreatic graft has been removed, include the development of abnormal glucose tolerance or diabetes mellitus itself, postoperative pancreatitis, and other possible complications related to the partial excision of the graft.

The complications encountered in the recipient are related to the type of operation (segmental versus whole pancreatic organ transplantation), the location of the pancreatic graft (extraperitoneal or intraperitoneal), the method of handling the pancreatic secretions, whether a synchronous or asynchronous kidney

Table 1 Postoperative Complications After Pancreatic Transplantation

Immediate postoperative complications
Rejection
Hemorrhage
Acute vascular occlusion
Sepsis
Late postoperative complications
Wound infection
Pancreatitis
Pancreatic fistula
Ascites
Vascular occlusion
Chronic rejection
Sepsis
Peritonitis
Abdominal abscesses
Peripancreatic collections
Massive hemorrhage
Mycotic aneurysms
Vascular stenosis
Myocardial infarction

and pancreatic transplant is performed, and complications related to the type of immunosuppressive therapy. We will not discuss the latter complications in this chapter since they are described in their various forms in other chapters of this book.

Immediate postoperative complications include rejection, hemorrhage, acute vascular occlusion, and sepsis. Late postoperative complications include wound infection, pancreatitis, pancreatic fistula, pancreatic ascites, vascular occlusion, chronic rejection, sepsis, peritonitis, abdominal abscesses, peripancreatic collections, massive hemorrhage, mycotic aneurysms, vascular stenosis, and myocardial infarction (Table 1).

The type of preservation solution, particularly the duration of the preservation, can be directly related to the pancreatic graft function. The ischemic injury during harvesting of the cadaveric pancreatic graft might result in early pancreatic damage with vascular thrombosis and/or various other complications.

II. COMPLICATIONS IN LIVING RELATED DONORS

Living related donors who undergo partial distal pancreatectomy could have complications associated with the operation itself or potential glucose intolerance related to the decrease of the pancreatic reserve. As of November 1985, 47 living related pancreas transplants had been performed at the University of Minnesota, and 3 had been performed at other centers [8]. Even though the development of diabetes mellitus is a real possibility, the University of Minnesota series has only reported a single patient who developed type II diabetes after donation [8]. All donors except one had normal glucose tolerance tests and metabolic profiles after donation. There was no incidence of prolonged graft ischemia or graft preservation, since in all the related donors the graft was immediately transplanted after removal. The complications occurring in living related donors can be easily recognized and should be managed aggressively by re-exploration if needed. In one patient, the spleen, which is left intact during surgery, infarcted and had to be removed in a second exploration. One donor had to be reoperated to ligate the pancreatic duct. Three donors had postoperative fluid collections necessitating percutaneous drainage. Pancreatitis, although a viable complication, is of a chemical nature and does not prolong hospitalization. Other potential complications, such as abscess, fistula, and pseudocyst, have not occurred yet [9].

III. COMPLICATIONS IN THE RECIPIENT

Various complications can be encountered in pancreatic transplantation, as in any other organ transplant, such as rejection, vascular thrombosis, and infectious complications. Complications that may occur after pancreatic transplantation include pancreatitis, pancreatic abscesses, fibrosis, and ascites. Other complications related to the management of the pancreatic duct may result in pancreatic fistula, intestinal leak, or urinary leak, depending on how the pancreatic secretions were handled.

A. Rejection

1. Hyperacute Rejection

Theoretically, pancreas transplant hyperacute rejection could occur, as it happens with other solid vascularized organs. In our experience, we have not seen a single case yet [10]. Others have not reported this complication either [11]. It is possible that the pancreas is less prone to humoral immunologic response than other solid organs or that this response has not been clearly documented. If this phenomena did occur, this would happen at the time of release of the vascular clamps following anastomosis, and probably it would be related to antibodies preformed to the donor pancreas, as in other organ transplants. A pancreatectomy would have to be done immediately and the recipient vessels repaired.

2. Acute and Chronic Rejection

These forms of rejection will cause graft failure following pancreatic transplantation. The most specific test to diagnose rejection is pancreatic histology, even though fibrosis can make the diagnosis difficult. Human C-peptide levels also decrease quickly during rejection; however, they are not always readily available. From the practical point of view, rejection is diagnosed by increased blood sugar levels and the need for exogenous insulin to maintain a normal glucose homeostasis, with an associated increase in pancreatic enzymes. An increase in serum amylase is not always a sign of rejection, and endocrine rejection is often present without modification of the exocrine function. Other means to aid in the diagnosis of rejection include ultrasound of the pancreatic graft, which might show an enlargement of the gland [12]. A pancreatic scan might show decreased uptake of the graft [13].

B. Vascular Complications

1. Hemorrhage

This complication following pancreatic transplantation can be immediate or delayed. Immediate hemorrhage may be from small vessels that have not been identified and have been left untied on the pancreatic surface or from a coagulation defect secondary to renal failure. The delayed hemorrhage following pancreatic transplantation is usually a secondary hemorrhage due to infection at the vascular anastomosis site. A spontaneous massive hemorrhage at the vascular anastomosis usually results in loss of the graft. Active bleeding in the immediate postoperative period can be controlled by immediate exploration, identification, and ligation of the bleeding foci. In case there is no active bleeder from the surface of the pancreas and the bleeding seems to be due to a coagulation defect, it should be treated by proper replacement therapy.

2. Vascular Thrombosis

Vascular thrombosis occurring after pancreatic transplantation can be arterial, venous, or combined and can be seen in the immediate or delayed postoperative period. Vascular thrombosis is more often seen in segmental pancreatic transplantation as it probably has a lower blood flow than the whole organ transplant. Arterial thrombosis at the time of surgery can be diagnosed directly or with an intraoperative angiogram. If, after taking off the clamp, the organ does not become pink or does not have pulsation, then an immediate intraoperative angiogram should be performed to determine the cause of the arterial thrombosis. In this situation, the thrombosis is usually due to technical factors associated with multiple vascular anastomosis. The thrombosis may be due to an intimal flap or intimal damage produced during donor pancreatectomy or at the time of vascular anastomosis. In the immediate postoperative period, a sudden and persistent increase in plasma glucose levels and the need for exogenous insulin to maintain a normoglycemic state may indicate either acute rejection or vascular thrombosis. The arterial thrombosis can be ruled out by performing an immediate angiogram of the pancreatic graft, which will diagnose any arterial or venous thrombosis in the delayed phase. An early exploration may avert the need for a pancreatectomy if there is a correctable problem.

A relatively high frequency of venous thrombosis has been reported by most centers performing pancreatic transplants. Simple mechanical factors may be responsible for venous thrombosis because of the angulation in the anastomosis of the portal vein to the external iliac vein. Therefore, the portal vein should be anastomosed as high as possible to maintain a wide angle between the portal vein and the pancreatic graft. Other factors that may be responsible for venous thrombosis can be extension of a venous thrombosis from the lower legs of the recipient or coagulopathy in the recipient. Venous thrombosis can also be related to the low vascular flow in segmental transplants or may occur following trauma during donor pancreatectomy or during the venous anastomosis procedure. Symptoms suggesting venous thrombosis include swelling of the graft and increased plasma glucose levels. The venous thrombosis may be partial, and conservative therapy may be helpful in a few cases in the form of anticoagulation therapy. Severe venous thrombosis might result in the loss of the pancreatic graft. Composite pancreas and spleen transplantation has been attempted in order to improve the hemodynamic status of the pancreatic graft and in this way to prevent vascular thrombosis [4,14]. On the other hand, distal arterial venous fistulas of the pancreatic graft have been tried with the same objective [15]. Since vascular thrombosis is one of the major factors of graft loss following pancreatic transplantation, several transplant centers have started to use heparin and/or low-molecular-weight dextran for the first few weeks posttransplantation [2].

3. Aneurysms

After pancreatic transplantation, the possibility of developing an aneurysm of the arterial anastomosis exists in long-term functioning grafts. However, the short duration of pancreas transplants has not allowed for identification of this complication postoperatively. If they occur, these aneurysms could be anastomotic, poststenotic, or mycotic. These could rupture, thrombose with distal embolization, or cause limb ischemia due to thrombosis and embolism of the iliac vessels. Anastomotic aneurysms are false aneurysms that result from partial or total separation of the anastomosis. They could be located at the junction of the splenic artery and the external iliac artery of the recipient, in the case of segmental pancreas transplants, or between the celiac and superior mesenteric artery and the external iliac artery of the recipient, in the case of whole-pancreas transplants. Anastomotic aneurysms can result from suture failure, because the integrity of the anastomotic line may have been in question at implantation or from damage of the suture material from careless handling. In addition, a hematoma surrounding the anastomosis could later become infected, leading to a communication with arterial lumen. Sometimes the pancreatic secretions from the surface of the transplanted pancreas collect in the form of peripancreatic collections, which may at times be associated with subsequent infection, resulting in a false aneurysm at the site of the anastomosis. Clinically, these aneurysms could present as a palpable pulsatile mass with such complications as rupture, distal embolization, or thrombosis. A definitive diagnosis is made by an angiogram, and surgical repair at times may be possible, although usually removal of the graft is necessary.

Mycotic aneurysms could develop as a result of septic embolization. They are evidenced by a rapidly enlarging tender, warm pulsatile mass, fever, and leukocytosis postoperatively. A systolic murmur may be heard over the mass. The diagnosis is made on a computed tomographic scan of the area, which shows gas bubbles, and can be confirmed by an arteriogram. Management of the mycotic aneurysm includes the removal of the graft and restoration of the vascular system. Antibiotics are continued for 4-6 weeks.

C. Wound Infection

Local wound infection has been seen predominantly in patients in whom the pancreas transplant has been placed extraperitoneally. Most of the wound infections are related to peripancreatic collections that have made their way to the surface by autodigestion of the local tissue. Usually these patients are not septic, and small amounts of pancreatic juices begin draining through one end of the wound. Proper management should include early exploration and drainage of the wound. It is also possible that the source of peripancreatic collections may be a small accessory duct that has not been either drained or occluded. The duct should be drained or occluded, and the wound should be drained externally so that it can be converted into a pancreatic fistula. Antibiotics should also be used to treat specific microorganisms (Figs. 1 and 2).

D. Sepsis

Lillehei and associates reported in 1973 that most of their pancreaticoduodenal transplant recipients died secondary to sepsis. The incidence of sepsis has decreased since then, but it is still a major cause for graft failure, mortality, and morbidity [11]. Sepsis can be in the peritoneal cavity in the form of peritonitis or intra-abdominal abscess, related to pulmonary sepsis in the already immunosuppressed individual, or a urinary tract infection in the case of ductocystostomy or ductoureterostomy. It is very important to identify the source of infection and to pursue aggressive surgical drainage of these abscesses, as well as complete

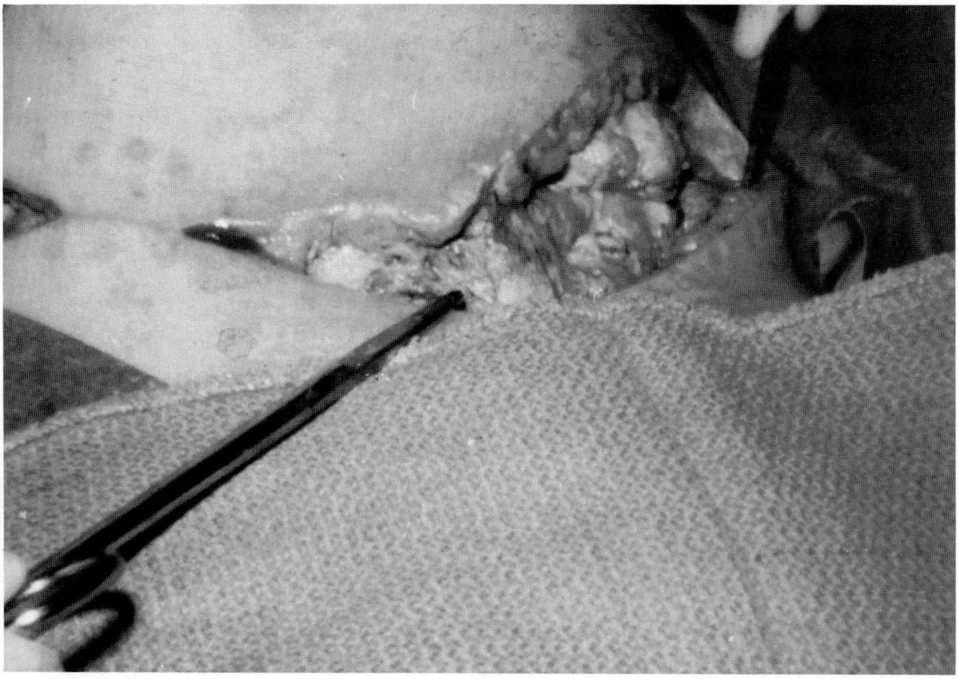

Figure 1 The pancreas transplant is seen in the deep areas of this wound. Infection and necrotic tissue from pancreatic secretions is evident. After debridement, drainage, and antibiotic irrigation, this wound healed satisfactorily.

antibiotic coverage. The initial approach is similar to that described in Chapter 13. Thereafter, specific treatment will be pursued when cultures have identified the microorganisms.

E. Myocardial Infarction

The incidence of myocardial infarction in juvenile diabetic patients is higher than in the general population, due to coronary vessel involvement secondary to diabetes mellitus. Immediately after pancreatic transplantation, we have found that myocardial infarction can be a cause of increased mortality unless careful selection of candidates is obtained through cardiac radionuclide imaging or hemodynamic measurements [16]. If the left ventricular ejection fraction is less than 50%, we are currently not recommending transplantation in these patients [16].

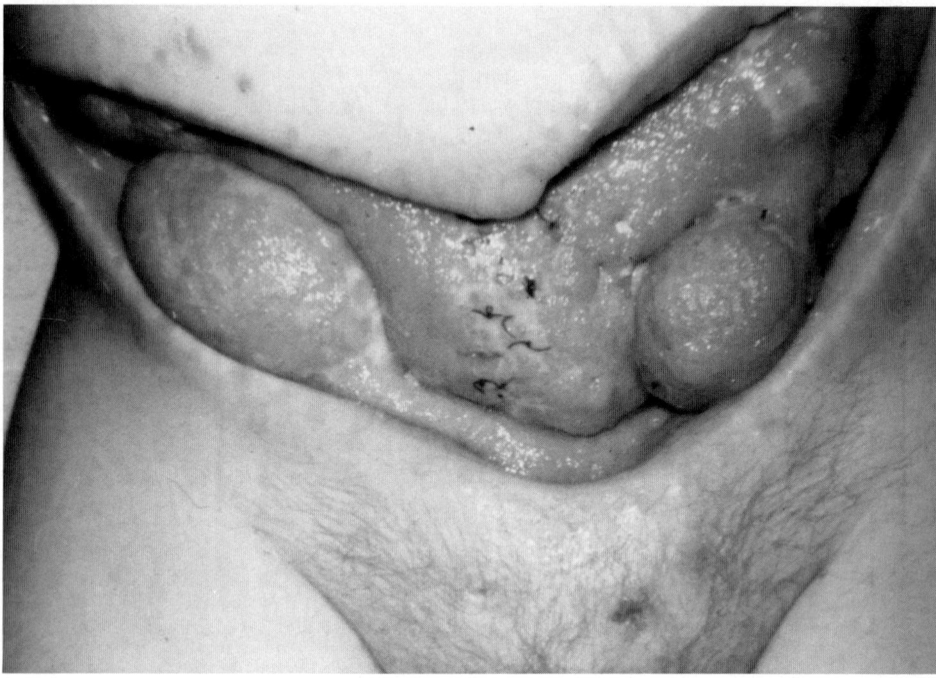

Figure 2A Kidney transplant on the right side (left side of figure) and pancreas transplant on the left side (right side of figure) are shown in this figure with granulation tissue covering them. The bladder is also exposed, with several suture lines present. Because of urinary leakage and subsequent leakage of the pancreatic secretions, the healing of the wound was impaired and the whole area had to be exposed to let it heal by second intention.

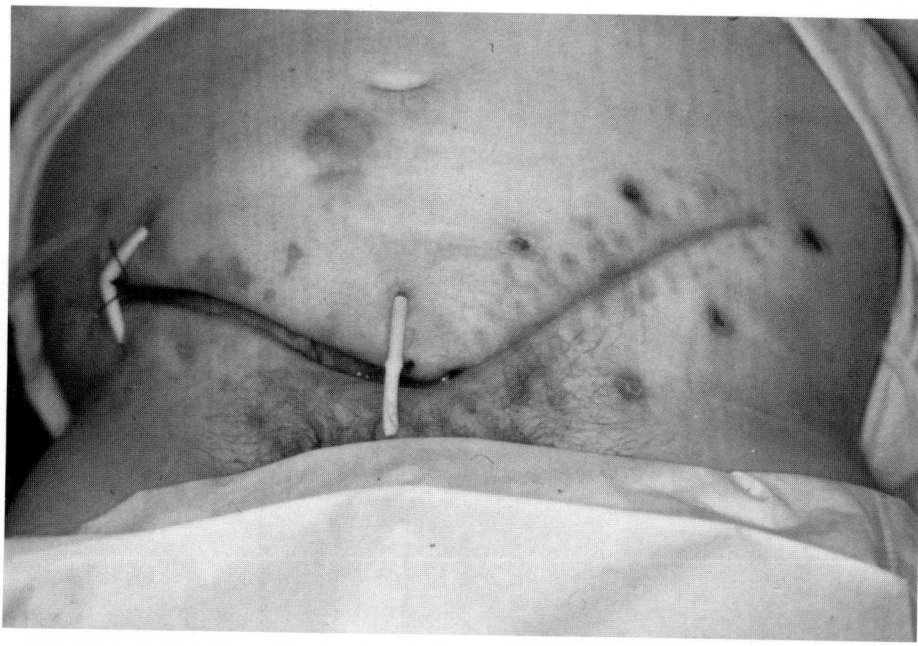

Figure 2B Pancreas transplant incision seen in Figure 2A is completely healed. Two retention sutures are evident on the kidney transplant side of the incision (left side of figure). This wound healed satisfactorily after 1 month more. The peritoneal catheter on the distal side of the incision can still be seen.

IV. COMPLICATIONS RELATED TO DUCTAL TECHNIQUE AND GRAFT PLACEMENT

Some of the postoperative pancreatic complications are directly related to the placement of the pancreas intraperitoneally or extraperitoneally and the management of the pancreatic duct. These include pancreatitis, peripancreatic fluid collections, pancreatic fibrosis, ascites, pancreatic fistula, leakage of the bowel or urine, and peritonitis.

A. Pancreatitis

This complication can be seen in the immediate postoperative period and can be diagnosed by increased serum and urine amylase levels and an enlarged and tender pancreas. The incidence of pancreatitis in the immediate postoperative period is quite high; however, it usually subsides with conservative management. If the symptoms of pancreatitis do not subside, one should consider the possibility that the pancreatic allograft may be undergoing an acute rejection episode. It is often difficult to differentiate between pancreatitis and rejection. Treatment should include both entities.

B. Peripancreatic Collections

This complication is more often seen with extraperitoneal placement of the pancreas than with the intraperitoneal position. The incidence of peripancreatic collections is also increased after duct ligation or polymer ductal occlusion compared with ductal drainage through the Roux-en-Y or into the bladder. The source of peripancreatic collections is secretions of pancreatic juice from the small unligated pancreatic duct or from the pancreatic surface. These collections can occur anywhere along the length of the transplanted pancreas and can develop into a pancreatic abscess if they become infected. Peripancreatic collections should be surgically drained promptly, once identified by ultrasound examination; otherwise they will usually present on the surface as wound infection. Following drainage, pancreatic fistulas may develop. These should be treated conservatively and should heal within a few weeks.

C. Pancreatic Fibrosis

When ductal ligation or polymer ductal occlusion is used, pancreatic fibrosis is frequently seen after transplantation. This complication is usually peri-insular and results in late graft failure. Open biopsies of long-term occluded grafts have demonstrated that the entire gland is replaced by loose fibrous tissue surrounding well-preserved islets [17-19].

D. Pancreatic Ascites

Ascites may develop after procedures involving open drainage into the intraperitoneal cavity and is often unresponsive to medical therapy. If the pancreatic ascites cannot be managed medically, the duct should be drained into a Roux-en-Y limb of the jejunum, into the urinary bladder, ligated, or occluded with polymer.

E. Pancreatic Fistula

The development of a pancreaticocutaneous fistula is usually related to an unidentified accessory pancreatic duct that secretes pancreatic juice and then collects in a peripancreatic form. Usually these fistulas heal by themselves over a period of time. If they do not heal within 4-6 weeks, the duct should be occluded with a polymer or drained into a Roux-en-Y loop.

F. Leakage

Leakage can result after pancreatic transplantation if the pancreatic duct is anastomosed to a Roux-en-Y of the jejunum, to the urinary bladder, or to the ureter. A small leak may go unidentified; however, a large leak may result in an intraperitoneal collection of fluid at the jejunojejunostomy of the pancreaticojejunostomy site and may lead to intra-abdominal sepsis or peritonitis. Usually, the pancreatic secretions are managed by putting a silastic catheter into the pancreatic duct, which is brought out through a separate incision in the abdominal wall as a controlled pancreatic fistula. The incidence of intestinal leak is low but has been documented in various series [14,20]. Once it is suspected, a prompt exploration of the pancreatic graft is advisable. An intestinal leak is properly managed by reinforcing the anastomosis, reanastomosing the duct to the Roux-en Y jejunal limb, or taking down the anastomosis and occluding the pancreatic duct.

Urinary leak can be encountered when the pancreatic duct is anastomosed to either the ureter to the urinary bladder. Leakage from the ureter or the bladder is directly related to improper technique or secondary to infection of pancreatic juices. In both these cases, the pancreatic duct should be cannulated and brought out into the urinary bladder either directly or through the ureter into the urinary bladder. Urinary leaks can be diagnosed by a cystogram, which will show extravasation of the urine at the site of the anastomosis or the site of the anterior cystotomy. The leak should be explored immediately, and its site should be repaired. A Foley catheter should be maintained for 4-6 weeks in either of these cases (Fig. 3).

A pancreatic leak may also come from an unidentified accessory pancreatic

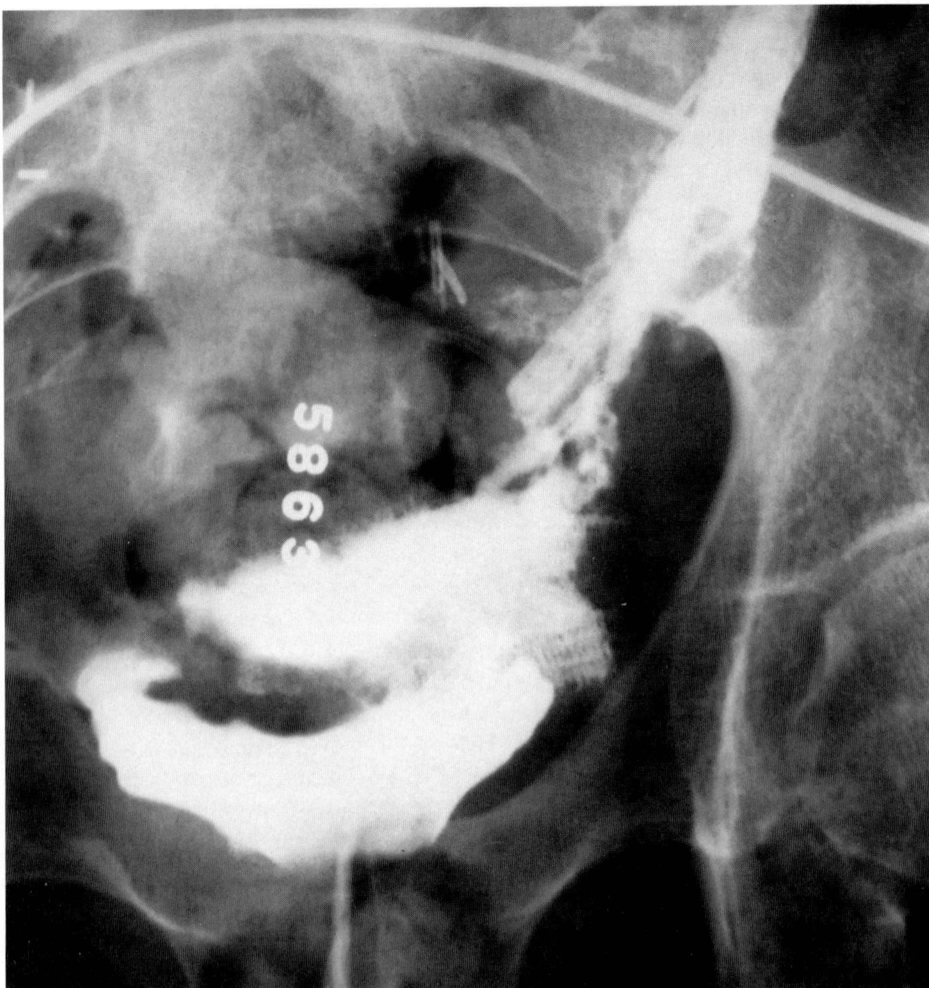

Figure 3 Persistent urinary leak at the pancreaticocystostomy site, which was treated conservatively.

duct or, in cases in whom the pancreatic duct has not been directly cannulated and erroneously brought out, either from the surface or from the urinary bladder. The pancreatic leak should be explored immediately and drained outside, or a pancreatic fistula will result.

G. Peritonitis

This complication can result following pancreatic transplantation from a leak after pancreaticojejunostomy or from infected pancreatic ascites. Peritonitis can also be encountered after pancreaticocystostomy if urine and pancreatic juice enter the abdominal cavity and become infected. Usually, the patient will have an acute abdomen. These patients should be promptly explored and managed by reimplanting the Roux-en-Y limb or by external drainage.

V. COMPLICATIONS OF PANCREATIC TRANSPLANTATION AT MAJOR INSTITUTIONS

A. University of Minnesota, Minneapolis

The first pancreatic transplant in a human was performed at the University of Minnesota [1], and over the next 7 years, 14 transplants were performed, including 1 whole-pancreas transplant. Of these 14 transplants, 3 grafts failed solely for technical reasons (1 from vascular thrombosis, 1 from donor ischemia, and 1 from duodenal necrosis). A single pancreas allograft was rejected. A total of 9 patients died with functioning grafts. Complications and causes of death in these patients included sepsis, septicemia, hyperkalemic cardiac arrest, abscess, stroke, perforation of grafted duodenum, infarction of graft duodenum and sepsis, and bleeding cecal ulcer and sepsis. A single recipient, in whom the graft was removed at 6 weeks, also had a pancreatic fistula. Only a transplant functioned for more than a year.

Between 1978 and 1983, 86 more pancreatic transplants were performed at Minnesota [11]. The 1-year actuarial patient survival rate after primary transplantation in these 86 patients was 85%, whereas the overall 1-year actuarial graft survival rate in these patients was 28%. Of the 60 technically successful pancreatic allografts, 41 had rejection episodes in the form of hyperglycemia interpreted as rejection. The various causes of graft loss were technical failures, rejection, sepsis, or death of a patient with a functioning graft. Of the grafts, 22 failed from technical reasons, which included 9 from vascular thrombosis, 4 from peritonitis, 3 from inadequate preservation, 2 from ascites, 1 from bleeding in a patient who had a concomitant myocardial infarction and died with a functioning graft, 1 from chemical peritonitis, and 2 from anastomitic leaks and peritonitis. A total of 35 functioned for 1-13 months before completely failing from rejection, fibrosis, or sepsis. A total of 5 patients died with functioning grafts. Outcomes of graft survival were related to ductal management, donor source, type of immunosuppression, and the treatment of rejection episodes. There was a 15% mortality in this report that included mainly myocardial infarction, sepsis, and peritonitis.

Transplant-related complications in the second series of 86 patients at Minnesota occurred in 16 patients [21]. These included bleeding requiring reoperation in 1 case, anastomotic leak requiring reoperation in 1 case, wound dehiscence requiring reoperation in 1 case, prolonged ileus in 1 case, severe ascites in 2 cases, peripancreatic graft pain attributed to graft pancreatitis in 2 cases, pancreatic graft fistula in 3 cases, and pancreatic pseudocyst or lymphocele treated by operative drainage in 4 cases.

In a recent review of 116 cases of pancreas transplantation at the University of Minnesota, the occurrences of postoperative infection were documented [22]. Of these, 26 recipients (22%) had intra-abdominal infections. In cases with enteric drainage, infections occurred in 19 of 57 patients. There was also a 33% rate of infection in the 15 pancreatic transplants managed by free intraperitoneal drainage. The infection rate was substantially lower (3%), however, in the 39 pancreas transplants managed by polymer injection. Of the 2 cases with pancreaticocystostomy, 1 developed an infection postoperatively. *Escherichia coli,* enterococci, Bacteroides, and several anaerobes were cultured from the patients with enteric drainage, and staphylococci were associated with open duct drainage. Fungal infections with *Candida* were found with all techniques.

B. Herriot Hospital, Lyon

A total of 59 pancreatic transplants were performed from 1976 to 1985 in Lyon [9]. In 44 cases, kidney and pancreas grafts from the same donor were grafted simultaneously, and in 12 cases only the pancreas was transplanted [7]. In most cases the duct was occluded by using neoprene. A total of 14 patients had pancreatic graft function varying from 3 to 42 months. Losses of pancreatic grafts were due to rejection in 11 cases and vascular thrombosis in 5 cases. Vascular thrombosis occurred generally early in the postoperative period. Postoperative local infections with or without residual pancreatic leakage were encountered in 28% of the patients. The local infections occurred more frequently in extraperitoneal grafts than in intraperitoneally placed grafts. All these were treated conservatively, and in most instances, this complication was resolved within 2 months. In the 12 patients who died, deaths were related to vascular problems in 4 cases, chronic hepatitis in 1 case, pulmonary embolism in 1, disseminated intravascular coagulation after irreversible kidney rejection in 1, lymphoproliferative syndrome in 3, acute graft pancreatitis in 1, and septicemia in 1. According to this group's experience, elimination of pancreatic ductal anastomosis by duct occlusion of the segmental pancreatic graft greatly simplifies pancreatic transplantation in end-stage diabetic patients, who are usually in a precarious condition. The Lyon group advocates simultaneous pancreatic and kidney transplantation in uremic diabetic patients because elevated serum creatinine values from kidney rejection can be used to diagnose rejection earlier than a rise in plasma glucose from pancreatic rejection.

C. Huddinge Hospital, Stockholm

A method including segmental pancreatic transplantation with enteric exocrine diversion in three patients was successfully reported by the Stockholm group [21]. Since then they have performed 29 combined renal and pancreatic transplants by draining the exocrine secretions into the Roux-en-Y limb of the jejunum, with temporary pancreatic duct tube drainage to the exterior. Of the 29 patients, 3 died of peritonitis, cardiovascular failure, and *Pneumocystic carinii* pneumonia, respectively. In 2 patients, the renal grafts were retained [2].

These 29 patients were divided into two subgroups based on the length of cold ischemia and the use of systemic anticoagulation. The first subgroup, with longer cold ischemia and no systemic anticoagulation used, were 13 transplants between 1981 and 1983. There were 7 early graft losses due to severe graft pancreatitis. Of these 7 transplants, 4 grafts underwent arterial or venous thrombosis: 1 patient had an exocrine pancreatic fistula, 1 had an arterial embolus in conjunction with myocardial infarction, and 1 had chronic rejection. In the second subgroup, transplanted between 1984 and 1985, 16 pancreatic transplants were performed. In this whole group, the ischemia time was less than 6 hr, and the patients were given systemic anticoagulation therapy with heparin. No grafts were lost from graft pancreatitis or thrombosis; however, there were two early graft failures, one attributable to intra-abdominal abscess formation and the other subsequent to severe bleeding from the cut end of the pancreatic graft. A single patient died with a functioning graft.

D. University of Munich

Through November 1985, 38 pancreas transplants were reported from this center to the International Pancreas Transplant Registry [9]. Posttransplant complications have been reported in 28, in whom the pancreatic duct was obliterated with Ethibloc [18]. All patients in this series received cyclosporine for immunosuppression. Posttransplant complications were related to the position of the transplant. In 22 pancreas allografts placed extraperitoneally, there were 2 wound hematomas, 4 peripancreatic fluid collections, 12 pancreatic fistulas, and 3 fistulas and wound infections. In the group of intraperitoneally placed grafts, small bowel obstruction in 2 patients required surgery. Actuarial patient survival in the entire group of 29 patients was 88%, and graft survival was 52.8%.

E. University of Wisconsin, Madison

Pancreatic transplantation was performed by the Wisconsin group with anastomosis of the pancreatic duct to the urinary bladder, an extension of Gliedman's earlier work in which the ureter was anastomosed to the pancreatic duct [4]. Through November 1985, this center reported 34 pancreas transplants to the

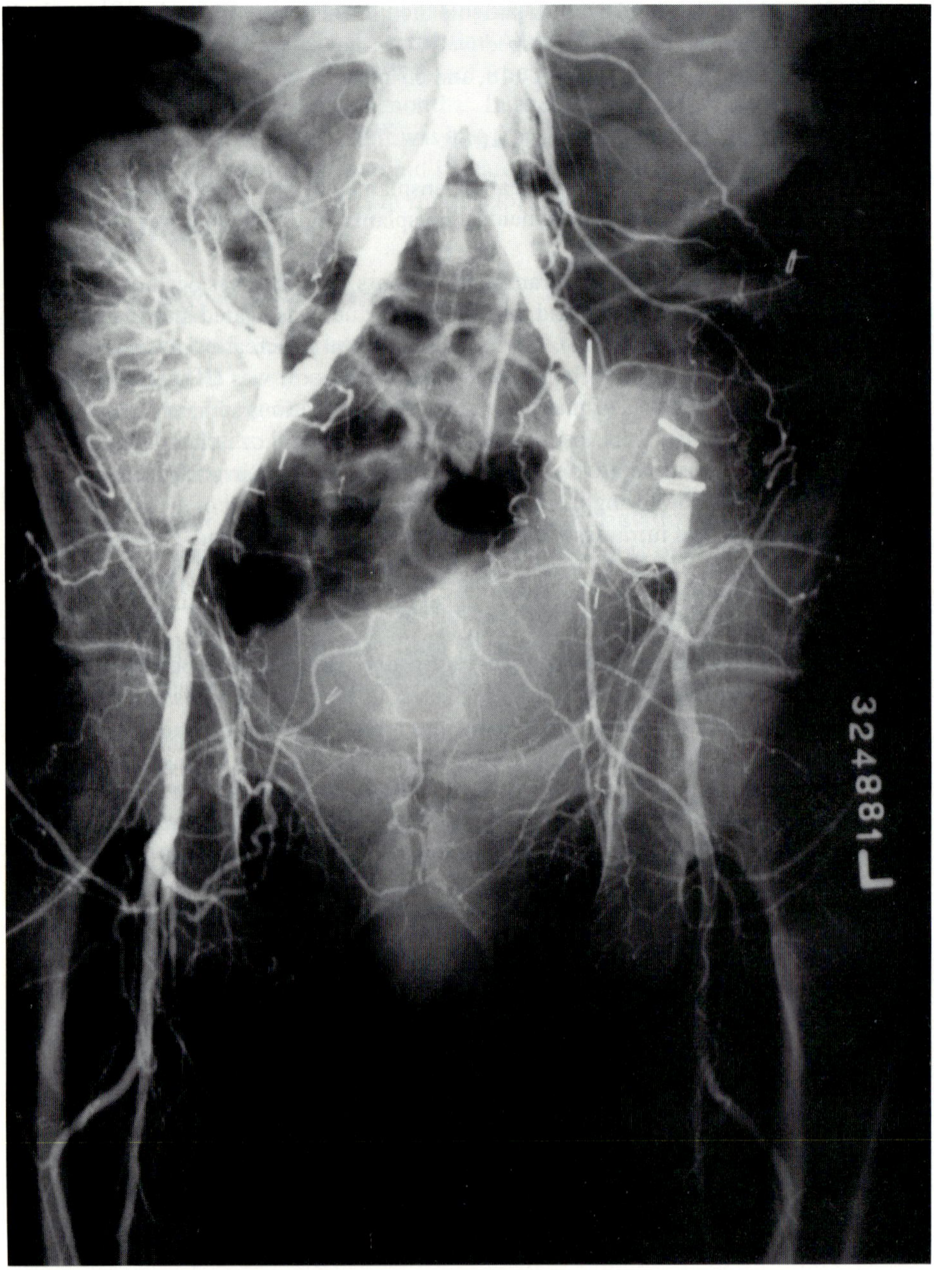

Figure 4 Distal femoral artery occlusion following combined kidney and pancreas transplantation.

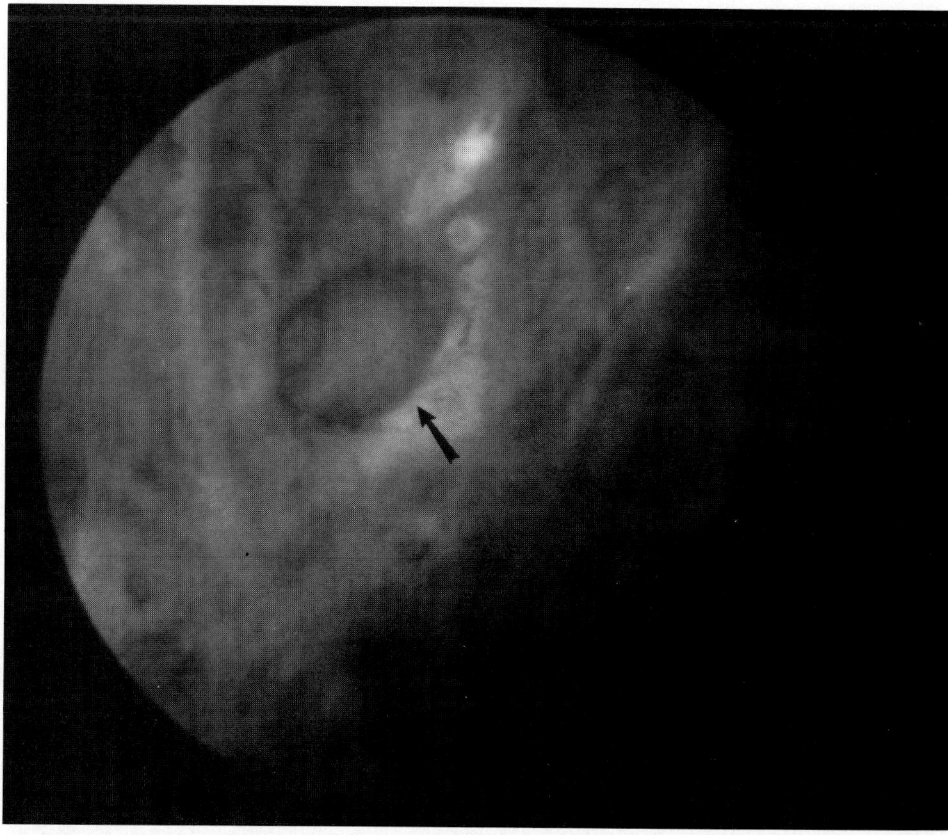

Figure 5 Cystoscopic view of the bladder mucosa and the pancreatic papilla (indicated by arrow). Note the cystitis evident in the bladder mucosa.

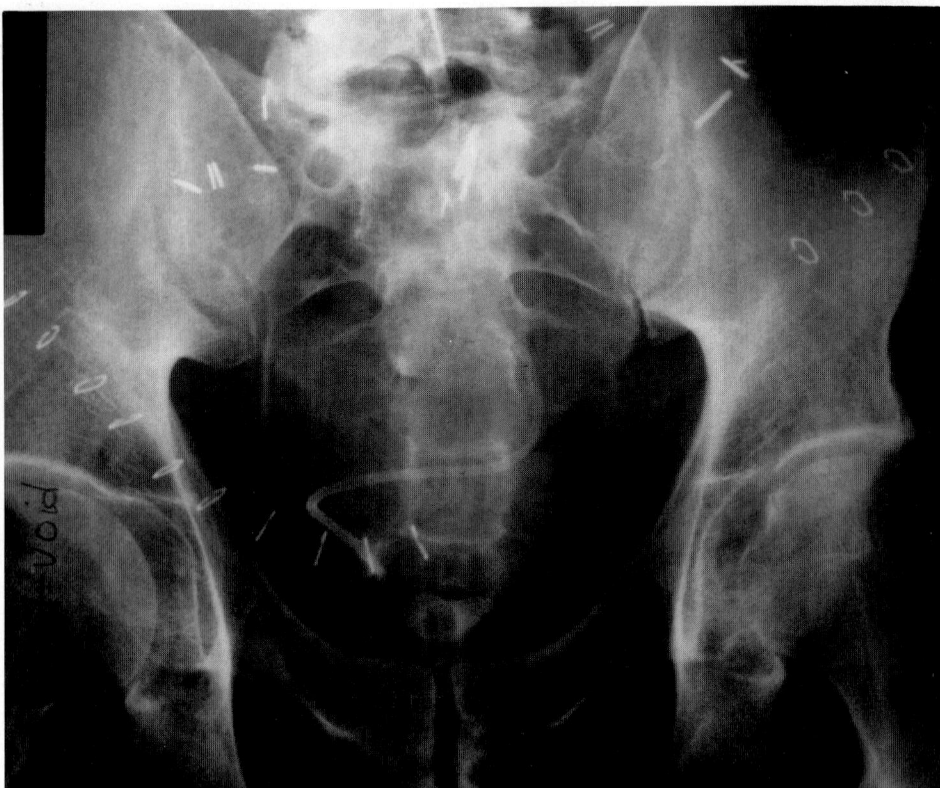

Figure 6 Silicone stent in bladder through the pancreaticocystostomy.

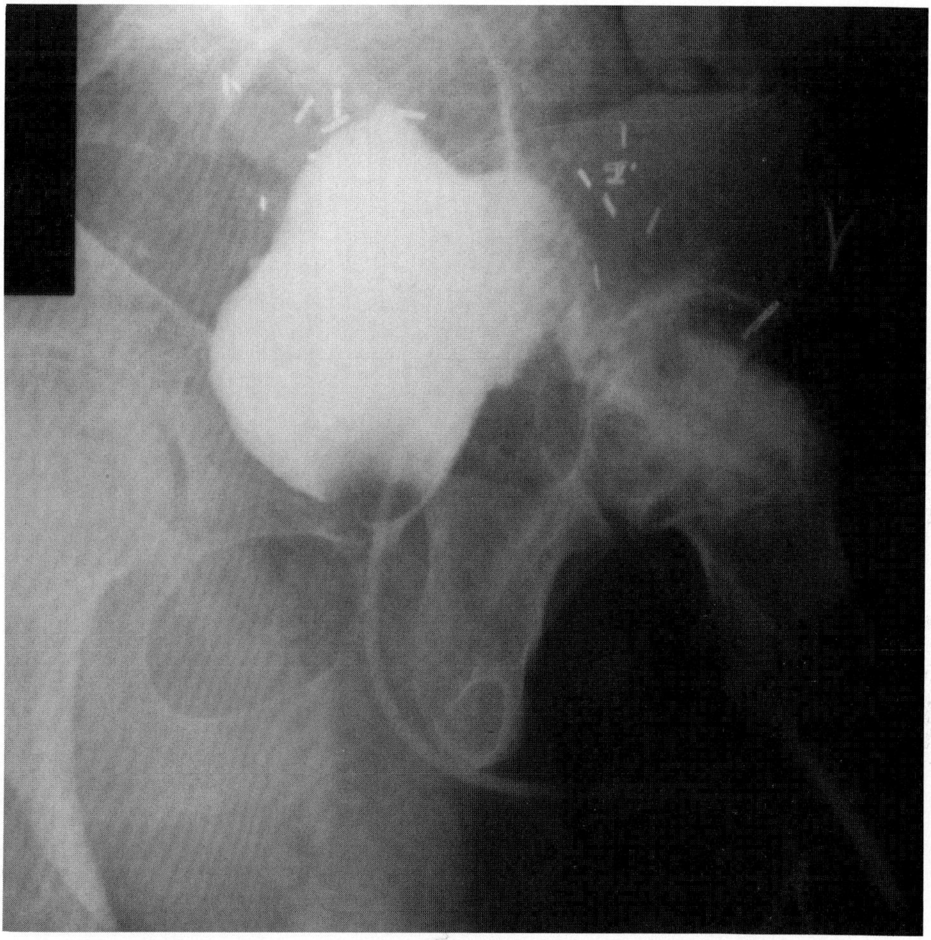

Figure 7A Cystogram showing the extravasation of the dye at the pancreatico-cystostomy site.

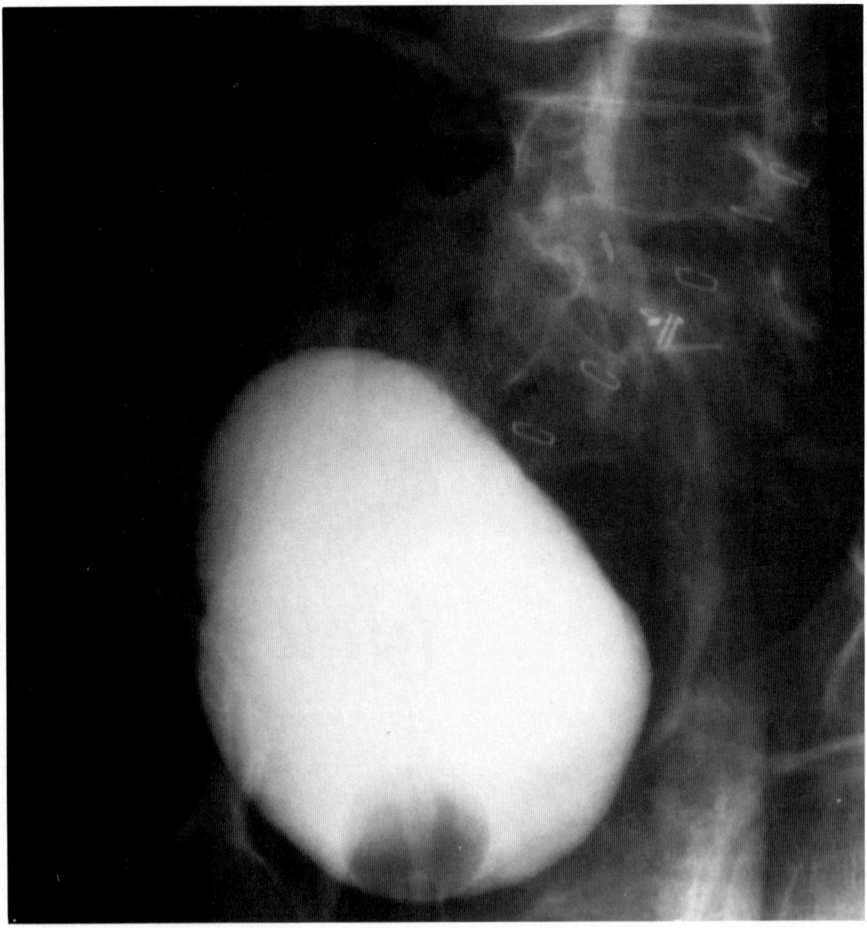

Figure 7B Normal cystogram following combined kidney and pancreas transplantation.

VI. SUMMARY

Although the technical aspects of pancreatic transplantation are important, the major cause of graft failure in all the reported series continues to be rejection and problems associated with the management of the exocrine pancreatic secretions. We hope that refinement of the various immunnosuppressive protocols for the treatment of rejection and management of the pancreatic duct will result in the development of a more effective, safe, and improved regimen for pancreatic transplantation.

REFERENCES

1. Kelly, W. D., Lillehei, R. C., Merkel, F. K., et al.: Allotransplantation of the pancreas and duodenum along with the kidney in diabetic nephropathy. Surgery 61:827-837, 1967.
2. Groth, C. G., and Tyden, G.: Strategy 2: Pancreatic transplantation with enteric drainage of the exocrine pancreas. Transplant. Immunol. Lett. 2(3): 1, 4-5, 1985.
3. Gliedman, M. L., Gold, M., Whittaker, J., et al.: Pancreatic duct to ureter anastomosis for exocrine drainage in pancreatic transplantation. Am. J. Surg. 125:245-252, 1973.
4. Sollinger, H. W., Kalayoglu, M., Hoffman, R. M., et al.: Results of segmental and pancreaticosplenic transplantation with pancreaticocystostomy. Transplant. Proc. 17:360-362, 1985.
5. Land, W., Liebe, W., Kuhlmann, H., et al.: Simultaneous kidney and pancreas transplantation using prolamine for duct obstruction. Transplant. Proc. 12:76-77, 1980.
6. Brynger, H., Blohme, G., Claes, G., et al.: Transplantation of a duct-ligated pancreatic allograft to a diabetic patient. Scand. J. Urol. Nephrol. 24(Suppl.); 59-62, 1975.
7. Dubernard, J. M., Traeger, J., Neyra, P., et al.: A new method of preparation of segmental pancreatic grafts for transplantation. Trials in dogs and in man. Surgery 81:633-639, 1978.
8. Sutherland, D. E. R., Goetz, F. C., Rynasiewicz, J. J., et al.: Segmental pancreas transplantation from living related and cadaver donors: A clinical experience. Surgery 90:159-169, 1981.
9. Sutherland, D. E. R.: Data from International Pancreas Transplant Registry, personal communication.
10. Toledo-Pereyra, L. H.: Pancreas transplantation. In: Toledo-Pereyra, L. H., ed. The Pancreas–Principles of Medical and Surgical Practice, New York: John Wiley & Sons, 1985, pp. 439-464.
11. Sutherland, D. E. R., and Najarian, J. S.: Pancreas and islet transplantation. In: Brooks, ed. Surgery of the Pancreas, Philadelphia: W. B. Saunders Co., 1983, pp. 434-471.

12. Toledo-Pereyra, L. H., Zeskind, H. J., and Mittal, V. K.: Ultrasound imaging of clinical pancreatic organ transplants. J. Clin. Ultrasound 10:121, 1982.
13. Toledo-Pereyra, L. H., Kristen, K. T., and Mittal, V. K.: Scintigraphy of pancreatic transplants. AJR 138:621-622, 1982.
14. Starzl, R. E., Iwatsuki, S., Shaw, B. W., et al.: Pancreaticoduodenal transplantation in humans. Surg. Gynecol. Obstet. 159:256-272, 1984.
15. Calne, R. Y., McMaster, P., Rolles, K., et al.: Technical observations in segmental pancreatic allografting: Observations on blood flow. Transplant. Proc. 12:51-57, 1980.
16. Toledo-Pereyra, L. H.: The importance of myocardial imaging as a selection criterion of patients prior to pancreas transplantation. Transplant. Proc. 16: 671, 1984.
17. Toledo-Pereyra, L. H., Baxter, J. R., Choudhury, S., et al.: Pancreatitis vs. rejection in human pancreatic transplantation. Unresolved pathological findings. Bol. Asoc. Med. P. R. 74:172, 1982.
18. Land, W., Landgraf, R., Illnew, W. D., et al.: Improved results in combined segmental pancreatic and renal transplantation in diabetic patients under cyclosporine therapy. Transplant. Proc. 17:317-324, 1985.
19. Blanc-Brunat, N., Dubernard, J. M., Touraine, J. L., et al.: Pathology of the pancreas after intraductal neoprene injection in dogs and diabetic patients treated by pancreatic transplantation. Diabetologia 25:97-107, 1983.
20. Lillehei, R. C., Ruiz, J. O., Aquino, C., et al.: Transplantation of the pancreas. Acta Endocrinol. (Copenh.) 83:303-321, 1976.
21. Groth, C. G., Collste, H., Lundgren, G., et al.: Successful outcome of segmental human pancreatic transplantation with enteric exocrine diversion after modifications in technique. Lancet 2:522-524, 1982.
22. Hesse, U. J., Sutherland, D. E. R., Simmons, R. L., et al.: Intra-abdominal infections in pancreas transplant recipients. Ann. Surg. 203:153-162, 1986.
23. Brekke, I. B., Bergan, A., Heen, L., et al.: Pancreatic endocrine function after duct occlusion in humans. Transplant. Proc. 16:739-740, 1984.
24. Baumgartner, D.: Simultaneous renal and intraperitoneal segmental pancreatic transplantation. Surg. Rounds December 1985, pp. 37-44.
25. Toledo-Pereyra, L. H., and Mittal, V. K.: Segmental pancreatic transplantation. Arch. Surg. 117:505-508, 1982.
26. Toledo-Pereyra, L. H., and Mittal, V. K.: Clinical segmental pancreatic transplantation. Am. Surg. 48:584-593, 1082.
27. Cederna, J., and Toledo-Pereyra, L. H.: Clinical pancreas transplantation. Contemp. Surg. 24:53, 1984.
28. Toledo-Pereyra, L. H.: Pancreas transplantation. Surg. Gynecol. Obstet. 157:49-56, 1983.
29. Sutherland, D. E. R., and Kendall, D.: Clinical pancreas and islet transplant registry report. Transplant. Proc. 17:307-311, 1985.

16
Complications of Islet Cell Transplantation

LUIS H. TOLEDO-PEREYRA
Mount Carmel Mercy Hospital, Detroit, Michigan

I. INTRODUCTION

Islet cell transplantation has been developed in the past decade with two major applications in mind, autotransplantation and allotransplantation. Autotransplantation has been used as a means of preserving the function of the islets of Langerhans when the pancreas must be removed for such reasons as intractable pain from chronic pancreatitis. Islet cell allotransplantation has been approached as a potential alternative to pancreas transplantation for patients with diabetes mellitus. This chapter presents the complications of both these procedures and summarizes their current clinical status.

II. PANCREATIC ISLET CELL AUTOTRANSPLANTATION

In cases of chronic pancreatitis requiring total or near-total pancreatectomy for relief of pain, islet cell autotransplantation has been used in an effort to avoid iatrogenic diabetes. As expected, however, the pancreatic tissue removed from these patients is often fibrous, necessitating more extensive processing than for pancreases from cadaver sources used for allotransplantation. Although there are no problems with histocompatibility, reintroduction of the pancreatic tissue into a suitable site has sometimes been associated with morbidity and even mortality.

A. Complications Associated with Patient Selection

Candidates for islet cell autotransplantation are carefully screened to assess their α- and β-cell reserves. Ideally, only those patients with normal carbohydrate tolerance are suitable as self-donors, since insulin-independent diabetes develops in 12-45% of the patients with chronic pancreatitis [1]. At our center, pretransplant metabolic evaluation is performed on two separate days before pancreatectomy. An oral glucose tolerance test, using 100 g glucose, is given and serial blood determinations of glucose, insulin, and human C-peptide are done. On the following day, evaluation of the α-cell reserve is carried out by administration of arginine (0.5 g/kg body weight, maximum dose 30 g), over 30 min, followed by serial measurements of plasma glucagon, glucose, insulin, and human C-peptide levels. Complications of patient selection include the potential for inaccurate assessment of α- and β-cell reserves resulting in transplantation of inappropriate candidates who do not have sufficient islet cell function to potentially maintain normoglycemia after autotransplantation. These patients would be unnecessarily exposed to the inherent risks of the procedure.

B. Islet Cell Autograft Preparation

As the pancreatectomy is being performed, the mobile islet cell laboratory at our center awaits receipt of the pancreatic tissue as soon as it is removed. As previously mentioned, the fibrous nature of these pancreases usually necessitates more extensive processing than for a cadaver pancreas. Often the surgeon will need to trim away areas, such as a pseudocyst, that cannot be used for processing. Once the workbench dissection has been performed under a laminar flow hood, the pancreas is mechanically minced, washed, and digested with collagenase. (The details of the method will be described in the islet cell allotransplantation section.) The collagenase is then removed by multiple centrifugal washes, and the islet preparation is ready for reimplantation. It is important to minimize processing time, since the patient and surgeon must wait for the return of the graft. An experienced team can usually process the pancreas in 1-1½ hr.

Complications associated with this technique are low islet cell yield, contamination of the preparation, potential preparation of thrombogenic material if not enough fibrotic fissure is removed, tissue damage if collagenase is not entirely removed, warm ischemia, and lack of viability (Table 1).

Table 1 Complications Associated with Islet Cell Preparation

Low islet cell yield
Microbial contamination
Injection of thrombogenic material
Tissue damage from collagenase
Tissue damage from warm ischemia
Loss of viability during processing

C. Choice of Transplant Site and Associated Complications

Postoperative complications after islet cell autotransplantation have been closely associated with the choice of transplant site (Table 2). The majority of cases have used intraportal injection as the chosen technique [2-12]. Intramuscular islet cell autotransplantation has also been used by Valente et al. in at least two patients [6]. Recently, we have also tested the use of the renal subcapsular region for islet cell placement [13].

A number of reports in the literature have documented postoperative complications after intraportal infusion of islet cell autografts. Transient elevations in portal pressure occur frequently at the time of islet cell infusion via the portal vein [1-4,7,11,12]. Often, the rise in portal pressures precludes infusion of the entire islet preparation. Experimental and clinical studies show, however, that the portal pressure returns to normal in the majority of cases after surgery. Changes in portal pressure during islet cell autotransplantation appear to be related to the rate of islet infusion and the amount of tissue being transplanted. More severe systemic hypotension and portal hypertension have been observed by ourselves and others in a limited number of cases [14,15]. It has been hypothesized that injection of the cellular suspension causes vasodilation, leading to hypotension and compensatory tachycardia [14]. Persistent portal hyperten-

Table 2 Postoperative Complications After Islet Cell Transplantation

Early
Transient elevations of portal venous pressure
Systemic hypotension
Shock
Temporary or permanent hepatic dysfunction
Hepatic infarction
Portal vein thrombosis
Disseminated intravascular coagulation
Bleeding
Infection
Rejection (allograft)
(Death)
Late
Rejection (allograft)
Sepsis
(Death)

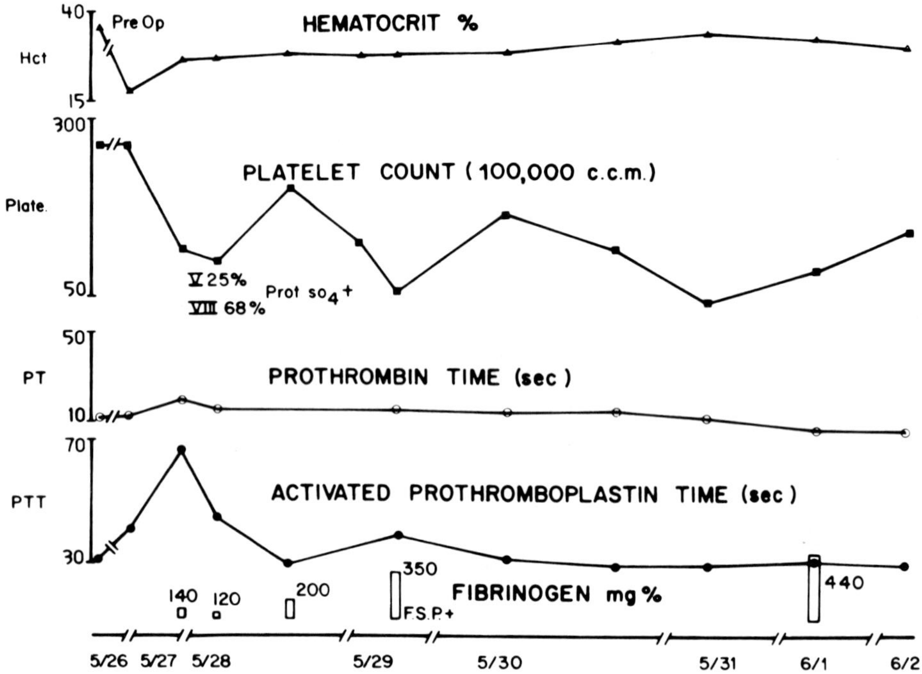

Figure 1 Sequential postoperative hematologic changes of disseminated intravascular coagulation (DIC) in a patient receiving an intraportal islet cell autotransplant after 85% pancreatectomy. After the islet cell infusion, the patient developed portal hypertension, systemic hypotension, and deep hemorrhagic shock. Military antishock trousers were applied for 30 hr while coagulation disturbances were being corrected. During the 16-day stay in the intensive care unit, the patient developed jaundice, confusion and agitation, high cardiac output failure, respiratory failure, and a subphrenic abscess. The patient expired 39 days after initial surgery. (From Mittal et al. [14], used with permission of Williams and Wilkins.)

sion has led to portal vein thrombosis and death in two patients [16,17]. Mesmic et al. [17] have reported bleeding esophageal varices together with portal vein thrombosis after islet cell autotransplantation, which required a mesocaval H graft to correct the portal pressure. The development of portal hypertension, shock, and disseminated intravascular coagulation after intraportal islet infusion has been observed by ourselves [15] and others [18,19] (Fig. 1). The addition of heparin and aprotinin (Trasylol) to the preparation prior to injection or systemic heparinization has proven useful for reducing the frequency of portal hypertension [4]. In addition, adequate washing of the islet cell preparation after collagenase digestion is important since the trypsin activity in the collagenase and trypsin released by damaged pancreatic cells may contribute to the pathogenesis of DIC. Other complications that have been observed after intraportal islet injection include temporary or permanent hepatic dysfunction and hepatic infarction (Fig. 2) [16,20].

D. Islet Cell Autotransplantation Results

When the worldwide results of islet autotransplantation for the major centers are compared, varying amounts of success have been obtained. The extent of pancreatectomy in these cases has ranged from about 70% to greater than 95%. When less than 90% of the pancreas is removed, there is a greater chance that the patient will be insulin independent because of the function of the remnant pancreas supplemented by the autotransplanted islets. As the extent of pancreatectomy increases, a greater burden of function is placed on the transplanted islet cells. This is observed in the differences between the results reported (Table 3) with total or near-total pancreatectomies versus those with partial pancreatectomy. Success for islet cell autotransplantation after pancreatectomy ranges from 25 to 40%. The details of our series of islet cell autotransplants are shown in Table 4 [12]. In summary, with the limited clinical experience in islet cell autotransplantation worldwide, there is still room for further developments in techniques of pancreas preparation and choice of sites for implantation.

E. New Approaches for Islet Cell Autotransplantation

The complications encountered with placement of islet cell autografts in the intraportal and intrasplenic sites have led us to investigate the use of the renal subcapsular region for islet cell engraftment. Our results obtained with the experimental use of this site for islet cell allotransplantation will be discussed in detail in that section. Thus far, we have used these techniques for two cases of autotransplantation following near-total pancreatectomy for chronic pancreatitis (Table 4). Both patients remained insulin independent up to 24 and 12 months, respectively.

III. PANCREATIC ISLET CELL ALLOTRANSPLANTATION

Initial difficulties encountered with the use of pancreatic transplantation led to the consideration of islet cell allotransplantation as an alternative procedure for the amelioration of diabetes mellitus. Experimental studies in rodents were very encouraging in this field [21-24]; however, subsequent work using larger animals has provided a more realistic view of the challenges to success in the clinical setting [25-29]. The problems of obtaining a sufficient yield to ameliorate diabetes

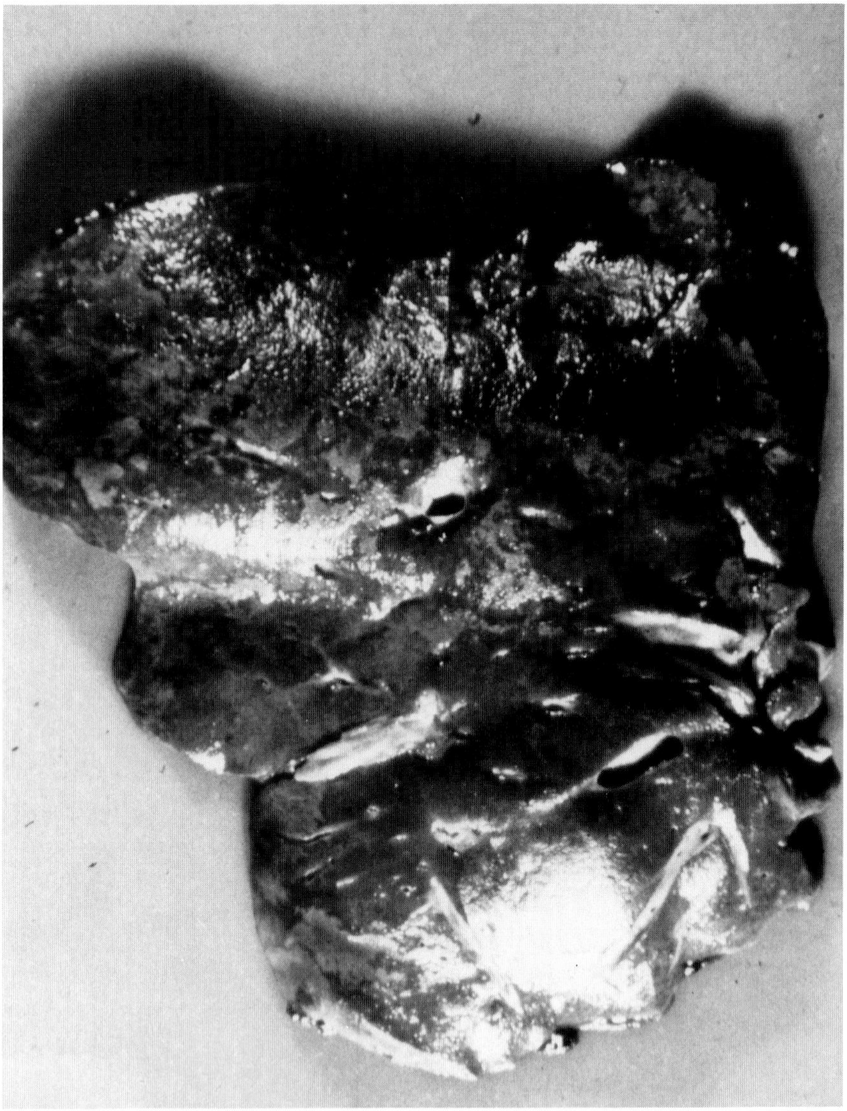

Figure 2 Postmortem liver specimen showing hepatic infarction following intraportal islet cell autotransplantation after a 95% pancreatectomy. Postoperatively the patient developed significant hypotension on day 5, DIC, and sepsis and expired 10 days after transplantation.

Table 3 Comparison of Results at Major Centers Reporting Islet Cell Autotransplantation

Authors	Year	No. patients, extent of pancreatectomy	% Insulin independent	Complications
Sutherland et al. [2,3]	1978	1 Total	25˙	Transient elevation in portal pressure in some patients during infusion
	1980	12 Near total (90%)		
Morrow et al. [4]	1985			
Dobroschke et al. [5]	1978	1 Near total	0	–
		3 Total		
Valente et al. [6]	1980	11 Partial	91[a]	None
Cameron et al. [7]	1980	8 Near total	37.5	Transient elevation in portal pressure during infusion
Lorenz and Wolf [8]	1980	6 Total	60	–
		4 Near total		
Nardi et al. (Sutherland [9])	1981	1 Partial (subcutaneous injection)	40	-
		2 Total (95%)–portal vein		
		2 Partial (70-80%)–portal vein		
Hinshaw et al. [10]	1981	5 Near total	40	None
Traverso et al. [11]	1981	4 Near total (95%)	40	Systemic hypotension, portal hypertension
Toledo-Pereyra et al. [12]	1983	1 Partial (80%)	33	DIC, hepatic infarction, transient increases in portal pressures, systemic hypotension
		8 Near total		

[a]Better results in this group could probably be attributed to the partial extent of the pancreatectomy.

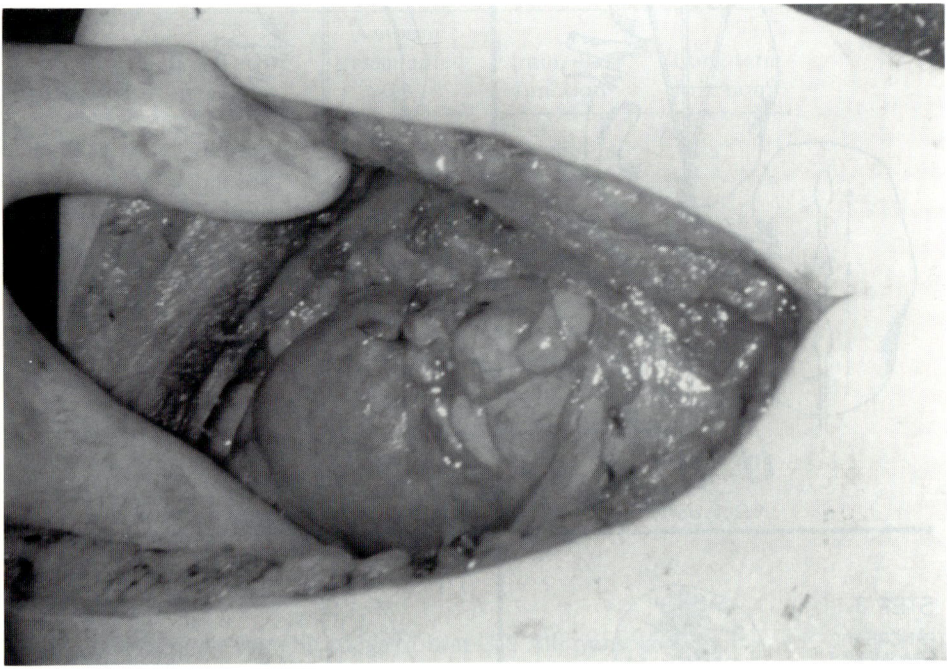

Figure 5 View of recipient kidney after injection of islet cell allograft.

shown that the canine renal subcapsular region provides a good location for islet cell engraftment. In addition, this site has an immunologically privileged character, since long-term islet cell allograft survival has been obtained in totally pancreatectomized animals. Thus far, we have attempted five clinical cases of islet cell allotransplantation in the renal subcapsular site (Fig. 5). Of five patients, two have a $>50\%$ reduction in exogenous insulin and serum C-peptide levels $\geqslant 0.9$ ng/mL at 2 weeks posttransplantation, indicating some immediate function of their islet cell allografts in the early postoperative period. However, long-term graft function has not been obtained.

Although long-term islet function has been achieved in some experimental settings, graft rejection and/or loss of function remain the major obstacles to success in human islet cell allotransplantation. As previously mentioned, the loss or lack of graft function may result from multiple factors, including donor source, tissue preparation, site of the graft, histocompatibility, and steroid administration. It is apparent that successful islet cell transplantation in humans will be dependent on the development of new approaches to solve these problems.

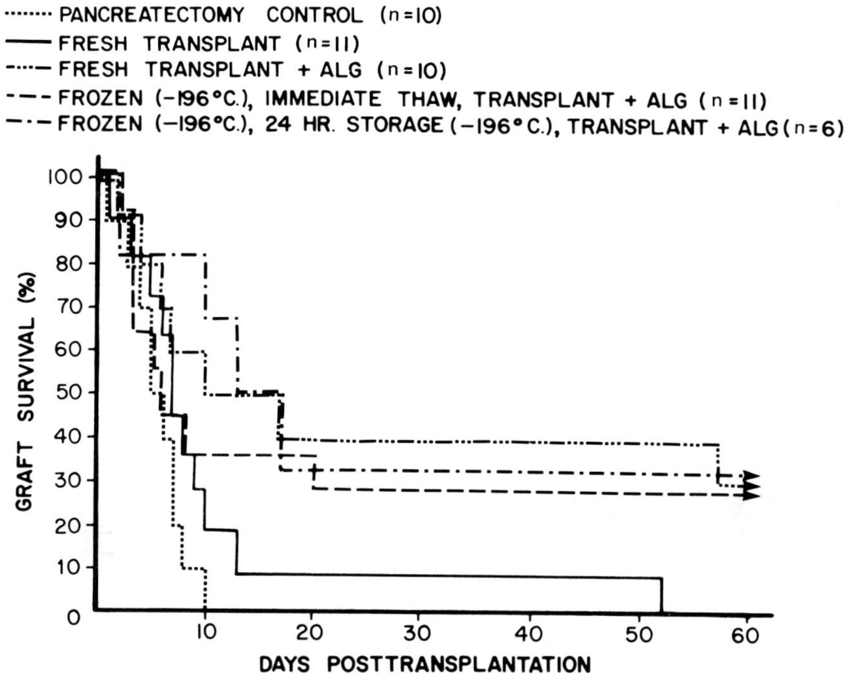

Figure 6 Comparative graft survival of fresh and cryopreserved islet cell allografts transplanted into pancreatectomized dogs. Significant prolongation of allograft survival was observed in all groups pretreated with ALG.

In our laboratories, graft pretreatment of islet cell allografts with various compounds has been tested as a means of altering the immunogenicity of the tissue [49]. Graft pretreatment of canine islet cell allografts with ALG (antilymphoblast globulin) resulted in significant prolongation of graft survival in totally pancreatectomized animals receiving only minimal immunosuppression with azathioprine (2.5-5.0 mg/kg per day) (Fig. 6). ALG graft pretreatment was also used clinically at our center in the first two cases [50]; however, the results were inconclusive because of the prolonged storage of the islet cell tissue prior to transplantation.

REFERENCES

1. Najarian, J. S., Sutherland, D. E. R., and Steffes, M. W.: Isolation of human islets of Langerhans for transplantation. Transplant. Proc. 7:611-613, 1975.

2. Najarian, J. S., Sutherland, D. E. R., Baumgartner, D., et al.: Total or near total pancreatectomy and islet autotransplantation for treatment of chronic pancreatitis. Ann. Surg. 192:526-542, 1980.
3. Sutherland, D. E. R., Matas, A. J., Goetz, F. C., et al.: Transplantation of dispersed pancreatic islet tissue in humans: Autografts and allografts. Diabetes 29(Suppl. 1):31-44, 1980.
4. Morrow, C. E., Cohen, J. I., Sutherland, D. E., and Najarian, J. S.: Chronic pancreatitis: Long-term surgical results of pancreatic duct drainage, pancreatic resection, and near-total pancreatectomy and islet autotransplantation. Surgery 96:608-616, 1984.
5. Dobroschke, J., Schwemmie, K., Langhott, G., et al.: Autotransplantation von Langerhansschen Inseln nach totaler Duodenopankreatokromie bei einer Pancreatitis. Dtsch. Med. Wochenshr. 103:1905-1910, 1978.
6. Valente, U., Ferro, M., Campisi, C., et al.: Report of clinical cases of islet autotransplantation. Transplant. Proc. 12(4, Suppl. 2):202-204, 1980.
7. Cameron, J. L., Mehigan, D. F., Harrington, D. P., et al.: Metabolic studies following intrahepatic autotransplantation of pancreatic islet grafts. Surgery 87:397-400, 1980.
8. Lorenz, D., Wolff, H., and Lippert, H.: The transplantation of islets of Langerhans in patients with chronic pancreatitis. In: Bretzol, R., Federlin, K., and Scholz, H., eds.) Proceedings of the 1980 Geissen Workshop on Islet Isolation, Culture, and Cryopreservation, Stuttgart: Thieme, 1981.
9. Sutherland, D. E. R.: Pancreas and islet transplantation II. Clinical trials. Diabetologia 20:435-450, 1981.
10. Hinshaw, D. B., Jolley, W. B., Hinshaw, D. B., et al.: Islet autotransplantation after pancreatectomy for chronic pancreatitis with a new method of islet of preparation. Am. J. Surg. 142:118-122, 1981.
11. Traverso, L. W., Abou-Zamzam, A. M., and Longmire, W. P.: Human pancreatic cell autotransplantation following total pancreatectomy. Ann. Surg. 193:191-195, 1981.
12. Toledo-Pereyra, L. H.: Islet cell autotransplantation after subtotal pancreatectomy. Arch. Surg. 118:851-858, 1983.
13. Toledo-Pereyra, L. H., Bandlien, K. O., Gordon, D. A., et al.: Renal subcapsular islet cell transplantation. Diabetes 33:910-914, 1984.
14. Torres, L. E., Traverso, L. M., and Sohn, Y. Z.: Intraoperative hemodynamic changes in patients undergoing mixed-cell intraportal autotransplantation of pancreatic tissue. Anesthesiology 53:427-429, 1980.
15. Mittal, V. K., Toledo-Pereyra, L. H., Sharma, M., et al.: Acute portal hypertension and disseminated intravascular coagulation following pancreatic islet autotransplantation after subtotal pancreatectomy. Transplantation 31:302-304, 1981.
16. Walsh, T. J., Eggleston, J. C., and Cameron, J. L.: Portal hypertension, hepatic infarction, and liver failure complicating pancreatic islet autotransplantation. Surgery 91:485-487, 1982.
17. Memsic, L., Busuttil, R. W., and Traverso, L. W.: Bleeding esophageal varices

and portal vein thrombosis after pancreatic mixed-cell autotransplantation. Surgery 95:238-242, 1984.
18. Mehigan, D. G., Bell, W. R., Zuidema, G. D., et al.: Disseminated intravascular coagulation and portal hypertension following pancreatic islet autotransplantation. Ann. Surg. 191:287-293, 1980.
19. Cameron, J. L., Mehigan, D. G., Broe, P. J., et al.: Distal pancreatectomy and islet autotransplantation for chronic pancreatitis. Ann. Surg. 193:312-317, 1981.
20. Toledo-Pereyra, L. H., Rowlett, A. L., Cain, W., et al.: Hepatic infarction following intraportal islet cell autotransplantation after near-total pancreatectomy. Transplantation 38:88-89, 1984.
21. Toledo-Pereyra, L. H.: Variations in dose and time of collagenase digestion for maximal islet cell separation for transplantation. Bol. Asoc. Med. P.R., 72:243-247, 1980.
22. Toledo-Pereyra, L. H., Valjee, K. D., and Zammit, M.: Important factors in islet cell transplantation: The role of pancreatic fragments, size, pH, potassium, concentration, and length of intraportal infusion. Eur. Surg. Res. 12: 72-78, 1980.
23. Ballinger, W. F., and Lacy, P. E.: Transplantation of intact pancreatic islets in rats. Surgery 72:175-186, 1972.
24. Toledo-Pereyra, L. H., Zammit, M., Malcom, S., et al.: Inconsistency of collegenase activity for isolation of islet cells for transplantation. Transplantation 27:222, 1979.
25. Mirkovich, V., and Campiche, M.: Successful intrasplenic autotransplantation of pancreatic tissue in totally pancreatectomized dogs. Transplantation 21:265-269, 1976.
26. Kretschmer, G. J., Sutherland, D. E. R., Matas, A. J., et al.: Autotransplantation of pancreatic islets without separation of exo- and endocrine tissue in totally pancreatectomized dogs. Surgery 82:74-81, 1977.
27. Kretschmer, G. J., Sutherland, D. E. R., Matas, A. J., et al.: Autotransplantation of pancreatic fragments to the portal vein and spleen of totally pancreatectomized dogs. A comparative evaluation. Ann. Surg. 187:79-86, 1978.
28. Kretschmer, G. J., Sutherland, D. E. R., Matas, A. J., et al.: The dispersed pancreas: Transplantation without islet purification in totally pancreatectomized dogs. Diabetologia 13:495-502, 1977.
29. Mehigan, D. G., Ball, W. R., Zuidema, G. D., et al.: Disseminated intravascular coagulation and portal hypertension following pancreatic islet autotransplantation. Ann. Surg. 191:287-193, 1980.
30. Toledo-Pereyra, L. H.: Criteria for patient selection for pancreatic transplantation. Diabetologia 22:298, 1982.
31. Toledo-Pereyra, L. H.: Pancreas transplantation. In: Toledo-Pereyra, L. H., ed., The Pancreas—Principles of Medical and Surgical Practice, New York: John Wiley & Sons, 1985.
32. Toledo-Pereyra, L. H., Valjee, K. D., Castellanos, J., et al.: 24-48 Hour pandreas preservation by hypothermic pulsatile perfusion prior to islet cell transplantation. Arch. Surg. 115:95-98, 1980.

33. Bank, H. L., Davis, R. F., and Emerson, D.: Cryogenic preservation of isolated rat islets of Langerhans: Effect of cooling and warming rates. Diabetologia 16:195-199, 1979.
34. Kemp, J. A., Mazur, P., Mullen, Y., et al.: Reversal of experimental diabetes by fetal rat pancreas. I. Survival and function of fetal rat pancreas fragments to –196°C. Transplant. Proc. 9:325-328, 1977.
35. Kemp, J. A., Mullen, Y., Weissman, H., et al.: Reversal of diabetes in rats using fetal pancreas stored at –196. Transplantation 26:260-264, 1978.
36. Mazur, P., Kemp, J. A., and Miller, R. H.: Survival of fetal rat pancreases frozen to –78 and –196 degrees. Proc. Natl. Acad. Sci. USA 78:4105-4109, 1976.
37. Payne, W. D., Sutherland, D. E. R., Matas, A. J., et al.: Cryopreservation of neonatal rat islet tissue. Surg. Forum 29:347-349, 1978.
38. Rajotte, R. B., Stewart, H. L., Voss, W. A. G., et al.: Viability studies on frozen-thawed rat islets of Langerhans. Cryobiology 14:116-120, 1977.
39. Toledo-Pereyra, L. H., Gordon, D., and MacKenzie, G. H.: Cryopreservation of islets of Langerhans. Cryobiology 18:483-488, 1981.
40. Toledo-Pereyra, L. H., Gordon, D., and MacKenzie, G.: Cryopreservation of whole pancreas versus islet cells. Trans. Am. Soc. Artif. Intern. Organs 27: 259-262, 1981.
41. Kramp, R. C., Cuche, R. Muller, W. A., et al.: Subcutaneous, isogeneic transplantation of duct-ligated pancreas in streptozotocin diabetic mice: Relationships between recovery of hormone contents in transplants or host pancreas. Metabolism 25:1007-1016, 1976.
42. Mangnall, Y., Smythe, A. Slater, D. N., et al.: Neonatal islet cell transplantation in the diabetic rat: Effect on hepatic enzyme activity and glucose homeostatis. J. Endocrinol. 74:231-241, 1977.
43. Matas, A. J., Sutherland, D. E. R., Payne, W. D., et al.: A mouse model of islet transplantation using neonatal donors. Transplantation 24:389-393, 1977.
44. Dafoe, D., Naji, A., Plotkin, S. A., et al.: Susceptibility to diabetogenic virus: Host vs. pancreatic factors. J. Surg. Res. 28:338-347, 1980.
45. Hegre, O. D., Leonard, R. J., Erlandson, S. L., et al.: Transplantation of islet tissue in the rat. Acta Endocrinol. (Copenh.) 83(Suppl. 205):257-278, 1976.
46. Gordon, D. A., MacKenzie, G. H., and Toledo-Pereyra, L. H.: Efficient pancreatic islet cell preparation utilizing a new tissue chopper prior to transplantation. Diabetologia 30:79-80, 1981.
47. Sutherland, D. E. R., and Kendall, D.: Clinical pancreas and islet transplant registry report. Transplant. Proc. 17:307-311, 1985.
48. Sutherland, D. E. R., and Najarian, J. S.: Pancreas and islet transplantation. In: Brooks, J. R., ed.), Surgery of the Pancreas, Philadelphia: W. B. Saunders Co., 1983, p. 434.

49. Toledo-Pereyra, L. H., Gordon, D. A., and MacKenzie, G. H.: Prolongation of pancreatic islet cell allograft survival by graft pretreatment with antilymphoblast globulin. Am. Surg. 48:282-286, 1982.
50. Toledo-Pereyra, L. H., Gordon, D. A., and Mackenzie, G. H.: Islet cell transplantation—experimental observations and initial clinical trials. In: International Symposium on Pancreas—Islet Cell Transplantation and Mechanical Pancreas—Normoglycemia for the Diabetic, May 6-7, 1981, Detroit, Michigan, p. 58-60.

and newer forms of immunosuppression. All these areas of improvement reflect better understanding of posttransplant complications. Early postoperative complications are, in many instances, similar to those experienced after routine cardiac surgery. Certain physiologic aspects of the early postoperative phase, particularly in reference to right ventricular function, are, however, unique to cardiac transplantation. Complications related to rejection and immunosuppression are manifested in the intermediate and longer term posttransplant course. Infection remains a major factor in posttransplantation morbidity and mortality. Malignancy related to immunosuppression is a consideration in cardiac transplantation, as it is in all organ transplantation, and improved understanding of this problem underscores the importance of maintaining the minimum effective level of immunosuppression.

II. PERIOPERATIVE PHASE

The immediate postoperative care of cardiac transplant patients is similar to that of other cardiac surgical patients. Early respiratory weaning and extubation are emphasized, as is the early ambulation of the patient. In our institution, patients are maintained on inotropic support, usually with isoproterenol, for 4-5 days postoperatively. This is based upon observed clinical efficacy and presumed graft intramyocardial edema and diminished high-energy phosphate stores during the early postoperative phase. Immediate postoperative hemorrhage and tamponade are managed with prompt re-exploration, as in the case of any other cardiac surgical patient. The cardiac transplant patient frequently has a large pericardial space into which the smaller, normal-sized donor heart is placed. Frequently, the postoperative chest radiograph does, therefore, show a large apparent cardiac silhouette. Substantial pericardial effusions are not uncommon in this setting and may or may not have hemodynamic significance. Postoperative echocardiography is frequently invaluable in assessing the need for pericardial drainage. In most instances, moderate fluid restriction and administration of diuretics will obviate the need for drainage.

Frequently, patients awaiting cardiac transplantation require insertion of mechanical assist devices. The most common of these is the intra-aortic counterpulsation balloon. Clearly, avoidance of complications related to balloon placement is of great importance in the postoperative care of the cardiac transplant patient. In particular, careful attention must be given to observance of strict aseptic technique at the time of balloon insertion and thereafter. Vigilance as to the status of the peripheral circulation and other aspects of routine intra-aortic balloon pump care must be stressed. Ordinarily, the intra-aortic balloon pump can be removed at the time of transplantation. This is best done in the operating room so that strict aseptic technique may be employed. Since reversal of anticoagulation may be incomplete, it is preferable to remove these devices, even those placed percutaneously, with direct visualization of the artery.

Increasing attention is being focused upon mechanical devices for augmentation or total assumption of cardiac output. Several left ventricular assist devices are available and being used clinically; we have used one such device as a bridge to transplantation in the unstable recipient awaiting a donor. The total artificial heart has received considerable publicity, and one pneumatic device has been employed in several cases recently as a permanent device. The use of such left ventricular assist devices and mechanical hearts may well prove to serve its principal function in the hemodynamic stabilization of patients awaiting cardiac transplantation. Here again, observance of strict aseptic technique in the implantation of such devices is of paramount importance, since the occurrence of prosthesis-related infection would ordinarily preclude transplantation and immunosuppression. Furthermore, the occurrence of thromboembolic phenomena must be studiously avoided, because of the adverse effect of such events on the operative and postoperative course of transplantation. In the case of the left ventricular assist device, removal of the device at the time of transplantation has not posed a significant problem. The device that we use (the Novacor solenoid, electrical pump) employs a porcine-valved inflow conduit from the left ventricular apex, a pumping chamber placed in the preperitoneal space, and a valved outflow conduit that may be anastomosed to the supraceliac abdominal aorta or to the ascending aorta. Removal of this device at the time of transplantation does not pose significant difficulties, except with respect to the outflow aortic anastomosis. The aortic repair is carried out after completion of the transplant and involves lateral closure of the aortic wall.

Early postoperative complications after cardiac transplantation in some instances reflect unique physiologic aspects of the cardiac allograft and its relationship with the pulmonary circulation. Patients with elevated pulmonary vascular resistance (greater than 8 Wood units) frequently evidence right ventricular failure in the early postoperative course. The normal donor right ventricle is unable to sustain circulation against elevated pulmonary pressure in the recipient, and right ventricular failure rapidly becomes apparent. When this complication is anticipated, it is often possible to ameliorate the problem through the use of on-site donors with relatively brief ischemic periods and through the use of donor allografts procured from donors larger in body mass than the recipients. Nonetheless, right ventricular dysfunction is still a frequent occurrence when elevated pulmonary vascular resistance pertains. We have employed direct pulmonary artery venting, using a sump catheter attached to a separate roller head suction, immediately after completion of the pulmonary arterial anastomosis, to provide absolute minimization of right ventricular work in the beating, decompressed heart on partial cardiopulmonary bypass.

This technique, employed for 20-30 min after completion of the pulmonary arterial anastomosis, may afford better recovery of right ventricular function. The use of pharmacological agents, particularly sodium nitroprusside, is essential in efforts to reduce pulmonary vascular resistance in the immediate postbypass phase. When right-sided dysfunction is anticipated in this setting, use of prostaglandins (particularly prostaglandin E_1) can prove very effective in the acute manipulation of pulmonary vascular resistance in the immediate postbypass period [4]. These vasodilatory agents are often best used in combination with central venous nitroglycerin for preload reduction. However, it is often necessary to simultaneously administer norepinephrine or another α agent. Because of the well-known metabolism and clearance of norepinephrine in the pulmonary circulation, it is preferable to administer the α agent through a direct left atrial infusion. These pharmacological maneuvers are frequently effective, and when the patient can be stabilized and safely transferred to the intensive care unit, gradual right ventricular compensation usually occurs.

When pharmacological maneuvers are ineffective, the use of mechanical devices, such as pulmonary artery balloon counterpulsation or right ventricular assist devices, may be contemplated [5]. This area remains investigational.

Cardiac allograft dysfunction may also occur in the setting of normal pulmonary vascular resistance, and such graft dysfunction may involve either or both ventricles. Such graft dysfunction is most often related to inadequate cooling or to the occurrence of ventricular distention at the time of graft procurement. We administer 500 mL crystalloid potassium cardioplegic solution at 4°C at the time of graft excision, used in combination with large volumes of topical saline at 4°C. Grafts are transported in plastic containers of cold saline packed in ice. The technique of surgical procurement should exclude the possibility of significant ventricular distention. Inflow occlusion, accomplished by ligation of both venae cavae, is performed first, and the heart is allowed to beat through several cycles to empty. The aorta is then cross-clamped, and cardioplegic solution is instilled via the aortic root. Simultaneously with this maneuver, the superior vena cava and right superior pulmonary vein are incised, to obviate the possibility of distention on either the right or the left side of the heart.

As in other areas of heart surgery, the postoperative course after transplantation may be complicated by the occurrence of supraventricular or ventricular arrhythmias. As noted previously, patients are supported with intravenous isoproterenol for the first few days after surgery. This drug is titrated to maintain a sinus rate of 110-120 beats per minute. In addition, we routinely place temporary epicardial pacing wires, which can be used when isoproterenol therapy is ineffective. These atrial pacing wires may also be used for diagnostic purposes and for rapid atrial pacing when atrial flutter complicates the postoperative course. Supraventricular arrhythmias are treated in a fashion similar to that used for routine cardiac surgical patients. Digoxin is frequently required, and quinidine sulfate is also used when appropriate. Occasionally, the use of calcium channel blockers is required for rate control, but β blockade is generally avoided because of its negative inotropic effects on the allograft.

Renal function is of critical importance after cardiac transplantation, particularly in the era of cyclosporine-based immunosuppression. Because of the well-known nephrotoxic effects of cyclosporine, which are frequently potentiated by prerenal azotemia, it is important to avoid overly vigorous diuresis in the early postoperative period. Patients may require judicious administration of intravenous diuretics, gradually, to achieve the desired weight, but it is important to recall that a normal or near-normal cardiac output can be expected and that adequate diuresis can be anticipated during the first postoperative week. In patients who have had preoperative renal dysfunction based on low output-related azotemia or intrinsic renal disease, early postoperative hemodialysis is often helpful. Again, because of the anticipated adequate cardiac output and renal perfusion in the early postoperative phase, the need for hemodialysis is often brief.

III. ADVERSE EFFECTS OF IMMUNOSUPPRESSIVE AGENTS

Immunosuppression for cardiac transplantation is currently centered around the use of the fungal metabolite cyclosporine. Despite its undoubted contribution to reduction in morbidity and improved survival, its use has been associated with several significant complications, including renal failure, hypertension, hepatotoxicity, malignancy, hirsuitism, neurological disturbances, and other less serious complications. Because of the considerable morbidity imparted by some of these problems, recent interest has focused on regimens employing lower dosages of cyclosporine in combination with other agents, including steroids, azathioprine, and antithymocyte globulin (Table 1).

Myers and his colleagues from our institution have analyzed the chronic nephropathy associated with cyclosporine administration [6]. A group of 17 cyclosporine-treated heart transplant recipients who had survived more than 12 months were compared with 15 survivors of 12 months or greater transplant who were treated with azathioprine immunosuppression. Glomerular filtration rate was significantly depressed ($P < 0.005$) in those patients treated with cyclosporine compared with the "conventional" immunosuppression group. Renal plasma flow was also significantly reduced, and trends toward loss of some specific glomerular transport mechanisms were also noted. Notably, cardiac output was nearly identical in the two groups.

In the Myers report, 5 of the cyclosporine-treated patients had renal biopsies and histopathologic examination. They found glomerulosclerosis and varying

Table 1 Current Immunosuppression Protocols for Cardiac Transplant Recipients at Stanford University

Protocol 1

1. Cyclosporine: 18 mg/kg PO as single preoperative loading dose; then 9-10 mg/kg per day, to achieve serum levels of 200-300 ng/mL during first 4-6 weeks
2. Azathioprine: 4 mg/kg PO as preoperative dose and approximately 2 mg/kg per day as maintenance, depending on WBC count
3. Equine antithymocyte globulin: 10 mg/kg per day IV for 7 days
4. Steroids: methylprednisolone, 500 mg IV at discontinuation of cardiopulmonary bypass and 125 mg IV every 8 hr, for three doses; then prednisone, 0.2 mg/kg per day as maintenance

Protocol 2: Same as 1 without maintenance prednisone

amounts of tubular and interstitial injury, of little specificity. Of the first 32 heart transplant patients treated with cyclosporine and surviving more than 12 months, 2 developed end-stage renal failure. This has lead us to reduce cyclosporine dosages and to monitor renal function closely, giving consideration to conversion to azathioprine-based regimens when moderate degrees of renal failure occur. Cyclosporine dosages are carefully adjusted according to levels in an effort to maintain levels in the 200-300 ng/mL range during the early phase (first 6 weeks), when rejection is most common and severe, and adjusting levels downward to achieve levels of 100-150 ng/mL in the long-term postoperative phase. The efficacy of these attempts to reduce nephrotoxicity is under study.

Hypertension is frequently seen in the early postoperative phase after cardiac transplantation, presumably on the basis of the product of normal cardiac output in the setting of chronically elevated peripheral vascular resistance. We have therefore employed vasodilator therapy, usually with hydralazine or prazocin, during the early postoperative phase. We have, however, avoided the use of β blockade because of deleterious effects on early graft function.

However, chronic arterial hypertension was a relatively infrequent complication among patients treated with azathioprine and steroid therapy, prior to the cyclosporine era [7]. When it did occur, it was presumed to be based on generalized atherosclerosis and physiology of decreased arterial capacitance. Among cyclosporine-treated patients, chronic arterial hypertension, usually presenting within 2-3 months postoperatively, is more common [7]. The mechanism of occurrence of cyclosporine-related hypertension is still not understood, and it is frequently difficult to treat, requiring a combination of agents, such as vasodilators and false neurotransmitters. In some instances of particularly refractory hypertension, discontinuation of cyclosporine, and institution of conventional immunosuppression may be required.

Myocardial interstitial fibrosis, apparently not related to rejection, has been observed in cyclosporine-treated patients, and the possibility of its leading to restrictive cardiomyopathic physiology has been raised [7]. However, such physiology has not been documented in follow-up catheterization studies, and the pathophysiologic significance of this histological finding remains unknown.

Hepatotoxicity related to cyclosporine has been extensively studied and observed in rats and has been reported in humans by Calne and others [8,9]. It is particularly important to follow serial liver function tests, particularly serum bilirubin, frequently after cardiac transplantation and to make appropriate dosage adjustments in the cyclosporine regimen. This is especially true in view of the significant preoperative passive congestion in many cardiac transplant recipients.

Malignancy has been observed with increased frequency in immunosuppressed patients, and the occurrence of malignant lymphomas has received particular attention [10,11]. In the first group of cardiac transplant recipients treated with cyclosporine in our institution, the incidence of diffuse histiocytic lymphoma was particularly high [12]. This and other experiences suggested an association between cyclosporine therapy and risk of lymphoma. Clinically, there were several distinguishing features to these lymphomas. All were of the large cell immunoblastic or diffuse histiocytic type, and all showed a relatively short induction period. Among six patients developing posttransplant lymphomas, the number of days after transplantation until diagnosis of lymphoma ranged from 85 to a maximum of 183. In addition, a predilection for the central nervous system was observed.

Partially in response to this problem, the overall immunosuppressive regimen among cyclosporine-treated patients was modified, to adjust cyclosporine dosages according to serum levels. This lead to an overall reduction in the quantity of cyclosporine administered. In addition, the routine use of prophylactic intramuscular rabbit antithymocyte globulin was discontinued. Since these modifications, only one posttransplant lymphoma has been diagnosed. Among the last 100 cardiac transplant recipients, there have been no lymphomas.

Recently, a retrospective quantitative analysis of measured parameters of immunosuppression has been carried out, comparing cardiac transplant patients who did and did not develop lymphoma [12]. Measured parameters during the first 3 months after transplantation included mean cyclosporine level, total dosage of rabbit antithymocyte globulin, number of days of T-cell suppression, and mean cyclosporine level during T-cell suppression. Interestingly, all these parameters were higher in the lymphoma group, and this difference achieves statistical significance in the instance of mean 3-month cyclosporine levels. This analysis supports the correlation between overall quantity of immunosuppression and

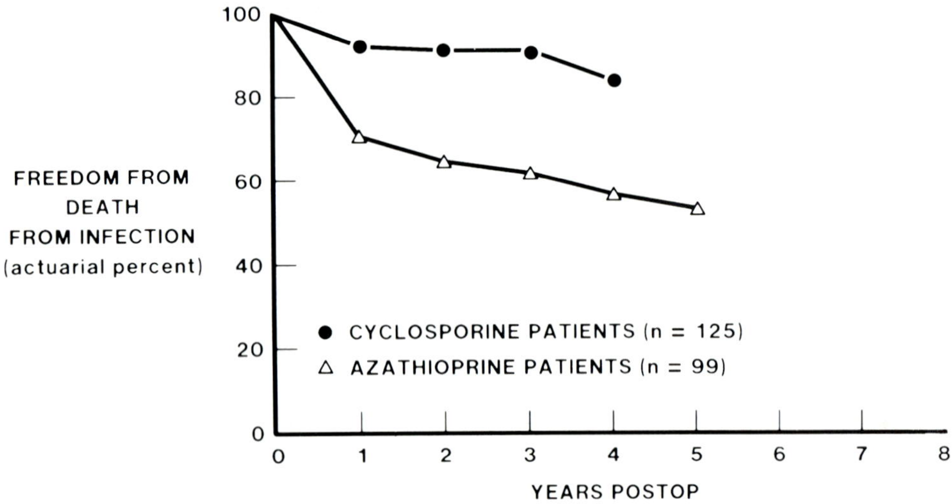

Figure 2 Probability of death from infection after cardiac transplantation.

cated and by the multiplicity of organ systems that may be involved (Tables 2 and 3). Although antimicrobial therapy must be prompt and definitive, its use must be carefully correlated with the immunosuppressive regimen, both in terms of the deleterious effect of unnecessarily stringent immunosuppression on infection and in terms of specific drug interactions. Well-known examples of the latter problem are the use of the aminoglycosides, trimethoprim-sulfa, and amphotericin in the setting of cyclosporine-related renal dysfunction.

VI. REJECTION

Despite improvement in immunosuppression techniques and the introduction of cyclosporine, rejection remains the second most common cause of death after cardiac transplantation and a very major clinical obstacle in successful implementation of cardiac transplantation. As cyclosporine has become the centerpiece for present-day immunosuppression, overall results have improved, and this does relate to the influence of the drug on the rejection phenomenon. However, as in the case of infectious complications, the introduction of cyclosporine has not significantly reduced the incidence of rejection when compared with results on conventional immunosuppression (Fig. 3). As will be noted, approximately one-half of patients will have experienced an episode of rejection requiring treatment by 1 month postoperatively on our current immunosuppressive regimen.

Table 2 Organisms Implicated in Infections After Cardiac Transplantation (December 15, 1980-May 1, 1985)

Organism	Number
Bacterial	
Acinetobacter	3
Anaerobic, mixed	4
Citrobacter	2
Enterobacter	6
Enterococcus	15
Escherichia coli	12
Klebsiella	9
Legionella sp.	7
Listeria	1
Pneumococcus	1
Proteus	2
Pseudomonas sp.	10
Salmonella	1
Serratia	12
Staphylococcus	8
Streptococcus	6
Fungal	
Aspergillus	12
Candida	5
Cryptococcus	2
Yeast, unidentified	1
Viral	
CMV	10
Titer rise	25
Herpes simplex	37
Herpes zoster	13
Protozoan	
Pneumocystis	2
Toxoplasma	2
Nocardia	3

Table 3 Location of Infections After Cardiac Transplantation (December 15, 1980–December 31, 1984)

Pulmonary	40
Urinary tract	23
Septicemia	18
Mediastinum	8
Empyema	1
CNS	1

During the early postoperative phase, surveillance for rejection in the cyclosporine-treated group is based entirely upon histological findings obtained from endomyocardial biopsy. Ordinarily, the first endomyocardial biopsy, performed under local anesthesia using the Caves bioptome introduced via the right internal jugular vein, is performed 1 week postoperatively. Subsequent biopsies are carried out on a weekly basis, unless overt clinical deterioration occurs. When rejection does occur, treatment is carried out with intravenous methylprednisolone, 1000 mg intravenously on a daily basis for 3 days. Endomyocardial biopsy is then repeated 4 days later, at which time histological resolution should have begun. In cases of persistent rejection, the therapy with intravenous methylprednisolone is repeated. Should rejection persist on a third consecutive endomyocardial biopsy, intravenous methylprednisolone therapy is combined with intramuscular antithymocyte globulin therapy. The later is ordinarily continued for 3 days, with serial monitoring of T-cell rosette counts, expecting levels to fall below 12%. In cases of persistent, severe, or fulminant rejection, retransplantation must be considered.

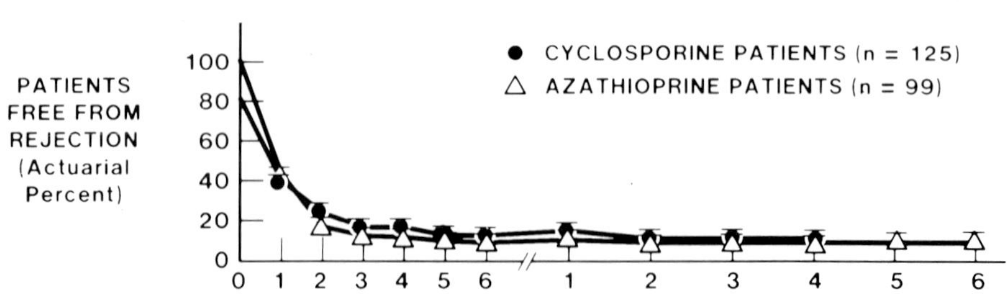

Figure 3 Rejection after cardiac transplantation: cyclosporine versus azathioprine immunosuppression.

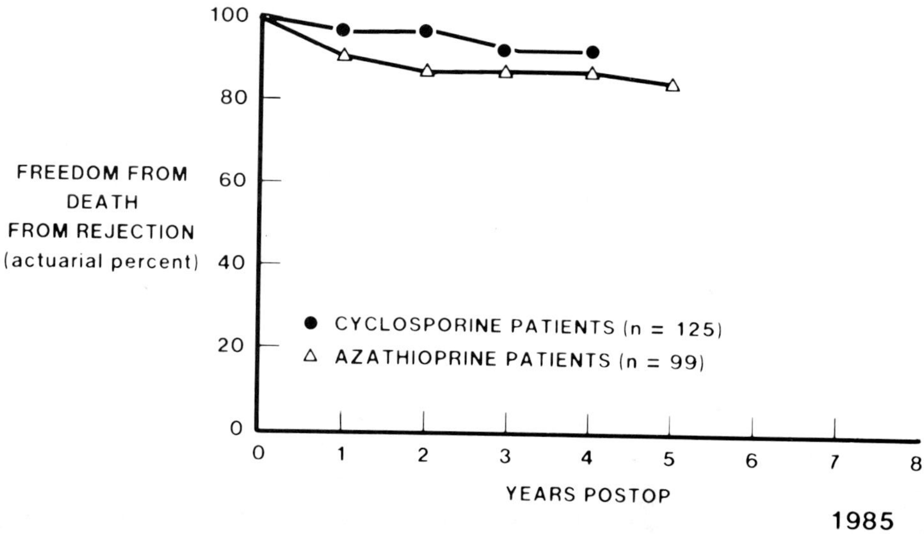

Figure 4 Probability of death from rejection.

Although it has been generally appreciated that rejection among cyclosporine-treated cardiac transplant patients is a more benign phenomenon than that observed with conventional immunosuppression, it is undoubtedly true that rejection may be severe and life threatening in this group. As shown in Figure 4, the actuarial probability of death from rejection is lower among cyclosporine-treated patients, but not significantly so.

VII. CONCLUSION

During the past few years, cardiac transplantation has emerged as a reliable mode of therapy for patients with end-stage congestive heart failure. There has been dramatic improvement in outlook for survival and qualitatively acceptable rehabilitation, and new areas for application of the technique in younger and older age groups and among patients with associated conditions previously contraindicating transplantation are being explored. Continued success and further improvement in results will depend upon recognition and early treatment of the array of recognized postoperative complications described in this chapter.

REFERENCES

1. Carrel, A., and Guthrie, C. C.: The transplantation of veins and organs. Am. J. Med. 10:1101, 1905.

2. Lower, R. R., and Shumway, N. E.: Studies on orthotopic transplantation of the canine heart. Surg. Forum 11:18, 1960.
3. Samuelsson, R. G., Hunt, S. A., and Schroeder, J. S.: Functional and social rehabilitation of heart transplant recipients under age thirty. Scand. J. Thorac. Cardiovasc. Surg. 18:97-103, 1984.
4. Naeije, R., Melot, C., Mols, P., and Hallemans, R.: Reduction in pulmonary hypertension by prostaglandin E_1 in decompensated chronic obstructive pulmonary disease. Am. Rev. Respir. Dis. 125:1-5, 1982.
5. Symbas, P. N., McKeown, P. P., Santora, A. H., and Vlasis, S. E.: Pulmonary artery balloon counterpulsation for treatment of intra-operative right ventricular vailure. Ann. Thorac. Surg. 39:437-440, 1985.
6. Meyers, B. D., Ross, J., Newton, L., Luetscher, J., and Perlroth, M.: Cyclosporine-associated chronic nephropathy. N. Engl. J. Med. 311:699-705, 1984.
7. Hunt, S. A.: Complications of heart transplantation. Heart Transplant. 3:70-74, 1983.
8. Ryffel, B.: Experimental toxicological studies with cyclosporine A. In: White, D. J. G., ed. Cyclosporine A, Amsterdam: Elsevier Press, 1982.
9. Calne, R. Y., Thiru, S., McMartin, P., Craddock, G. N., White, D. J. G., Evans, D. B., Durin, D. C., Pentlow, B. D., and Roller, K.: Cyclosporine A in patients receiving renal allografts from cadaver donors. Lancet 2:1323-1327, 1978.
10. Penn, I.: Malignancies associated with immunosuppressive or cytotoxic therapy. Surgery 83:492-502, 1978.
11. Penn, I.: Malignant lymphomas in organ transplant recipients. Transplant. Proc. 13:736-738, 1981.
12. Brumbaugh, J., Baldwin, J. C., Stinson, E. B., Oyer, P. E., Jamieson, S. W., Bieber, C. P., Henle, W., and Shumway, N. E.: Quantitative analysis of immunosuppression in cyclosporine-treated heart transplant patients with lymphoma. Heart Transplant. 4:307-311, 1985.
13. Atkinson, K., Biggs, J., Darveniza, P., et al.: Cyclosporine A associated central nervous system toxicity after allogeneic bone marrow transplantation. N. Engl. J. Med. 310:527, 1984.
14. Rolles, K., White, D. G., Thiru, S., et al.: Cyclosporine A initially as the only immunosuppressant in 34 recipients of cadaveric organs: 32 kidneys, 2 pancreases, and 2 livers. Lancet 2:1033-1036, 1979.
15. Shah, D., Rylance, P. B., Rogerson, M. E., Beewick, M., and Parsons, V.: Generalized epileptic fits in renal transplant recipients given cyclosporine A. Br. Med. J. 209, 1984.

The technique of bypass has been discussed elsewhere and is beyond the scope of this discussion [2-4]. The advantages of the system include

1. Maintenance of mean arterial pressure, central venous pressure, and pulmonary artery wedge pressure at prehepatectomy levels with a decreased incidence of cardiac arrhythmias, hypotension, and organ hypoperfusion
2. Elimination of the need for excessive volume preloading of the patient and therefore less risk of pulmonary edema at the time of liver revascularization
3. Protection of the kidneys from renal venous hypertension and hypoperfusion with a significant reduction in postoperative renal dysfunction
4. A significant decrease in the mean operative and early postoperative blood replacement requirements
5. A significant improvement in 30-day patient survival

The routine use of venovenous bypass has converted the anhepatic phase of liver transplantation into a controlled, calm procedure, but it is not without inherent problems. A major risk of using a nonheparinized bypass system is the development of thrombus in the bypass tubing and in the cannulated veins, which could result in pulmonary embolization. Although this has been an infrequent occurrence, both pulmonary emboli and deep venous thrombosis have been documented and have been a rare cause of patient death. The case report below is one example. One effort to alleviate this problem has led to the development of a commercially produced, heparin-bonded single-circuit polyvinyl chloride tubing system that incorporates the bypass pump head. The system is primed before use with Ringer's lactate containing dilute (1:1000) heparin. In patients with small veins, smaller caliber chest tubes can be adapted to the ends of the tubing to facilitate cannulation.

During bypass, the rotation of the centrifugal blood pump is kept to the minimum revolutions per minute required to maintain an acceptable flow of at least 1000 mL/min. Usually flows of 2-3 L/min are obtained. In children, using heparin-bonded and dilute heparin-primed tubing, flows down to 500 mL/min may be acceptable. Maintenance of adequate flow reduces the risk of thrombus formation. The use of one-piece tubing systems, careful priming of the system to eliminate air bubbles, and moderate pump speed minimizes the risk of introducing air into the bypass.

Certain patients may present special risks for use of the venovenous bypass. One patient with polycystic disease of the liver who was transplanted to relieve massive hepatomegaly and inferior vena cava obstruction suffered a fatal pulmonary embolus soon after initiating bypass. Two patients with Budd-Chiari syndrome had attempts at thrombectomy of the clotted portal vein and vena cava followed by establishment of bypass. Flows in the circuit were critically low with great risk of thrombus formation in the bypass circuit. Bypass was abandoned in both patients without further incidence. Such conditions, with preexisting thrombus in the venous beds, are contraindications to the use of bypass.

Wound hematomas, seromas, or lymphoceles in the access wounds in the groin or axilla have occurred in approximately 25% of patients. Usually these are mild, self-limited problems, but surgical exploration and drainage are occasionally required. There has been one significant brachial plexus injury in a child. Meticulous dissection and gentle handling of neural tissues are essential to minimize these complications.

The following case report illustrates the risk of thrombotic complications associated with the use of venovenous bypass.

Case Report

A 30-year-old female was admitted in fulminant hepatic failure from B virus hepatitis. She failed to improve after 12 hr of vigorous medical therapy. An appropriate liver donor was found within 24 hr. At surgery, the hilum and ligaments of the liver were dissected without incident. The patient was placed on venovenous bypass. Heparin-bonded Gott shunts were used to cannulate the vena cava via the saphenofemoral system, the axillary vein, and the portal vein. Bypass flow was 3 L/min. During anastomosis of the suprahepatic vena cava, there was a sudden rise in pulmonary artery pressure followed by a cardiac arrest. All efforts at resuscitation failed, and the patient expired on the operating table. The right atrium was opened and approximately 100 mL of soft clot was found. Thrombus was also found in the bypass tubing.

IV. GRAFT-VERSUS-HOST DISEASE

Whenever possible, liver transplantation is carried out between ABO blood group matched donors and recipients. In kidney transplantation, ABO matching is essential, since the presence of ABO isoagglutinating antibodies against a renal graft almost always result in hyperacute rejection of the graft. The liver, however, is privileged, and hyperacute rejection has not been observed when liver transplantation is performed between ABO-mismatched donor and recipients. The use of ABO-mismatched grafts, such as transplantation of a group O liver to an non-group O recipient or a group A or B liver to a AB recipient, is done frequently for patients in urgent need of transplantation and for small children, for whom the supply of available donors is especially limited.

The liver graft, a reticuloendothelial organ, can produce isoagglutinating antibodies against the ABO blood determinants of the recipient. A large number of lymphocytes accompany the liver from donor to recipient in both the lymphatics of the liver and the lymph nodes in the hepatic hilum. Therefore, the graft contains a significant number of B lymphocytes with the potential to produce anti-ABO group determinant antibodies. Ramsey et al. [5] were able to detect such

ABO antibodies in 27.6% of recipients of ABO-mismatched livers. No such antibodies were found in 180 recipients of ABO-matched transplants. In five of the eight patients with detectable antibodies, there was clinical evidence of significant hemolysis occurring well after the period of perioperative transfusion requirement. Antirecipient ABO antibodies were first detected 8-16 days after transplantation and were last seen 11-41 days after surgery. Hemolysis, when present, was seen between 5 and 8 days after surgery and lasted 7-19 days.

The hemolytic graft-versus-host reaction that occurs with transplantation of an ABO-mismatched graft is usually self-limited and treatment with immunosuppression is already in place. The following case report illustrates the clinical course.

Case Report

An 11-year-old male, blood group A, with type II homozygous hypercholesterolemia was admitted for hepatic transplantation to reverse his life-threatening enzyme deficiency. His disease was manifested by cutaneous xanthomas, atypical angina pectoris with demonstrable coronary artery stenosis, and two right parietal cerebrovascular accidents. The best available donor, blood group O, had a larger liver requiring a left lateral segmentectomy at transplantation.

The patient made a prompt recovery from surgery but developed enzyme and electrocardiographic findings of acute myocardial infarction. This resulted in mild, transient pulmonary edema. The patient improved, but a drop in hematocrit from 32 to 18% occurred on postoperative day 10 with no evidence of external bleeding. Direct Coombs test was positive, and circulating anti-A blood group antibody was detectable. The patient was treated with a 2-unit packed red blood cell transfusion and an intravenous bolus of 500 mg methylprednisolone. He developed a severe thrombocytopenia (platelet count 4000 mm^3) and epistaxis 14 days after transplantation. He received another bolus of 500 mg methylprednisolone followed by a 5-day burst of steroids starting at 200 mg methylprednisolone on the first day and tapering by 40 mg/day until reaching a maintenance dose of 20 mg/day. Azathioprine, 50 mg/day, was added. The platelet count remained below 10,000 mm^3 for the next 6 days, and a splenectomy was performed. Over the next 10 days the platelet count slowly recovered.

The self-limited hemolytic anemia experienced by this patient was typical of the findings in the graft-versus-host response seen with ABO-mismatched donor and recipient. The thrombocytopenia is unusual but could also have been related to antibody coating and damage to platelets, which were then removed from the circulation by the spleen and possibly also by the liver. This case is exceptional in that previously we have not had to perform a splenectomy in patients with ABO-mismatched grafts.

V. VASCULAR THROMBOSIS

Technical complications remain an important cause of morbidity and mortality after liver transplantation. Thrombosis of the hepatic artery is one of the most common and most serious complications. In a recent review of 244 patients who received 309 liver transplants at the University of Colorado and the University of Pittsburgh from March 1980 to June 1984, 22 cases (7.1%) of hepatic artery thrombosis were identified [6]. Of these, 14 cases occurred in children (11.8%) and 6 in adults (3.4%). Mortality was 37.5% in children and 50% in adults. A total of 66 liver retransplants were performed during this period: 13 (19.7%) were for hepatic artery thrombosis; 9 patients (62.9%) survived. Only 27.3% of the patients not retransplanted survived. A specific anatomic cause of thrombosis was identified in only 3 cases: an intimal dissection of the hepatic artery in 2 and medial necrosis and intramural hemorrhage of the celiac axis in 1.

The clinical presentation of hepatic artery thrombosis usually follows one of three patterns:

1. *Fulminant hepatic necrosis* (8 patients) with frank hepatic gangrene characterized by a rapid rise in serum transaminase levels and rapid clinical deterioration between 9 and 33 (mean 16.4) days after transplantation (Fig. 1)
2. *Delayed biliary leak* (7 grafts in 6 patients) at 7-65 (mean 29.0) days after transplantation from ischemic necrosis of the bile duct manifested by subhepatic fluid collections, drainage of bile through abdominal drains, frank bile peritonitis, bacteremia, and changes in the clinical liver profile (bilirubin and transaminases) often similar to those seen with graft rejection
3. *Relapsing bacteremia* in 7 cases characterized by an indolent clinical course presenting 15-45 (mean 26.7) days after transplantation, usually with only minor abnormalities in the liver function profile

Case Report

A seriously ill 4-year-old male with α_1-antitrypsin deficiency received a liver transplant with a double hepatic arterial supply. The left hepatic artery arose from the celiac axis and the right hepatic artery from the superior mesenteric artery. Reconstruction required the use of donor throacic aorta left attached to the celiac and superior mesenteric arteries and implanted into the right common iliac artery. The patient had *Klebsiella* septicemia with moderate elevations of liver function studies 4 weeks after surgery. No obvious source of sepsis was found, but the patient responded well to antibiotic therapy. The patient had a second episode of *Klebsiella* septicemia 1 week later. A CT scan of the abdomen suggested the presence of thrombus in the thoracic aortic conduit, and an arteriogram was obtained that confirmed arterial thrombosis. Initially the patient was managed conserva-

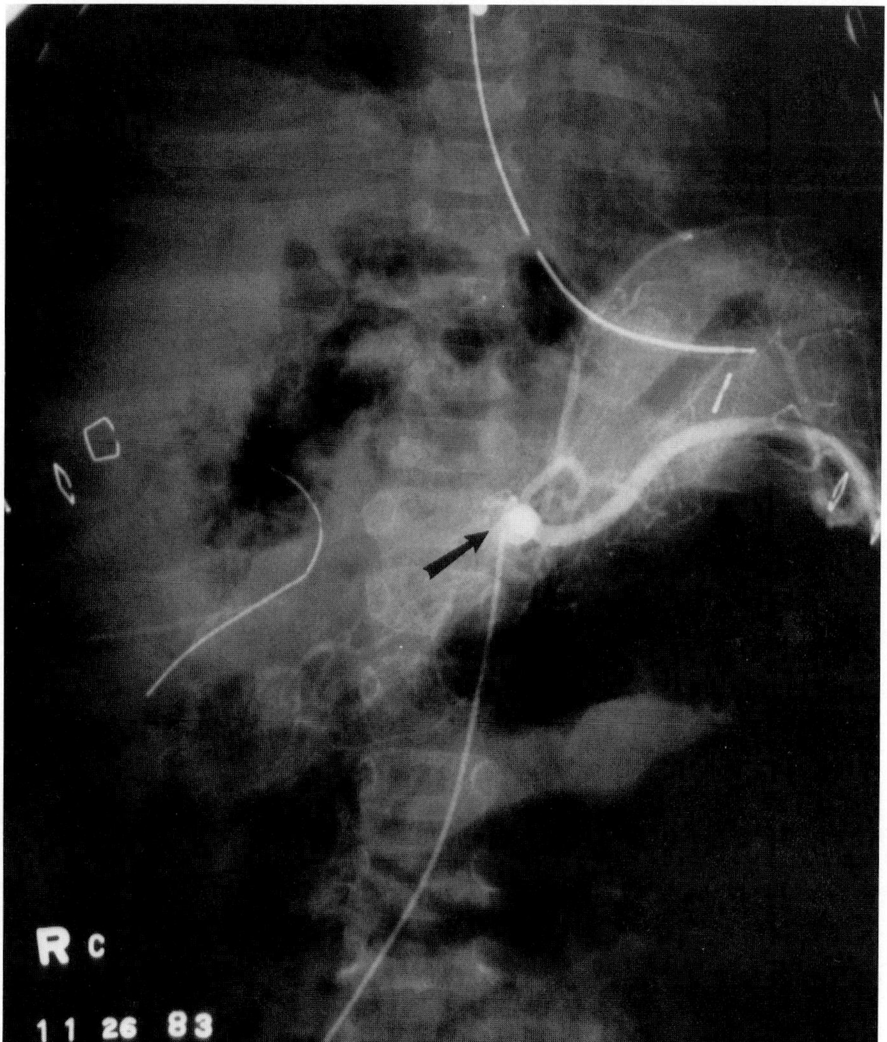

Figure 1 Complications of hepatic artery thrombosis. Selective celiac angiography demonstrating hepatic artery thrombosis (arrow) and resulting in air in the liver.

tively since he remained clinically stable. However, when antibiotics were discontinued he again became septic and developed gastrointestinal bleeding. He was retransplanted at 53 days. The bile ducts in the first graft were impacted with inspissated bile and old blood clots. Disimpaction of this material resulted in vigorous hemorrhage from a portobiliary fistula. The patient died 15 days after retransplantation of hemorrhage caused by rupture of a mycotic aneurysm at the suture line between the new aortic conduit and the native aorta.

Hepatic artery thrombosis must be considered in all patients presenting with fever and a positive gram-negative blood culture after transplantation. If hepatic arterial pulsations cannot be detected with the Doppler ultrasound, arteriography is indicated (Figs. 1 and 2). Laparotomy is a potentially dangerous diagnostic maneuver. Manipulation of the devascularized liver may result in severe hemorrhage and septicemia. Evaluation of the hepatic artery is sometimes difficult since an artery with a palpable pulse may be thrombosed at a more distal level or a transmitted pulse in an occluded vessel may be misinterpreted as a sign of vessel patency.

Although patients with arterial thrombosis may have a fulminant clinical course, many patients have a subtle and indolent course. The principal injury of hepatic arterial thrombosis is ischemic necrosis of intrahepatic or extrahepatic bile ducts. If the extrahepatic ducts are involved, extrahepatic bile abscess or frank bile peritonitis occurs, which requires laparotomy for drainage and eventual liver replacement. If the intrahepatic ducts are involved, hepatic abscess is common. In milder cases, late biliary strictures may develop. CT scans are useful in detecting bile collections inside or outside the liver (Fig. 3a). Percutaneous or T-tube cholangiography may be necessary to define the biliary tract anatomy (Fig. 3b). Percutaneous transhepatic catheter manipulation can drain intrahepatic collections and permit dilatation of strictures. In the occasional case this may be sufficient to permit healing and avoid the need for retransplantation.

Hepatic artery thrombosis must be differentiated from primary graft failure and primary biliary tract technical complications. Herpetic hepatitis, a rare complication, can attack the biliary system and result in disruption of the bile duct. Bile duct stricture, intra-abdominal abscess, or other undetected sources of persistent infection must also be excluded.

Most patients with hepatic arterial thrombosis require retransplantation. Children and some young adults appear to tolerate hepatic arterial thrombosis more readily than older patients and are more likely to present with an indolent course. Younger patients are better able to develop hepatopedal arterial collaterals (Fig. 2). Although a limited number of patients have been initially managed successfully with antibiotics and, as indicated, percutaneous transhepatic manipulation, the long-term durability of such management remains to be established.

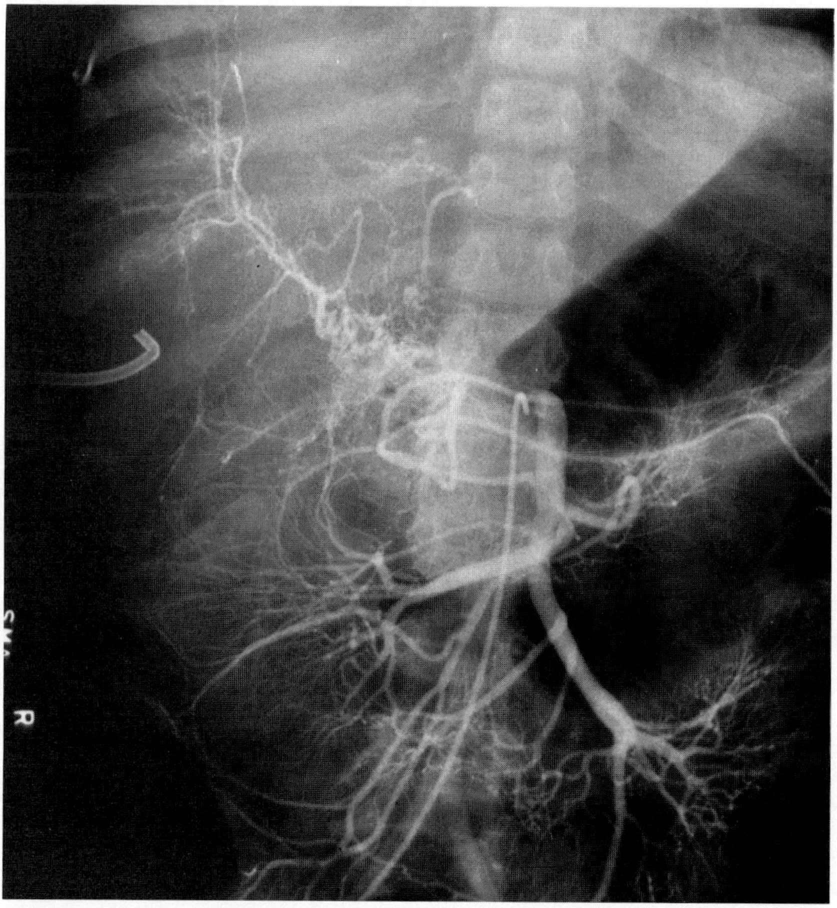

Figure 2 Selective superior mesenteric arteriography showing the extensive collateral circulation that has developed in the right upper quadrant following thrombosis of the hepatic graft artery.

Portal vein thrombosis (Fig. 4) is much less common after liver transplantation and has occurred in only 6 of 313 recipients. The majority of cases occurred in patients with previous surgery for portal hypertension, such as portacaval shunting or splenectomy. Other potential causes include technical mistakes, such as stricture, misalignment, or excessive length (Fig. 5), hypercoagulable states, and thrombus formation resulting from the presence of the venovenous bypass cannula.

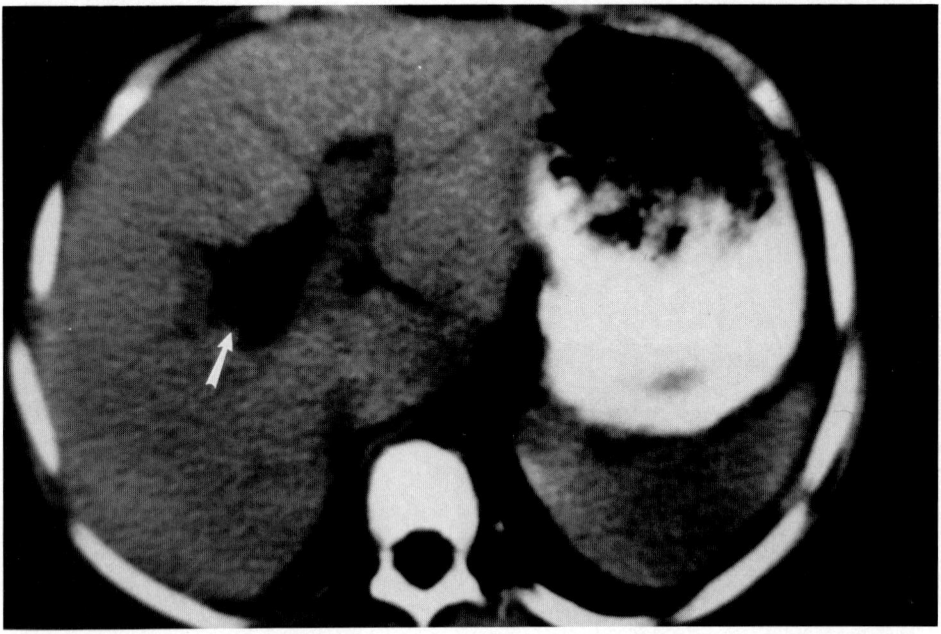

(A)

Figure 3 Biliary tract complications after hepatic arterial thrombosis (same patient as Fig. 2). (A) CT scan demonstrating a single hypodense zone (arrow) in the transplanted liver. (B) Percutaneous transhepatic cholangiogram demonstrating a significant biloma (arrow) that corresponds to the findings on the CT scan.

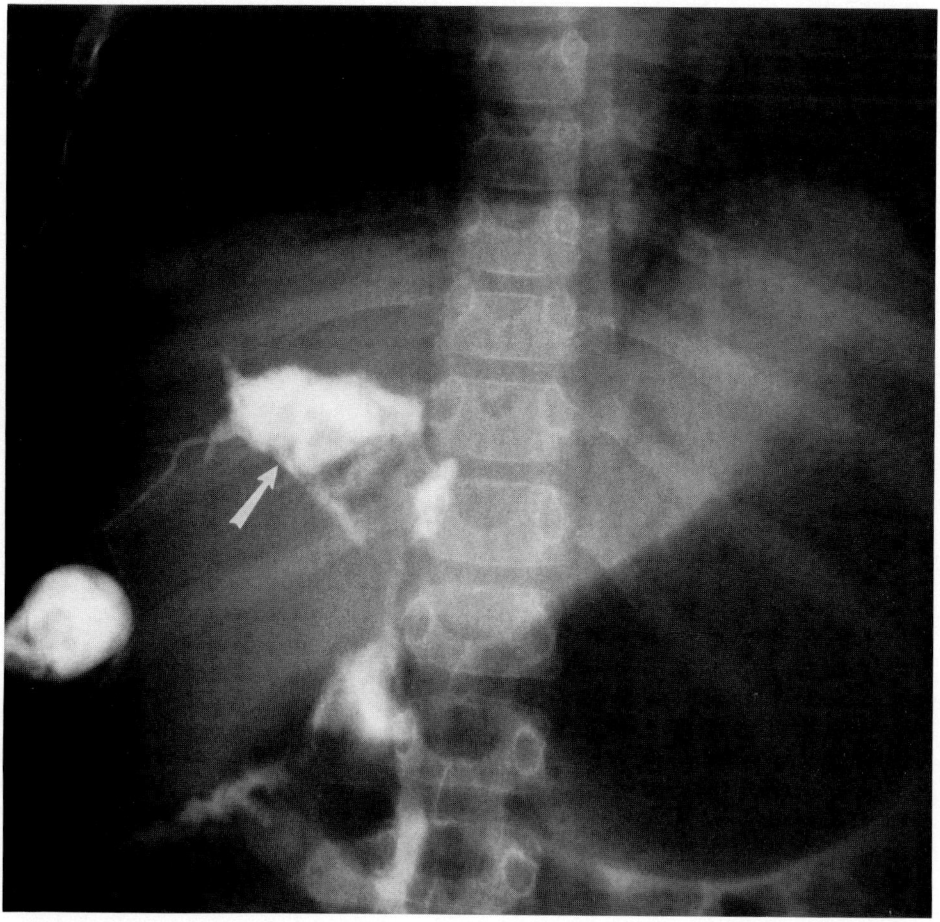

(B)

Figure 3 (continued)

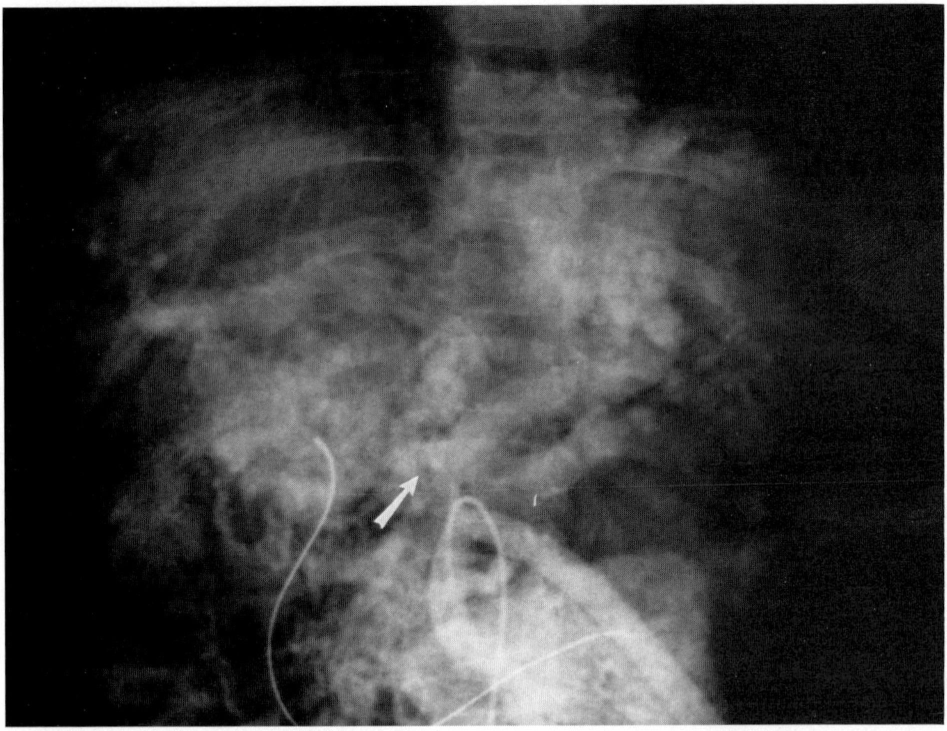

Figure 4 Venous phase of a selective superior mesenteric arteriogram demonstrating thrombosis of the portal vein (arrow) and formation of secondary venous collaterals.

Clinical presentation of portal vein thrombosis is variable. It may present acutely with hepatic failure, intestinal swelling, and massive ascites or, more often, with chronic ascites and variceal hemorrhage. The diagnosis is confirmed by arteriography and has been made at laparotomy. Treatment is retransplantation or, when feasible, conservative management of portal hypertension.

Other vascular complications that may have a similar clinical presentation and require retransplantation are mycotic aneurysms and pseudoaneurysms. In small children and in patients with significant disease of the native hepatic artery, it is often necessary to use donor aortic or iliac arterial segments as grafts for rearterialization of the liver. These grafts are usually sewn into the recipient infrarenal aorta and tunneled under the pancreas to reach the hepatic hilum. A short tunnel can be made above the left renal vein and superior mesenteric artery and under

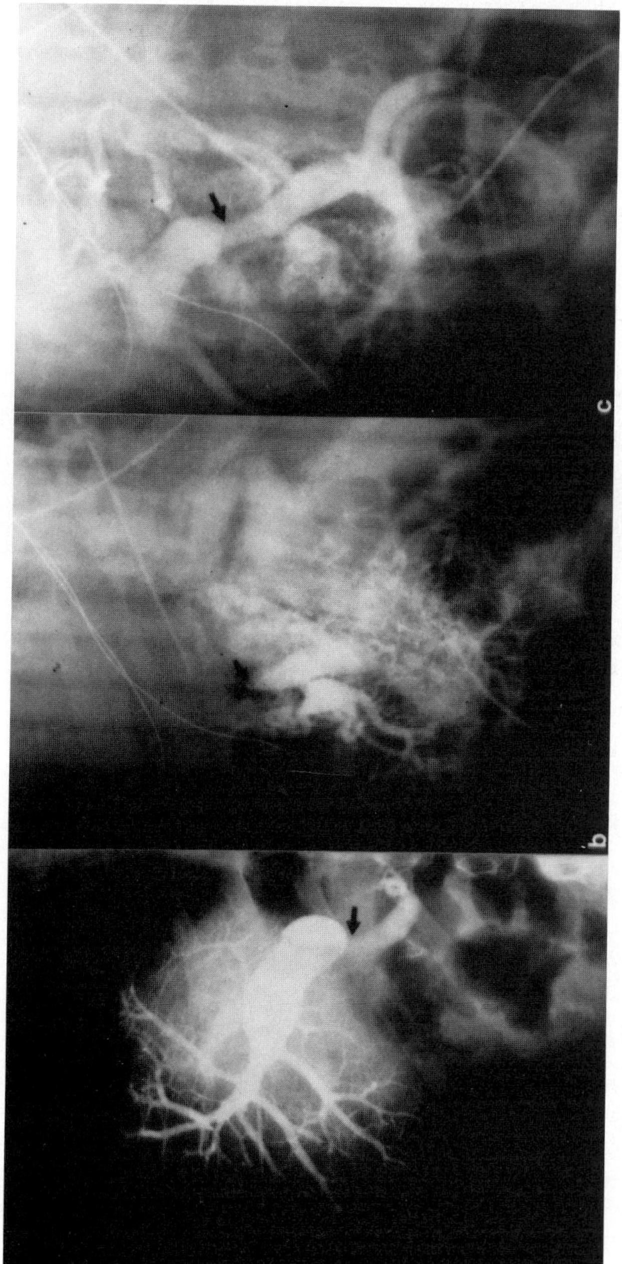

Figure 5 Portal vein thrombosis resulting from technical error. (a) Stenosis of the portal vein anastomosis (arrow) diagnosed at transhepatic portography. (b) Operative venogram through a mesenteric vein demonstrates complete portal obstruction (arrow). (c) Management of this problem consisted of resection of the stenosis, thrombectomy, and reanastomosis (arrow).

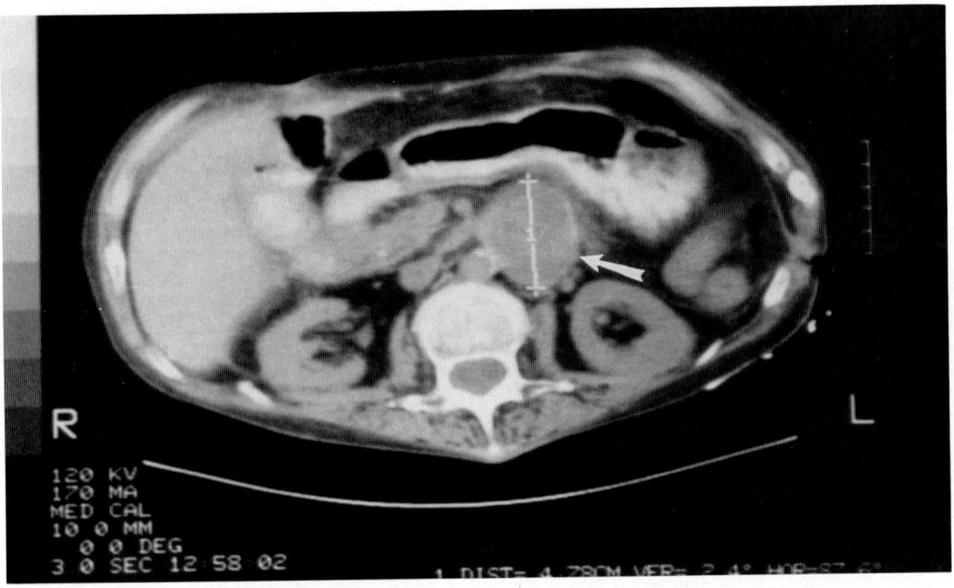

(A)

Figure 6 Pseudoaneurysm (arrows) of an aortic graft in a pediatric liver transplant recipient demonstrated by both CT scan (A) and aortography (B).

the neck of the pancreas, or a longer tunnel can be made crossing over the inferior vena cava and under the superior mesenteric artery, head of the pancreas, and duodenum. The anastomosis between the donor arterial conduit and the recipient aorta has been the most frequent site of pseudoaneurysm or mycotic aneurysm formation (Fig. 6). Ultrasound and CT scanning have been helpful in making the diagnosis.

VI. BILIARY TRACT COMPLICATIONS

The two principal technical advances in liver transplantation in recent years have been the development of a reliable, effective venovenous bypass technique and standardization of the techniques for biliary reconstruction. Direct duct-to-duct (choledochocholedochostomy) over a T-tube stent in adults is the preferred method of reconstruction when possible. In children with biliary atresia and other patients with disease rendering the recipient bile duct unsuitable for direct

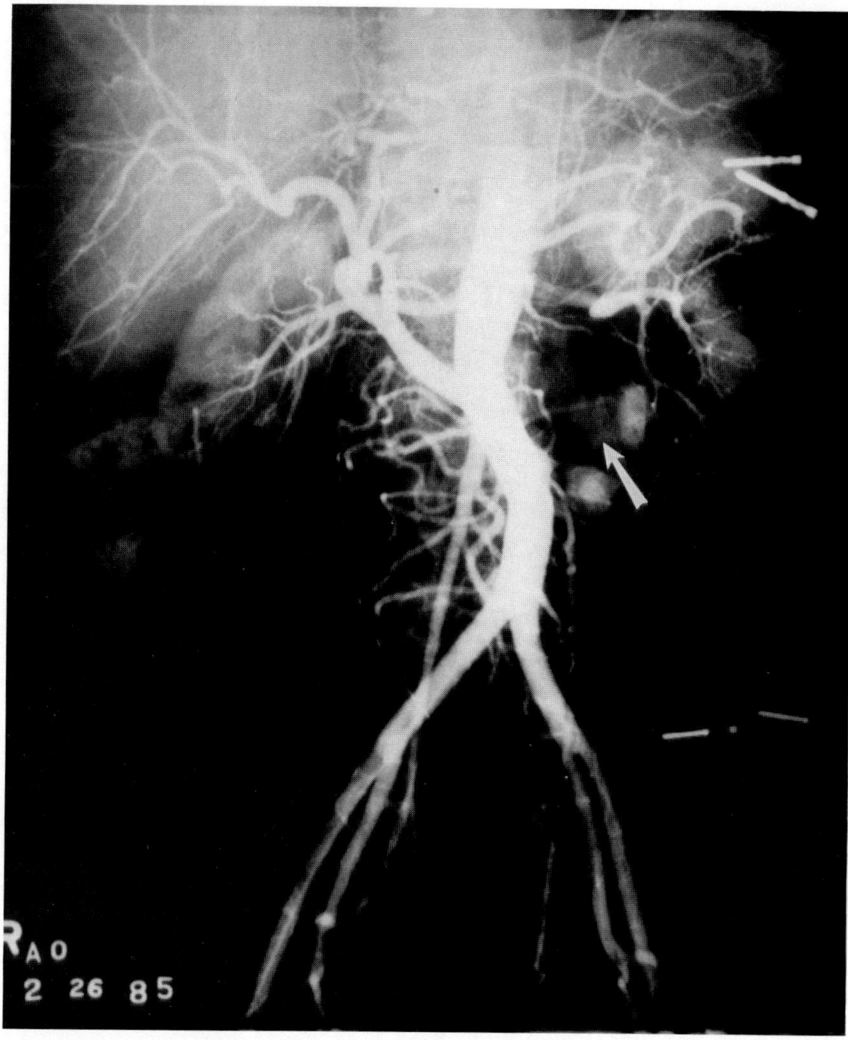

(B)

Figure 6 (continued)

reconstruction, anastomosis of the donor bile duct to Roux-en-Y limb of jejunum (choledochojejunostomy) is the reconstruction of choice. These reconstructions are now successful in over 90% of cases.

In 313 patients between March 1, 1980, and December 31, 1984, biliary tract complications occurred in 52 patients [7]. Of these patients, 5 (9.6%) died as a direct result of the complication. Prior to this period, the incidence of biliary tract complications was even higher. It had been thought that a deficient blood supply of the graft duct system was responsible for the high incidence of complications, but, in fact, the majority of problems were probably the result of inappropriate surgical techniques, such as choledochoduodenostomy, and the failure to diagnose complications promptly. With the advent of cyclosporine-steroid immunosuppression in 1980, frequent use of postoperative cholangiography, standardization of choledochocholedochostomy and Roux-en-Y choledochojejunostomy, and prompt operative intervention for complications, the incidence of complications and morbidity and mortality have decreased markedly.

It has already been emphasized that primary biliary tract complications must be differentiated from those secondary to arterial insufficiency. Other less common and unusual biliary tract complications include bile cast syndrome, transplantation of a traumatized liver, and unexplained changes in the peripheral intrahepatic bile ducts not related to the biliary anastomosis.

Case Report

A 34-year-old female received a liver transplant for chronic aggressive hepatitis. The operation went without incident, and a direct duct-to-duct biliary reconstruction over a T tube was performed. Completion and postoperative cholangiography demonstrated a normal biliary tree and patent leak-free anastomosis. The early postoperative course was complicated by pneumonia and several episodes of acute rejection treated with corticosteroids.

A cholangiogram performed on postoperative day 53 showed a stricture at the confluence of the hepatic ducts of the graft and dislocation of one T-tube limb out of the biliary tract. The tube was replaced percutaneously by a straight tube stent. The stricture was treated by seven percutaneous balloon dilatations. The stricture was dilated to 12 mm, resulting in a patent duct with no detectable pressure gradient across the site of the stricture.

The patient was again hospitalized 18 months later with an abnormal liver function profile. A liver biopsy showed moderate allograft rejection. Percutaneous transhepatic cholangiography and ERCP demonstrated recurrence of the stricture. Percutaneous balloon dilatation was unsuccessful, and the patient was reconstructed with a Roux-en-Y hepaticojejunostomy. Histology showed only mild fibrosis of the duct. The patient made an uneventful recovery. Ultrasound of the liver prior to hospital discharge showed no dilatation of the biliary tree.

This case demonstrates several important aspects of biliary tract reconstruction in liver transplantation (Fig. 7). First, the differential diagnosis between rejection and biliary tract complications can be difficult. Second, T tubes and stents may dislocate or migrate out of proper position predisposing to stricture. Third, biliary tract obstruction need not involve the anastomosis even in the absence of ischemic injury to the graft ductal system. Fourth, percutaneous transhepatic dilatation is only an interim method of management. Definitive management usually requires resection of the obstruction and mucosa-to-mucosa repair of the bile duct to a Roux-en-Y jejunal loop.

The biliary tract reconstruction is no longer the "Achilles heel" of liver transplantation. The use of standard reconstructive techniques, appropriate postoperative investigation, and aggressive intervention when a complication is identified can minimize morbidity and mortality and save most grafts.

VII. VIRAL HEPATITIS

Infection still accounts for much of the morbidity and mortality after liver transplantation. The differential diagnosis of liver dysfunction after transplantation is complicated by the difficulty of distinguishing rejection from postoperative viral hepatitis. Cytomegalovirus (CMV) infection of the liver is a particularly troublesome and still frequent occurrence. Between March 1980 and September 1985 we have identified 17 patients with pathologically proven CMV hepatitis after liver transplantation.

CMV hepatitis tends to occur relatively late after transplantation (15-132 days; mean, 44 days). It is characterized by elevation of bilirubin and transaminases with a prolonged clinical course of spiking temperatures (ranging 5-68 days in 15 of the 17 patients). Since the management of viral infection and rejection is radically different, the establishment of the correct diagnosis is essential. Percutaneous liver biopsy is the method of choice and is performed frequently on our service. Prior to our liberal use of biopsy, three patients had liver retransplantation for an incorrect diagnosis of rejection based only on liver function abnormalities. All three patients had been overimmunosuppressed because of the mistaken diagnosis. All three patients ultimately died. At autopsy CMV hepatitis, not rejection, was found.

More striking evidence of the need for liver biopsy is found in further evaluation of the 17 confirmed cases of CMV hepatitis in our series. Of the first 8 patients, 5 were diagnosed at the time of retransplantation. The next 9 patients were all diagnosed by percutaneous biopsy. Only 4 of 12 patients diagnosed by biopsy have died compared with 4 of the 5 patients diagnosed at reoperation.

CMV infection is diagnosed by serological changes and/or isolation of the virus. Liver biopsy may show the typical inclusion bodies in the hepatocytes,

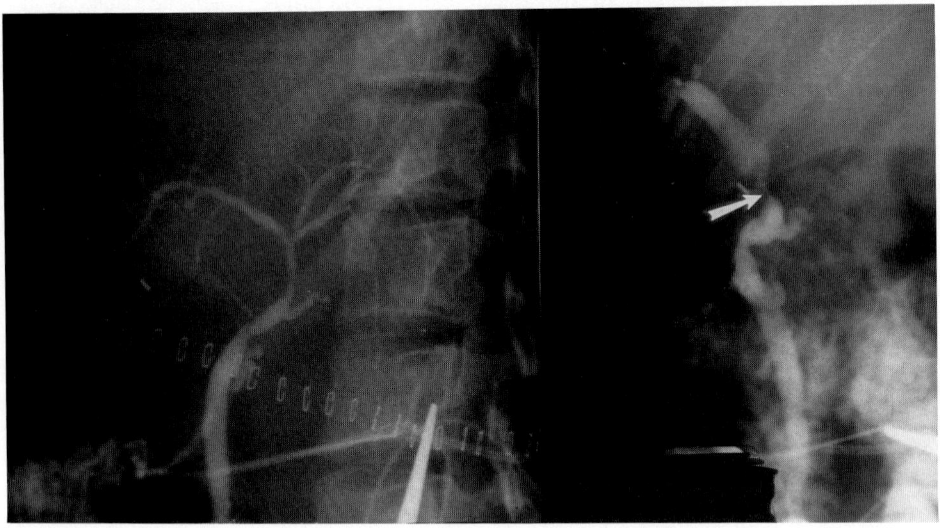

(A)

Figure 7 Bile duct stricture after liver transplantation. (A) Operative cholangiogram (left) demonstrating normal biliary tree after the initial reconstruction. Cholangiography (right) demonstrating stricture of the donor common hepatic duct. (B) Cholangiogram showing a dislodged T tube lying outside the biliary tree, which was subsequently replaced with a straight tube stent. (C) The dislodged T tube has been replaced with a straight tube stent passed up toward the hepatic duct bifurcation. (D) Cholangiography showing resolution of the stricture after repetitive percutaneous transhepatic balloon dilatations. No pressure gradient was detectable across the stricture site. (E) Cholangiography showing recurrence of the stricture 2 years later subsequently treated by conversion of the choledochocholedochostomy to a Roux-en-Y choledochojejunostomy.

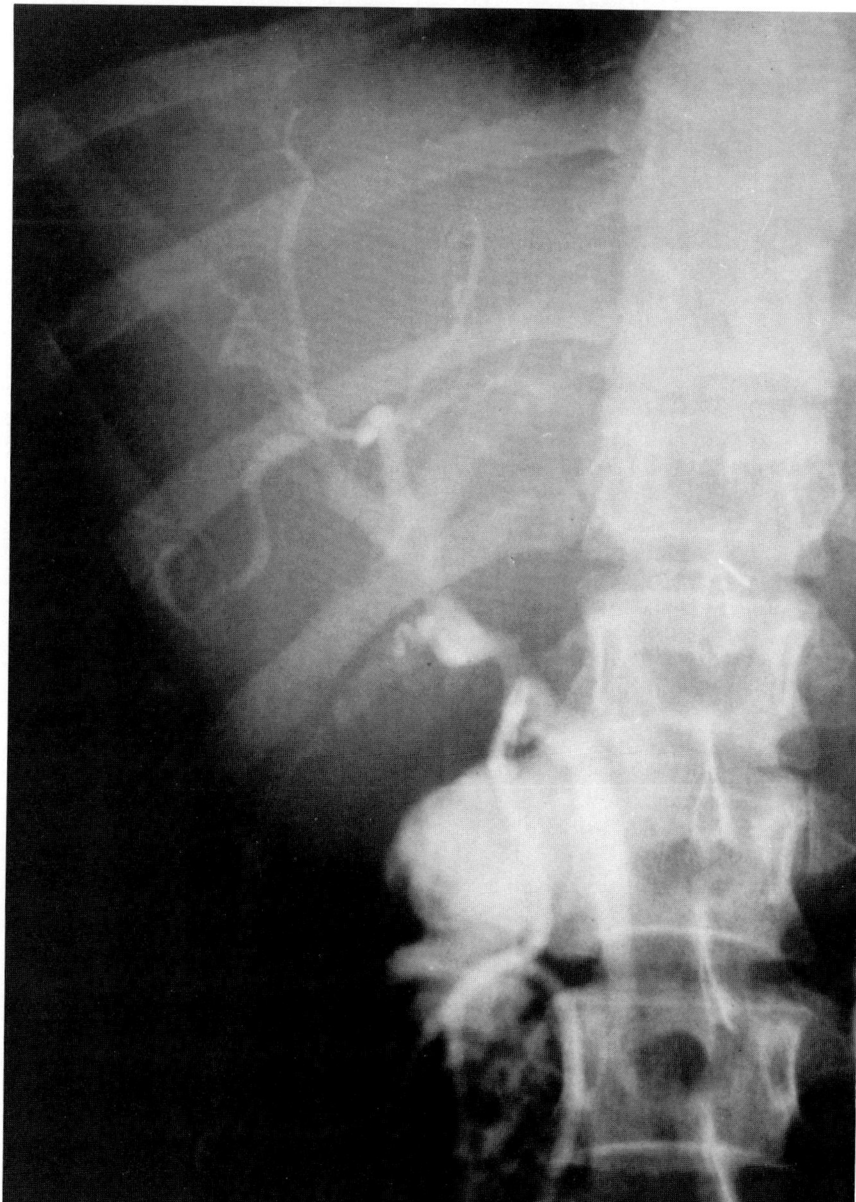

(B)

Figure 7 (continued)

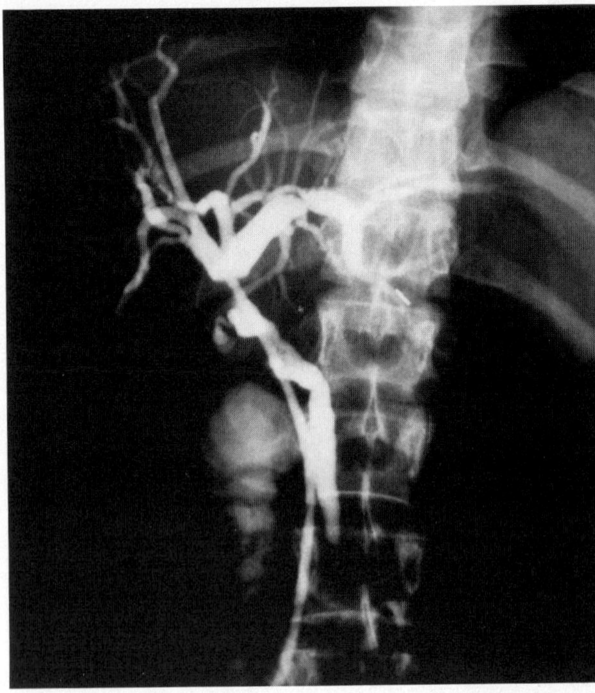

(C)

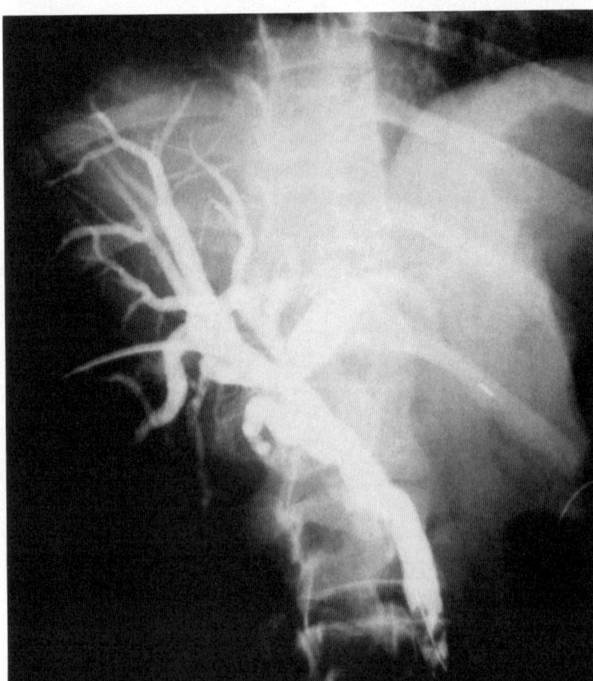

(D)

Figure 7 (continued)

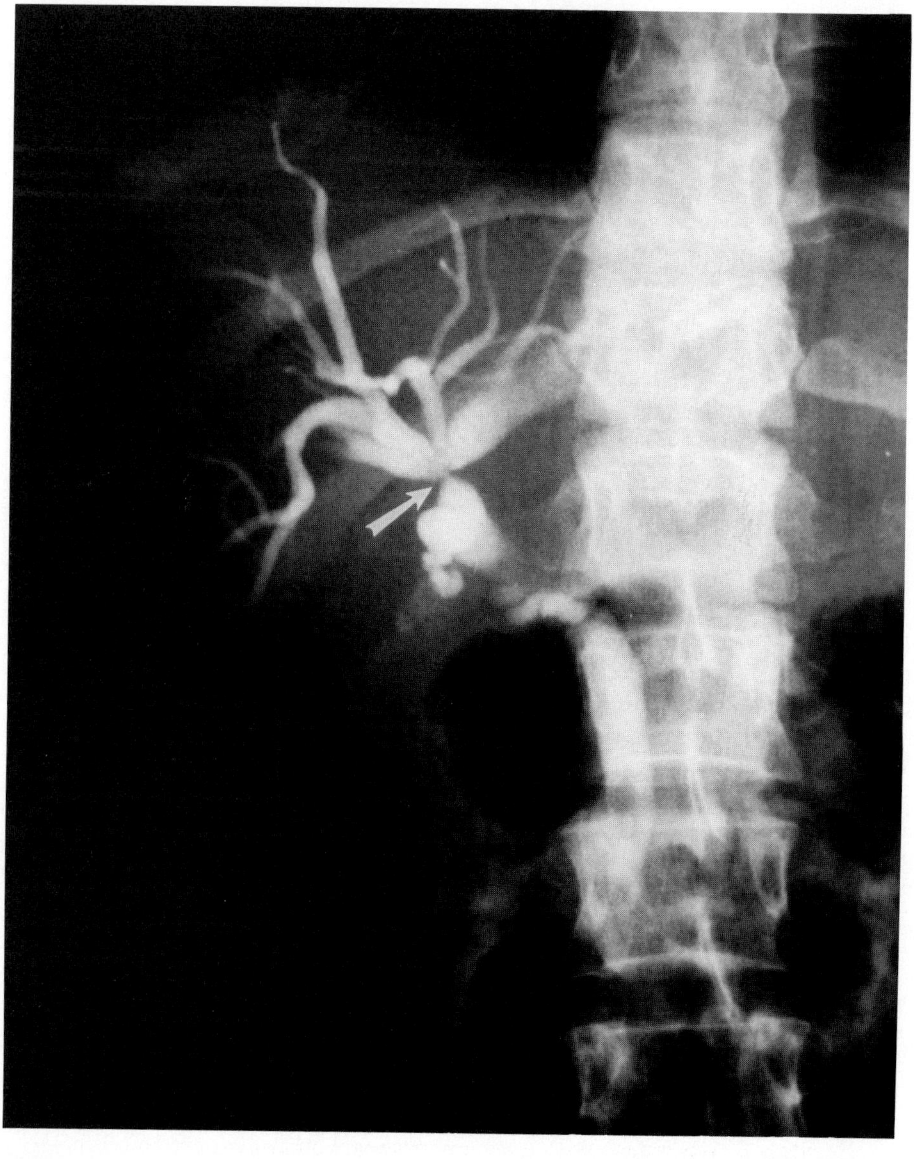

(E)

Figure 7 (continued)

but biopsy material should always be cultured since isolation of virus is the best way to establish the diagnosis. CMV infection can occur primarily, as established by seroconversion, or by reactivation of prior infection, as documented by a fourfold or greater rise in antibody titer. Reactivation is promoted by immunosuppression. Primary infection in the transplant patient can originate from many sources, including the graft itself and blood products. Greater than 35% of the U.S. population is serologically positive for CMV and thus the virus is frequently transmitted from donor to recipient. Of the 17 cases we reviewed, 8 patients had primary infection and 1 had definite and 5 had probable reactivation of infection. In 3 cases, insufficient serum samples were available to make a determination.

The finding of primary infection in 8 of 14 (57%) patients with CMV hepatitis is higher than one would expect and suggests that patients with primary infection are more at risk of developing significant hepatitis [8]. It is well known that primary CMV infections tend to be more symptomatic and result in higher morbidity and mortality in immunocompromised patients, such as kidney transplant patients [7]. It is important to note, however, that in the group of 17 patients with CMV hepatitis we recently reviewed, we found no difference in clinical prognosis between primary infection or reactivated infection.

Most CMV infections are self-limited if immunosuppression is managed with restraint. It is also worth noting that CMV infection is by itself immunosuppressive. Full maintenance of immunosuppressive agents in the face of CMV infection may easily result in dangerous overimmunosuppression and increase susceptibility to other opportunistic infections.

Once the diagnosis of CMV hepatitis is established, our management strategy includes reduction of cyclosporine to achieve moderate blood levels (400-500 ng/mL by whole-blood RIA) and reduction of maintenance steroids from 20 to 10 mg/day or less. As the disease resolves, cyclosporine is increased to maintain blood levels in the usual therapeutic range (800-1000 ng/mL).

The management of the occasional patient with both rejection and CMV hepatitis is difficult. We often reduce the daily maintenance dose of steroids but supplement therapy with boluses of 0.5-1.0 g of methylprednisolone or hydrocortisone every 4-5 days. CMV hepatitis may worsen after therapy for rejection, requiring judicious lowering of immunosuppression. Finally, in some cases, only retransplantation can save the patient.

Hepatitis B virus, adenovirus, and herpesvirus are other less common offenders. Hepatitis B is also often self-limited and managed by conservative immunosuppressive therapy. Herpes and adenovirus hepatitis are rare but often ominous and severe.

Case Report

A 23-year-old male underwent an uneventful orthotopic liver transplant in December 1983 for end-stage sclerosing cholangitis. He did well postoperatively until about day 16, when he developed significant elevations in bilirubin and hepatic transaminases. His temperature reached 39°C, and fever lasted for 6 days. A cholangiogram and an arteriogram were normal. Liver biopsy was not performed. He was treated for rejection with steroids and antilymphocyte globulin without significant improvement in liver function.

The patient suddenly deteriorated with disorientation, hypoxia, and bilateral pulmonary infiltrates requiring intubation and high-pressure ventilatory support. Retransplantation was performed, but the patient died 7 days later. Pathological examination of the first liver graft showed severe cytomegalovirus hepatitis without evidence of rejection. CMV was also identified in the spleen, which had also been removed at surgery. CMV was isolated in urine and from buffy coat blood. In addition, *Clostridium difficile* was isolated from the spleen and *Staphylococcus aureus* and *Enterobacter* were isolated from blood.

This case demonstrates the severe penalty for treating viral hepatitis as rejection. A liver biopsy can be especially helpful in this situation and prevent inappropriate immunosuppressive treatment.

VIII. CONCLUSION

Just a few years ago, the patient with end-stage liver disease had little to hope for. Liver transplantation was still an experimental procedure with a high morbidity and mortality. Today, the surgical technique, though still demanding, has become standardized and operative mortality is below 10%. Cyclosporine and monoclonal antibody therapy have made rejection more manageable. Nonetheless, the majority of patients undergoing liver transplantation will experience at least one major complication and many will require at least one additional operation. Fortunately, our experience in recognizing and managing the complications of liver transplantation has also grown in recent years, and this also has contributed significantly to the improved survival now being enjoyed by our patients.

REFERENCES

1. NIH Consensus Development Conference Statement: Liver transplantation. June 20-23, 1983. Hepatology 4:1075-1095, 1984.
2. Shaw, B. W., Martin, D. J., Marquez, J. M., Kang, Y. G., Bugbee, A. C., Iwat-

suki, S., Griffith, B. P., Hardesty, R. L., Bahnson, H. T., and Starzl, T. E.: Venous bypass in clinical liver transplantation. Ann. Surg. 200:524-534, 1984.

3. Griffith, B. P., Shaw, B. W., Hardesty, R. L., Iwatsuki, S., Bahnson, H. T., and Starzl, T. E.: Veno-venous bypass without systemic anticoagulation for transplantation of the human liver. Surg. Gynecol. Obstet. 160:270-272, 1985.
4. Starzl, T. E., Iwatsuki, S., Shaw, B. W., Gordon, R. D., Esquivel, C. O., Todo, S., Kam, I., and Lynch, S.: Factors in the development of liver transplantation. Transplant. Proc. 17(Suppl. 2):107-119, 1985.
5. Ramsey, G., Nusbacher, J., Starzl, T. E., and Lindsay, G. D.: Isohemagglutinins of graft origin after ABO-unmatched liver transplantation. N. Engl. J. Med. 311:1167-1170, 1984.
6. Tzakis, A., Gordon, R. D., Shaw, B. W., Iwatsuki, S., and Starzl, T. E.: Clinical presentation of hepatic artery thrombosis after liver transplantation in the cyclosporine era. Transplantation 40:667-671, 1985.
7. Ho, M.: Cytomegalovirus: Biology and Infection. New York: Plenum, 1982.
8. Ho, M., Wajszczuk, C. P., Hardy, A., Dunmer, J. S., Starzl, T. E., Hakala, T. T., and Bahnson, H. T.: Infections in kidney, heart and liver transplant recipients on cyclosporine. Transplant. Proc. 15:2768-2772, 1983.
9. Lerut, J., Gordon, R. D., Iwatsuki, I., Shaw, B. W., Jr., Esquivel, C. O., Tzakis, A., and Starzl, T. E.: Biliary tract complications in 393 human liver transplantations. Transplantation (in press).

19

Complications of Lung Transplantation

LUIS H. TOLEDO-PEREYRA
Mount Carmel Mercy Hospital, Detroit, Michigan

I. INTRODUCTION

For the last three decades, lung transplantation has been considered a potential treatment for patients with end-stage lung disease [1]. Although there has been considerable growth in other areas of transplantation, application of this procedure in the clinical setting has been limited [2]. In spite of experimental work studying various techniques and problems associated with lung transplantation [3-7], only 38 transplants were performed in patients with end-stage disease between 1963 and 1980 [2]. Of these, only 2 patients survived long-term, for 6 and 10 months, respectively. The use of new immunosuppressive agents, such as cyclosporine, however, may improve these statistics [8,9]. Recently, lung transplants have again resurged as a modality of treatment for patients with irreversible pulmonary disease. In this chapter we review the complications associated with this procedure.

II. LUNG PROCUREMENT AND PRESERVATION COMPLICATIONS

A major problem in lung transplantation has been the scarcity of available donors meeting the necessary criteria for lung procurement (Table 1) [10]. Often patients with end-stage lung disease die while waiting for a donor lung or are in suboptimal condition by the time an organ is procured. As in other types of organ transplantation, complications can result during organ procurement and preservation (Table 2). The donor and recipient should be of compatible blood groups

Table 1 Criteria for Single Lung Donation

Negative cross-match
Compatible size for donor and recipient hilar structures
Donor free of lung infiltrates on chest roentgenogram
Lung secretions—nonpurulent and relatively free of gram-negative organisms
Donor arterial O_2 tension $>$250 torr
FIO_2 = 1.0
Donors may be excluded because of
Pulmonary edema
Pneumonia
Tracheal intubation
Aspiration of blood or gastric contents

Table 2 Complications of Lung Procurement and Preservation

Procurement complications
Nonideal donor
Poor ventilation
Undetected infection
Fluid overload
Harvesting complications
Injury to hilar vessels
Ischemic damage
Other surgical mishaps
Preservation complications
Preservation or perfusion injury
Edema
Reperfusion injury
Contamination

and the recipient must have a negative cross-match prior to transplantation. The size of the donor lung must be compatible with that of the recipient so that the hilar structures may be properly anastomosed. The donor should be free of infection and lung infiltrates and have normal lung function. Many potential donors are excluded because of pulmonary edema, pneumonia, tracheal intubation, or aspiration of blood or gastric contents. Ideally, the donor and recipients should be located in the same hospital, so that ischemia may be minimized. Experimental work has shown that lung allografts can tolerate only about 30 min of normothermia in a deflated state [11]. Exposure to longer periods results in alveolo-capillary edema and disruption, mitochondrial swelling, interstitial hemorrhage, significantly depressed pulmonary function, elevation of pulmonary vascular resistance, and a considerable drop in glucose, phospholipid, and adenosine triphosphate levels [12].

Several investigators have attempted experimentally to preserve lung allografts for 24 hr or longer by hypothermic storage, hyperbaria, and hypothermic pulsatile or nonpulsatile perfusion using a variety of solutions [13-15]. Clinically, preservation has been limited to a few hours prior to implantation in an effort to prevent preservation injury. The complications that arise during lung preservation are dependent on the type and the duration of preservation, whether hypothermic storage or perfusion are used, edema, preservation injury, and contamination can be observed as complications (Table 2). In the clinical setting, however, until more experience is gained, we continue to recommend that preservation times be minimized to less than 6 hr to obtain optimal functional results.

III. TECHNICAL CONSIDERATIONS

Some transplant surgeons have advocated using cardiopulmonary bilateral lung transplants rather than single-lung transplants to simplify the technical aspects of the procedure. When the heart and lungs are transplanted as a unit, the bronchial anastomosis is eliminated and substituted with a simpler tracheal anastomosis. Also, transplantation of the cardiopulmonary graft as a unit avoids the possibility that the emphysematous contralateral native lung will overexpand, causing compression of the transplanted lung, which has occurred occasionally in clinical lung transplantation.

IV. REIMPLANTATION RESPONSE

After transplantation, changes occur in the lung within 3 days after surgery and usually regress within 3 weeks. They are independent of the rejection process and have been termed the "reimplantation response" [16]. It is thought that this phenomenon is induced primarily by ischemia followed by increased capillary permeability. However, surgical trauma, denervation, lymphatic interruption, and other processes, which may damage the lung, may also be involved. The reimplantation response occurs because of the presence of edematous fluid within the airspaces of the lung. It can be identified histologically as alveolar edema and on plain chest roentgenogram as alveolar infiltrates. Functionally, a temporary impairment of transplant ventilation is observed with decreased compliance and a diminished ventilation-perfusion ratio. Some transient impairment of blood flow may also be encountered. In general, the reimplantation response can be minimized by avoiding ischemia and postmortem damage and trauma to the donor lung. Some investigators have found that flushing the lung with intracellular solutions may reduce this response [14].

V. BRONCHIAL ANASTOMOTIC DISRUPTION AND ASSOCIATED COMPLICATIONS

In the preliminary lung transplant experience, using standard steroid immunosuppressive therapy, defective healing of the bronchial anastomoses has been a frequent problem [1,2]. This has been associated with the additional problems of air leakage, infection, bleeding, stenosis, and mucosal necrosis with aspiration pneumonia. The primary cause of bronchial anastomotic disruption appears to be ischemia of the transplanted bronchus. To prevent this, it has been suggested that the transplant bronchial arteries be revascularized by implantation of a button of donor aorta into the recipient aorta [17,18]. This would obviously add technical difficulty and operative time to the transplant procedure. Another approach has been to shorten the donor bronchial stump. Experiments studying the effect of donor bronchial length on healing have indicated that less mucosal ulceration occurs when the left main bronchus is divided close to the lobar bronchus than when the division is closer to the carina [19]. Other solutions for improving bronchial healing have included reinforcing the anastomosis with surrounding vascularized tissue, using an intussuscepting anastomotic method for the bronchus, and omental wrapping of the bronchial anastomosis (Fig. 1) [2]. The recent use of cyclosporine, without high-dose steroids, would also contribute to improved bronchial healing, since this has already been observed in the experimental setting [20,21].

VI. VASCULAR COMPLICATIONS

There have not been enough clinical cases so far to account for a definite number and variety of vascular complications. However, this can be related to thrombosis of the arterial or venous anastomosis. It is not infrequent to obtain deposits

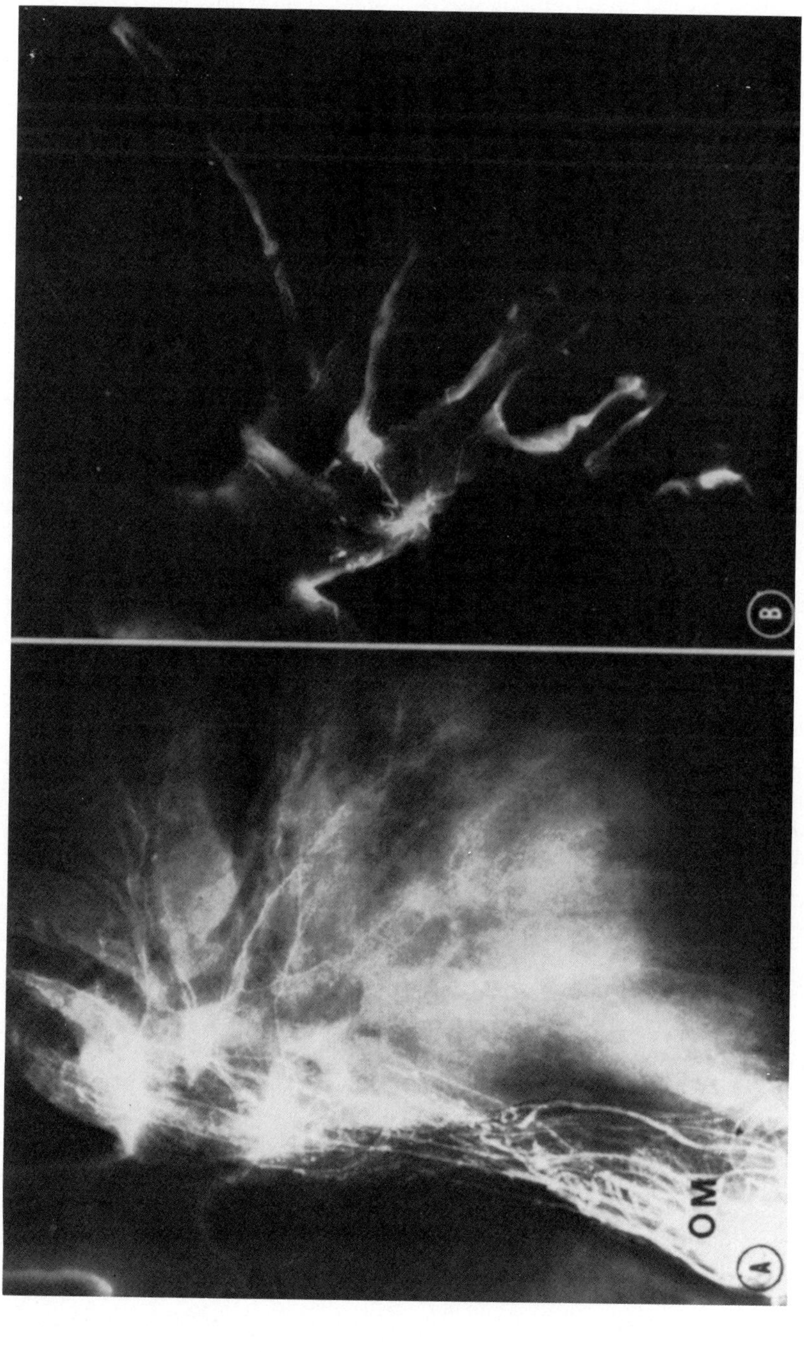

Figure 1 Using the technique of omental wrapping to prevent bronchial anastomotic disruption, the collateral circulation is established to the distal bronchus from the omental vessels. (A) Postmortem canine lung with the omentum still in place. (B) Radiograph of the dissected bronchial specimen stripped of omentum with contrast material in the bronchial vessels. (From Morgan et al. J. Thorac. Cardiovasc. Surg. 85:134-139, 1983. Used with permission of C. V. Mosby Co.)

of platelets with development of small thrombi at the anastomosis of the atrium if the suture line has not been properly placed. Arterial thrombi are not as frequently encountered as those on the venous side. Surgical technique is important to minimize these complications, as well as consideration of the moderate use of anticoagulants and/or platelet inhibitors.

VII. INFECTIOUS COMPLICATIONS

In experimental lung transplantation, major infectious complications are usually absent initially because of the generally healthy condition of the canine allograft recipients [1]. In human lung transplantation, however, patients with chronic pulmonary insufficiency usually have chronic pulmonary infection in both lungs. After transplant, when immunosuppression is added to prevent rejection, the bacteria remaining in the unremoved lung frequently cause bilateral pneumonitis. The lung is also always subjected to some bacterial contamination; therefore, in immunosuppressed patients, the potential for pulmonary infection is great after lung transplantation. In the original series of 38 clinical patients receiving lung allografts, 10 of the 19 recipients surviving greater than 1 week after transplant died with pneumonia or other signs of infection [1]. As the length of graft and patient survival is increased with the use of cyclosporin, one would additionally expect other opportunistic infections, such as cytomegalovirus (CMV) and herpes, in lung transplant recipients.

VIII. LUNG ALLOGRAFT REJECTION

Several experimental studies have analyzed the immunologic response of the transplanted host to the lung allograft [22-25]. Without immunosuppression, rejection proceeds rapidly with survival of one-stage bilateral allotransplants between 4 and 12 days. The clinical symptoms appear on or around postoperative day 2, beginning with a cough, frothy sputum, and listlessness. On plain chest roentgenograms, the presence of lung infiltrates is gradually observed as progressive opacification.

With immunosuppressive therapy, such as azathioprine, steroids, and antilymphocyte serum, lung allograft survival is prolonged; still, fewer than 10% of the transplanted canine recipients survive greater than 2 months. The recent use of cyclosporin for immunosuppression has resulted in improved allotransplant results and milder manifestations of rejection [20-22].

In humans, the process of lung rejection has been systematically analyzed. Veith et al. [2] attempted to histologically evaluate changes occurring during rejection of the first 25 lung transplant cases. Based on these studies, three types of pulmonary rejection have been described: classic, atypical or alveolar, and vascular (Fig. 2, Table 3).

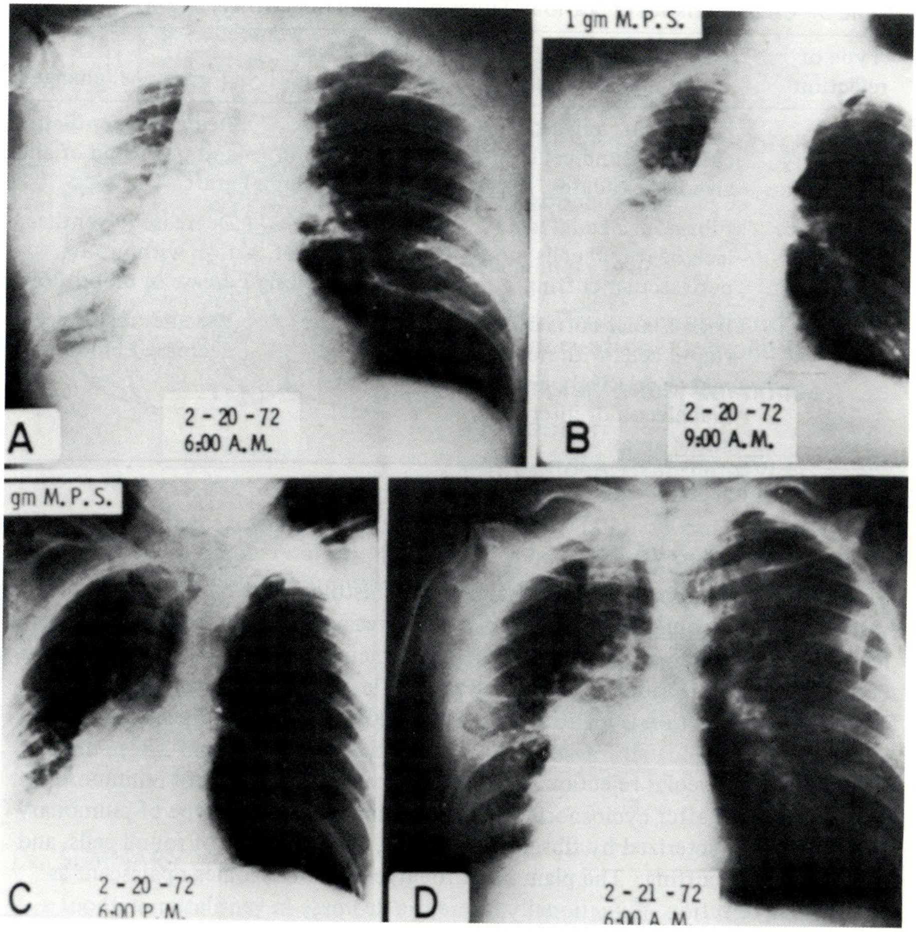

Figure 2 Sequential plain chest roentgenogram of lung allograft recipient. In the first chest x-ray (A), the patient's symptoms included slight dyspnea and increased sputum production. As the symptoms worsened over the next 3 hr, the infiltrate in the right lung became more apparent. Methylprednisolone (1 g) was given, and a decrease in the patient's symptoms was observed within 2 hr. By 9 hr after treatment (C), the chest roentgenogram was improved, and these changes were even greater 12 hr later (D). (From Veith et al. Ann. Thorac. Surg. 16:172, 1973. Used with permission of Little, Brown & Co.)

2. Veith, F. J., Kamholz, S. L., Mollenkopf, F. P., and Montefusco, C. M.: Lung transplantation 1983. Transplantation 35:271-278, 1983.
3. Reitz, B. A., Burton, N. A., Jamieson, S. W., et al.: Heart and lung transplantation: Auto- and allotransplantation in primates with extended survival. J. Thorac. Cardiovasc. Surg. 80:360, 1980.
4. Veith, F. J., Norin, A. J., Montefusco, C. M., et al.: Cyclosporin A in experimental lung transplantation. Transplantation 32:474, 1981.
5. Alican, F., Isin, E., Cockrell, J. V., and Hardy, J. D.: One stage allotransplantation of both lungs in the dog. Ann. Surg. 177:193, 1973.
6. Veith, F. J., Sinha, S., Torres, M., and Richards, K.: Bilateral simultaneous canine lung allotransplantation. Ann. Surg. 174:48, 1971.
7. Blumenstock, D. A., and Kahn, D. R.: Reimplantation and transplantation of the canine lung. J. Surg. Res. 1:40, 1961.
8. Reitz, B. A., Wallwork, J. L., Hunt, S. A., et al.: Heart-lung transplantation: Successful therapy for patients with pulmonary vascular disease. N. Engl. J. Med. 306:557, 1982.
9. Reitz, B. A., Hunt, S. A., Gaudiani, V., et al.: Clinical heart-lung transplantation. Transplant. Proc. 15:1256, 1983.
10. Veith, F. J.: Lung transplantation. Transplant. Proc. 9:203, 1977.
11. Blades, B., Pierpont, H. C., Samadi, A., et al.: The effect of experimental lung ischemia on pulmonary function. Surg. Forum 4:255, 1953.
12. Toledo-Pereyra, L. H., Hau, T., Simmons, R. L., and Najarian, J. S.: Lung preservation techniques. Ann. Thorac. Surg. 23:487, 1977.
13. Veith, F. J., and Montefusco, C. M.: Lung preservation, in Basic Concepts in Organ Procurement, Perfusion and Preservation for Transplantation, New York: Academic Press, 1982, pp. 279-299.
14. Veith, F. J., Crane, R., Torres, M., et al.: Effective preservation and transportation of lung allografts. J. Thorac. Cardiovasc. Surg. 72, 97, 1976.
15. Toledo-Pereyra, L. H., and Condie, R. M.: Lung transplantation. Hyperthermic storage for 24 hours in a colloid hyperosmolar solution. J. Thorac. Cardiovasc. Surg. 76:846, 1978.
16. Siegelman, S. S., Sinha, S. B. P., and Veith, F. J.: Pulmonary reimplantation response. Ann. Surg. 177:30, 1973.
17. Haglin, J. J., Ruiz, E., Baker, R. C., and Anderson, W. R.: Histologic studies of human transplantation. In: Wildevuur, C., ed. Morphology in Lung Transplantation, Basel: Karger, 1973, Vol. 13.
18. Mills, N. L., Boyd, A. D., and Gheranpong, C.: The significance of bronchial circulation in lung transplantation. J. Thorac. Cardiovasc. Surb. 60: 866, 1970.
19. Siegelman, S. S., Sinha, S. B. P., and Veith, F. J.: Serial bronchography following pulmonary autotransplantation. Chest 62:475, 1972.
20. Veith, F. J., Norin, A. J., Montefusco, C. M., et al.: Cyclosporin A in experimental lung transplantation. Transplantation 32:474, 1981.
21. Goldberg, M., Lima, O., Morgan, E., et al.: A comparison between cyclosporin

A and methylprednisolone plus azathioprine on bronchial healing following canine lung autotransplantation. J. Thorac. Cardiovasc. Surg. 85:821, 1983.
22. Kamholz, S. L., Veith, F. J., Mollenkopf, F. P., et al.: Single lung transplantation with cyclosporin immunosuppression. J. Thorac. Cardiovasc. Surg. 86:537-542, 1983.
23. Veith, F. J., Hagstrom, J. W. C.: Alveolar manifestations of rejection: An important cause of the poor results with human lung transplantation. Ann. Surg. 175:336, 1972.
24. Kahn, D. R., Abell, M. S., Vontz, F. K., and Sloan, H.: Rejection response on canine lung transplantation. Ann. Thorac. Surg. 1:650, 1965.
25. Halasz, N. A., Cantazaro, A., Trummer, M. J., et al.: Transplantation of the lung. Correlation of physiologic, immunologic, and histologic findings. J. Thorac. Cardiovasc. Surg. 4:581, 1973.

20

Complications of Small Bowel Transplantation

LUIS H. TOLEDO-PEREYRA
Mount Carmel Mercy Hospital, Detroit, Michigan

I. INTRODUCTION

Although the development of experimental techniques for small bowel transplantation was begun almost a quarter of a century ago, technical and immunologic obstacles have made significant progress in this area extremely slow [1-9]. To date, we have been able to document nine cases from published reports and personal communications (Table 1) [10-17]. Early clinical results were disappointing; however, recent results of small bowel transplants in humans have been encouraging, with improved survival using cyclosporine for immunosuppression. This chapter will overview the complications associated with small bowel transplantation and the considerations for achieving long-term graft and patient survival.

II. PROCUREMENT AND PRESERVATION—CONSIDERATIONS AND COMPLICATIONS

The criteria for considering cadaver donors for small bowel allograft procurement have not been standardly established because of the limited number of clinical cases. From experimental work, however, we know that the basic parameters observed for donor maintenance of other organs are also important for small bowel transplantation (Table 2). In addition, obviously, prior intestinal surgery or abdominal trauma would be relative contraindications to donation. It is important, of course, that the donor be free of infection, and donor pretreatment with antibiotics is recommended. Ideally, the donor's and recipient's weights should be within close range to facilitate vascular and intestinal anasto-

Table 1 Summary of Clinical Small Bowel Transplantation

Author, year	Recipient, condition	Donor	% Small bowel resected	Surgical technique	Graft survival	Cause of death
Deterling et al., 1964 [10]	Infant, mesenteric thrombosis	Mother (ileum)	Entire	Mesenteric artery to aorta, mesenteric vein to vena cava	12 hr	Not specified
	Child, mesenteric thrombosis	Cadaver	Entire	Not specified	2 days[a]	Patient died a few weeks later
Lillehei et al., 1967 [11]	46-year-old female, massive intestinal infarction; diffuse mesenteric venous thrombosis	Cadaver	Entire (jejunum to rectum)	Superior mesenteric to iliac vein and artery (end to side), jejunostomy and colostomy (total orthotopic)	12 hr	Pulmonary infarction, extensive pulmonary congestion, portal vein thrombosis, shock; anastomosis patent
Okumura [12] 1968 [12]	36-year-old female, superior mesenteric artery thrombosis	Cadaver	Entire (jejunum, ileum, and left colon)	Mesenteric to iliac vessels end to end and enterostomies (partial heterotopic 1.7 m)	6 days	Early rejection, necrotic bowel, renal failure
Oliver et al., 1969 [13]	35-year-old male, Gardner's syndrome, colonic polyposis, and mesenteric fibromas	Cadaver	Entire (jejunum to transverse colon)	Mesenteric to mesenteric vessels, end to end, colostomy (total orthotopic)	26 days[b]	Rejection began at 14 days, necrotic bowel at 23 days, septic shock

Alican et al., 1970 [14]	10-year-old male, gangrenous small bowel secondary to strangulation by mesenteric band	Mother (1 m of ileum)	Entire (jejunum to ileocecal valve)	Mesenteric to renal vein, end to side, mesenteric artery to aorta, end to side, enterostomies (partial heterotopic)	7 days[c]	Intra-abdominal sepsis and gastrointestinal bleeding, 32 days
Forter et al., 1972 [15]	37-year-old female, massive intestinal resection for polyposis (Gardner's syndrome)	HLA-identical sister (1.7 m), lower colon)	Entire (jejunum to right colon)	Mesenteric to right iliac vessels (partial orthotopic)	79 days[d]	Shock, renal failure, rejection, sepsis
Cohen [16]	26-year-old female on home TPN preoperatively	Cadaver	Entire	End to side	10 days	Sudden neurological event, CyA toxicity?
Butt [17]	59-year-old female, intestinal obstruction secondary to adhesions from cholecystectomy	Living related (twin)	Entire	End to side, inferior mesenteric vein and artery	3 days	Sepsis, patient reexplored 2 days postoperatively. Total dehiscence of arterial anastomosis, bowel necrosis; patient died 7 days posttransplant

[a] Antemortem autolysis of allograft prior to harvesting.
[b] Immunosuppression (azathioprine, ALG + 6-mercaptopurine and steroids for rejection).
[c] Graft removed (rejection or poor perfusion), necrotic bowel, immunosuppression (azathioprine, ALG, and prednisone).
[d] Rejection at 75 days, immunosuppression (ALG, azathioprine, and prednisone).

Table 2 Considerations for Small Bowel Allograft Donation

Adequate donor maintenance
No prior intestinal surgery or abdominal trauma
Free of infection
Antibiotic donor pretreatment suggested
Donor and recipient of compatible weights
Multiple organ harvesting acceptable except whole pancreas

moses, as well as to maintain adequate space for bowel positioning. Age criteria for small bowel donation are similar to that used for kidney donation. Small bowel procurement from cadaver donors is generally compatible with multiple organ harvesting procedures, except for obtaining whole-pancreas allografts from the same donor. Also, special anatomic considerations should be kept in mind when livers are simultaneously harvested for orthotopic transplantation, since the portal vein could be limited in length and the hepatic artery could originate from the superior mesenteric artery in some cases.

As with other organs, it is important to minimize the exposure of the small bowel to warm ischemia, since prolonged warm ischemia will result in compromise of function after transplantation [8,9,18-27]. Care should be taken to prevent damage to the bowel lumen during harvesting, as tears will result in spillage of the bowel contents and the potential for infection and/or sepsis after transplantation. As soon as the bowel has been removed, it should be thoroughly flushed with a cold (4°C) preservation solution via the aorta and superior mesenteric artery until the venous effluent is clear. Based on our experimental experience in small bowel preservation [22-26], we recommend colloid solutions for flushing. However, no definitive solution has yet been established.

Numerous studies have attempted to prolong preservation periods and to optimize small bowel preservation techniques (Table 3) [8,9,18-27]. Results have shown great variability, depending on the method used and the type of preservation solution chosen (Fig. 1). For clinical small bowel transplantation, preservation methods have not been standardized. In the reported clinical cases, the ischemic times were short (usually less than 1½ hr) [10-17]. Our general recommendations, at present, however, would be to minimize preservation times until more clinical experience is gained. The major complication resulting from inadequate preservation of small bowel allografts is temporary or permanent loss of viability after transplantation. If function is only transiently compromised, hyperalimentation may be used to support the nutritional needs of the recipient.

Table 3 Complications of Small Bowel Preservation

Bacterial contamination (spillage of bowel contents)
Ischemic damage
Vascular damage from cannulation
Damage to bowel lumen during perfusion or storage

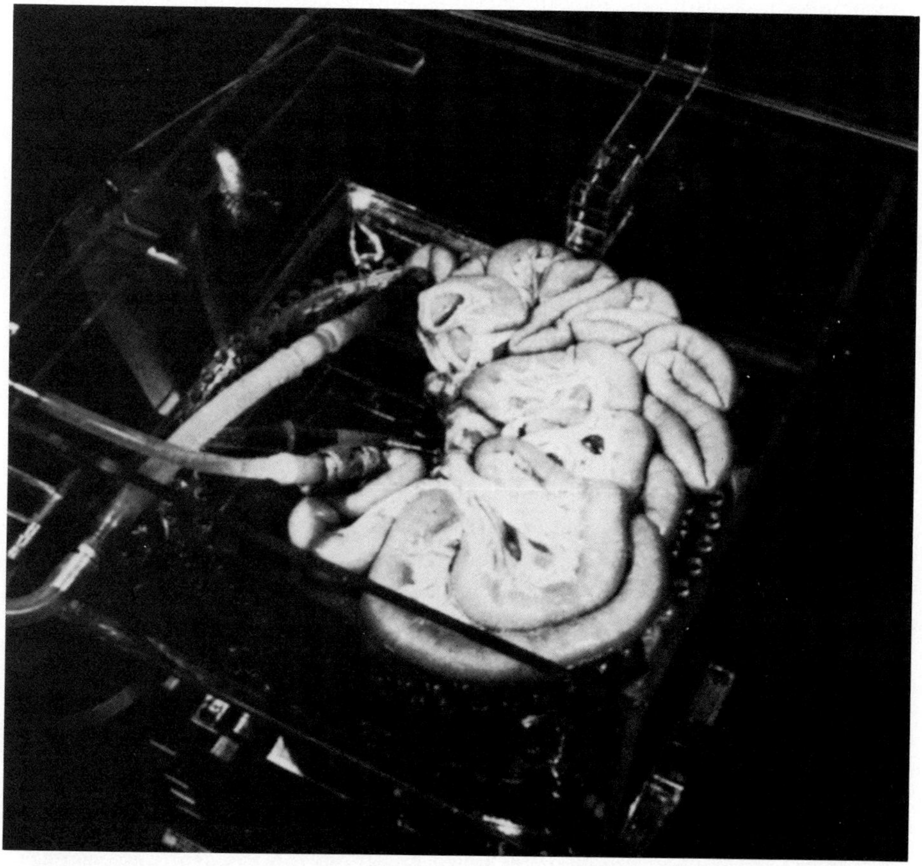

Figure 1 Hypothermic pulsatile perfusion of entire canine small intestines. The mesenteric artery is cannulated for perfusion, and a tubing or a cannula is inserted in each end of the bowel to drain intraluminal contents.

III. TECHNICAL COMPLICATIONS

A. Venous and Arterial Thrombosis

Most of the canine small bowel allograft studies have observed a high incidence of early arterial and/or venous thrombosis in the first week after transplantation [1-9]. One report has indicated that almost 40% of their transplants had thrombotic complications [28]. It has been theorized that edema in the transplanted bowel leads to a low-flow situation that promotes thrombosis. Poor preservation techniques may also contribute to subsequent thrombosis formation.

In the clinical setting, the most important and frequent indication for extensive small bowel resection is vascular thromboembolic disease. Therefore, special efforts should be made to overcome this complication. Diminishing ischemia, proper technique, and utilization of initial moderate heparinization followed by dextran compounds is important. Location of anastomosis to prevent vascular kinking is also significant. Even though a mesocaval shunt has been created in almost all clinical cases, this procedure may not be required. In human cases, thrombosis has not evidenced itself as a complication, to the degree that it has been observed with experimental studies; however, we should be aware of the potential for this complication. Early angiography would be used for confirmatory diagnosis, with a prompt follow-up exploratory procedure if necessary.

B. Hemorrhagic Infarction

This complication has been identified by Stauffer et al. [29] as one of the major complications in experimental small bowel allotransplantation, occurring within 48 hr after transplant. Previous experimental work in our laboratories indicated that the appearance of hemorrhagic necrosis after transplantation was associated with sepsis [30]. When donor and recipient animals were given perioperative antibiotics, sepsis could be prevented and the incidence of associated infarct could be decreased. In human small bowel recipients, similar perioperative antibiotics are advised; however, if preliminary symptomology (i.e., diarrhea, pain, or fever) is indicative of bleeding, follow-up angiography or, perhaps, scintigraphy scans using technetium-labeled erythrocytes to diagnose bleeding are indicated.

C. Anastomosis Leakage

Compromised vascular supply of the bowel anastomosis is frequently associated with anastomosis breakdown with subsequent leakage. Special attention should be given to this particular complication since it can carry a high rate of morbidity and mortality.

D. Herniation

Lack of proper positioning of the small bowel can account for the development of intestinal hernias, particularly when partial small bowel transplants are performed. Even though there are not enough clinical cases to accurately document the frequency of this complication, its potential occurrence after small bowel transplantation should be recognized.

IV. IMMUNOLOGIC COMPLICATIONS

A. Graft-Versus-Host Disease (GVHD)

In early experimental small bowel transplantation, in nonimmunosuppressed animals, recipients of entire small bowel allografts were observed to die within 6-9 days after transplant, with gross enlargement of their mesenteric lymph nodes but without evidence of cellular infiltration [8]. The cause of death in these animals was thought to be severe graft-versus-host disease rather than allograft rejection, since the grafts appeared viable at autopsy. The etiology of this graft loss was additionally confirmed by the finding that short segments of small bowel, without lymph nodes, followed a typical pattern of rejection within 1 week after transplant, without evidence of GVHD [8]. The addition of immunosuppression with azathioprine and steroids has extended small bowel allograft survival in canine recipients to about 3-5 weeks [1]. During the period of graft function in these animals, it appears there is a balance between GVHD and rejection. Interestingly, however, there have been no confirmed reports of GVHD in canine recipients given cyclosporin for immunosuppression [26,28,31,32]. It is possible that it is too early in our experience using cyclosporine for immunosuppression in small bowel transplantation to determine whether GVHD will be a long-term problem. There have not been enough procedures performed in humans to indicate if GVHD will be a complication, even though, at present, it appears that GVHD might not be a serious problem.

B. Small Bowel Allograft Rejection

As previously discussed, canine small bowel allograft recipients given azathioprine and prednisone experienced graft rejection at about 3-5 weeks posttransplant [1,4]. This was characterized by sloughing of the mucous membrane, mucosal bleeding, villous atrophy, thickening of the bowel wall, perforation, and perivascular round cell infiltration of the muscular and serosal layers [33].

In clinical small bowel transplants, the majority of the allografts have been lost to rejection [10-17]. Most early human recipients prior to the cyclosporine era also died after rejection of their grafts. One difficulty in clinical intestinal transplantation has been the development of tests that could accurately monitor the graft for early diagnosis of rejection. Early diagnosis would allow removal of the graft before the subsequent death of the recipient. Serial mucosal biopsies have been most commonly applied to evaluate the status of the small bowel allograft. This is only practically possible when proximal and/or distal enterostomies are performed. Several investigators have also attempted to correlate physiologic parameters, such as absorption of various sugars, with the onset of functional changes indicative of rejection [7]. Possibly these could be standardized for future clinical use. However, in the immediate postoperative period, absorption tests will likely be impaired, and with GVHD the tests may be normal [34].

V. NUTRITIONAL COMPLICATIONS

The short duration of the majority of the clinical small bowel transplants has not allowed for extensive studies of the functional status of the allografts after transplant. In the experimental work with canine autografts by Ballinger et al. [35], a decreased capacity for fat absorption and loss of mucosa and villi was observed after autotransplantation. These changes have also been seen in small bowels after denervation without ischemia. It is thought, therefore, that these changes may be induced primarily by denervation.

As previously discussed, there is at least a transient compromise of function after most small bowel allografts; therefore, nutritional requirements will probably have to be supplemented with intravenous hyperalimentation for at least the first few weeks after transplantation.

VI. INFECTIOUS COMPLICATIONS

The obvious risks from infectious complications after small bowel transplantation may be minimized by strict aseptic technique during donor harvesting, subsequent preservation, and transplant procedures. Donor pretreatment with antibiotics is recommended, as well as perioperative antibiotic coverage of the recipient. In the clinical small bowel transplant experience, sepsis and septic shock have been reported in the three cases surviving a week or greater. The most common microorganisms found postoperatively are *Escherichia coli, Bacteroides, Pseudomonas,* and *Proteus.* These infectious complications are probably secondary to technical problems and steroid immunosuppression and may decrease with the more recent use of cyclosporine as the primary immunosuppressant.

VII. CONCLUSIONS

At the present time, small bowel allotransplantation and total parenteral nutrition (TPN) are the only alternatives for patients undergoing entire small bowel re-

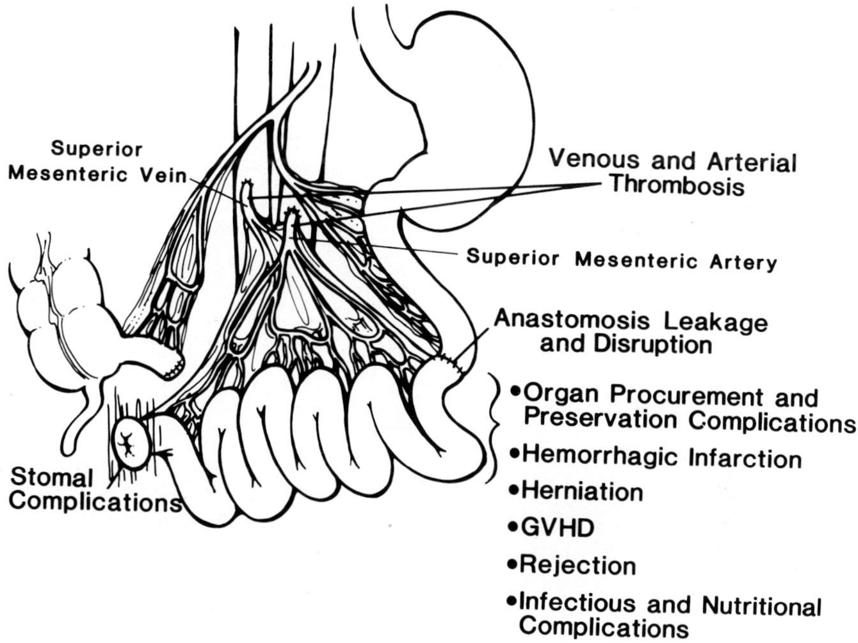

Figure 2 Detail of one of the anastomosis techniques that may be used for small bowel transplantation. An end-to-side vascular connection between the superior mesenteric artery and the aorta and the superior mesenteric vein and the vena cava has been created. Common postoperative complications of this procedure are noted.

section. The long-term effects of TPN are not yet known. The limited number of human small bowel transplants has been restricted extensive investigation of all the complications of this procedure in humans. However, the large amount of experimental investigations in the literature provide more realistic expectations for the transplant surgeon. In general, although some positive results have been obtained experimentally, the clinical experience with small bowel transplantation has been disappointing and postoperative complications remain (Fig. 2). The recent implementation of cyclosporine as an immunosuppressive agent may provide some new hope for prolonging graft survival and minimizing post-transplant complications. In addition, further work is needed to develop consistent preservation techniques and better methods for prognosticating rejection that may be used clinically.

REFERENCES

1. Taylor, R. M. A., Watson, J. W., Walker, F. C., and Watson, A. J.: Prolongation of survival of jejunal homografts in dogs treated with azathioprine (Imuran). Br. J. Surg. 53:134, 1966.
2. Preston, F. W., Macalalad, F., Wachowski, T. J., et al.: Survival of homografts of the intestine with and without immunosuppression. Surgery 60: 1203, 1966.
3. Monchik, G. J., and Russell, P. S.: Transplantation of small bowel in the rat: Technical and immunological considerations. Surgery 70:693, 1971.
4. Ruiz, J. O., and Lillehei, R. C.: Intestinal transplantation. Surg. Clin. North Am. 52:1075, 1972.
5. Lillehei, R. C., Boott, B., and Miller F. A.: Homografts of the small bowel. Surg. Forum 10:197, 1959.
6. Holmes, J. T., Yeh, S. D. J., Winawer, S. J., et al.: Absorption studies in canine jejunal allografts. Ann. Surg. 174:101, 1974.
7. Cohen, W. B., Hardy, M. A., Quint, J., and State, D.: Absorptive function in canine jejunal autografts and allografts. Surgery 65:440, 1969.
8. Lillehei, R. C., Goott, B., and Miller, F. A.: The physiological response of the small bowel of the dog to ischemia including prolonged in vitro preservation of the bowel with successful replacement and survival. Ann. Surg. 150:543-560, 1959.
9. Eyal, Z., Manax, W. G., Bloch, J. H., and Lillehei, R. C.: Successful in vitro preservation of the small bowel, including maintenance of mucosal integrity with chlopromazine, hypothermia, and hyperbaric oxygenation. Surgery 57:259-268, 1965.
10. Deterling, R.: Comments to Alican, F. A. Am. J. Surg. 121:159, 1971.
11. Lillehei, R. C., Idezuki, Y., Feemster, J. A., et al.: Transplantation of the stomach, intestine, and pancreas: Experimental and clinical observations. Surgery 62:721-741, 1967.
12. Okumura, M., Fujimura, I., Ferrari, A. A., et al.: Transplante de intestine delgado. Apresentacao de um caso. Rev. Hosp. Clin. Fac. Med. S. Paulo 24:39-54, 1969.
13. Olivier, C. H., Olivier, C. L., and Rettori, R.: Les conséquences de l'interruption lymphatique et de l'enervation lors de l'homotransplantation totale du grele chez l'homme. J. Chir. 98:341-348, 1969.
14. Alican, F., Hardy, J. D., Cayirli, M., et al.: Intestinal transplantation: Laboratory experience and report of a clinical case. Am. J. Surg. 12:150-159, 1971.
15. Fortner, J. S., Sichuk, G., Litwin, S. D., and Beattle, E. J.: Immunological responses to an intestinal allograft with HL-A-identical donor-recipient. Transplantation 14:531-535, 1972.
16. Cohen, Z.: Personal communication, 1985.
17. Butt, K.: Personal communication, 1985.
18. Barnett, W. O., Truett, G., and Stone, J.: Experimental small-bowel homografts. Am. J. Dig. Dis. 7:833-838, 1962.

19. Austen, W. G., and McLaughlin, E. D.: In vitro small bowel perfusion. Surg. Forum 16:359-361, 1965.
20. Lyons, G. W., Manaz, W. G., Largiader, F., and Lillehei, R. C.: Intestinal absorption of ileum preserved by hypothermia and hyperbaric oxygen. Surg. Forum 16:357-359, 1965.
21. Ruiz, J. O., Shultz, L. S., Hendricks, J., and Castelfranchi, P. L.: Trans. Am. Soc. Artif. Intern. Organs 17:42-48, 1971.
22. Toledo-Pereyra, L. H., Simmons, R. L., and Najarian, J. S.: Comparative effects of chlorpromazine, methylprednisolone, and allopurinol during small bowel preservation. Am. J. Surg. 126:631, 1973.
23. Toledo-Pereyra, L. H., and Najarian, J. S.: Small bowel preservation:Comparison of perfusion and nonperfusion systems. Arch. Surg. 107:875-877, 1973.
24. Toledo-Pereyra, L. H., Simmons, R. L., and Najarian, J. S.: Prolonged survival of canine orthotopic small intestinal allografts preserved for 24 hours by hypothermic bloodless perfusion. Surgery 75:368-376, 1974.
25. Toledo-Pereyra, L. H., Simmons, R. L., and Najarian, J. S.: Two-to-three day intestinal preservation utilizing hypothermic pulsatile perfusion. Ann. Surg. 179:454-459, 1974.
26. Toledo-Pereyra, L. H., unpublished data.
27. Toledo-Pereyra, L. H.: Small bowel preservaion. In: Toledo-Pereyra, L. H., ed. Basic Concepts of Organ Procurement, Perfusion, and Preservation for Transplantation, New York: Academic Press, 1982, pp. 317-331.
28. Resnick, R. K., Craddock, G. N., Langer, B., et al.: Structure and function of small bowel allografts in the dog: Immunosuppression with cyclosporin A. Can. J. Surg. 25:51-55, 1982.
29. Stauffer, U. G., Becker, M., Hirsig, J., et al.: The risks of small intestinal transplantation for the recipient: Experimental results in the young minipigs. J. Pediatr. Surg. 13:465, 1978.
30. Toledo-Pereyra, L. H., Raif, L., Simmons, R. L., and Najarian, J. S.: Role of endotoxin and bacteria in long-term survival of preserved small-bowel allografts. Surgery 73:474-481, 1974.
31. Diliz-Perez, H. S., McClure, J., Bedetti, C., et al.: Successful small bowel allotransplantation in dogs with cyclosporine and prednisone. Transplantation 32:126-129, 1984.
32. Raju, S., Didlake, R. H., Cayirli, M., et al.: Experimental small bowel transplantation 38:561-566, 1984.
33. Preston, F. W., Macalalad, F., Graber, R., et al.: Function and survival of jejunal homotransplants in dogs with and without immunosuppressive treatment. Transplantation 3:224, 1965.
34. Hardy, M. A., Quint, J., and State, D. L.: Effect of antilymphocyte serum and other immunosuppressive agents on canine jejunal allografts. Ann. Surg. 171:51-60, 1970.
35. Ballinger, W. F., Christy, M. S., and Ashby, W. B.: Autotransplantation of the small intestine: The effect of denervation. Surgery 52:151-164, 1962.

21

Corneal Transplantation: Medical and Surgical Complications

JOHN W. COWDEN
Kresge Eye Institute, Wayne State University, Detroit, Michigan

I. INTRODUCTION

Most ophthalmic microsurgeons are able to do a satisfactory penetrating keratoplasty (corneal transplant); however, the successful corneal surgeon is the one who is able to correctly identify and manage the multitude of postoperative complications that can arise. There is no other ocular procedure fraught with so many problems that extend over such a long period of time.

The following is an attempt to help the reader identify and successfully manage the complications that may arise at the time of, or following, a corneal transplant. There has been an attempt to mention the complications to chronological sequence; however it should be pointed out that in some cases complications arise at times other than those under which they are listed here.

II. MEDICAL COMPLICATIONS

The medical complications of corneal transplantation include the early findings of primary graft failure, infections, healing disorders, and glaucoma. The late complications include corneal decompensation, of which the allograft rejection reaction is the most significant cause, as well as vascularization and glaucoma. Recurrent corneal disease and other medical complications preventing good vision are also discussed.

A. Early Medical Complications

1. Primary Graft Failure

A primary graft failure is the presence of a hazy, thickened graft from postoperative day 1 that fails to improve over the next week, despite the absence of other factors that may complicate the graft, such as low intraocular pressure or excessive inflammation. If the intraocular pressure is very low, because of a wound leak or ciliary body shutdown, the cornea will appear thickened and hazy, like a primary graft failure, but will thin and clear when the pressure is normalized.

A primary graft failure is due to an inadequate number of endothelial cells needed to keep the corneal detergested or endothelial cell dysfunction because of trauma, age, inflammation, or toxic medications. Poor donor tissue may be the cause of a graft failure, which can occur because of excessive time between donor death and storage or transplantation and diseased or aged donor endothelium. Poor storage or handling techniques, including a traumatic donor excision or trephination, excessive intraocular irrigation, excessive movement of an intraocular lens, or other surgical trauma, may cause the loss of endothelial cells resulting in a primary graft failure [1].

The treatment for such a condition if there is no improvement over a several-day period (providing other factors have been excluded) is to replace the corneal graft within 2 weeks. Procrastination will result in a more difficult surgical procedure complicated by hemorrhage or partial wound healing and only delay the time of visual restoration.

2. Infection

A fulminating bacterial infection, either endophthalmitis or corneal ulceration, is a dreaded complication of corneal transplantation. The possibility of an infection transmitted by the donor cornea has been decreased by careful modern eyebanking procedures using technicians trained in sterile techniques for cornea excision, enucleation procedures, and the processing of the donor tissue. Despite the use of antibiotics in the storage media and careful screening of the donor for contagious conditions; it is impossible to eliminate all cases of donor-transmitted infection. The most common bacterial organism cultured from the donor rim in storage media is *Staphylococcus epidermitis.* Because most patients are given antibiotics at the time of surgery, this rarely causes an endophthalmitis [2]. The development of a donor-transmitted streptococcal endophthalmitis or a gram-negative endophthalmitis, which may have been resistant to prophylactic antibiotics used in the storage media or irrigating solutions, will occasionally continue to occur despite the most careful eyebanking procedures [3]. The use of intraoperative and postoperatively antibiotics reduces the changes for endophthalmitis since not all organisms will be covered by gentamicin, which is the most commonly used in antibiotic in the storage media. Although rare in its occurrence, the development of a fungal or viral infection may also occur [4,5].

The treatment for endophthalmitis following a corneal transplant in an aphakic eye is an emergency total vitrectomy with the infusion of intraocular antibiotics and replacement of the cornea graft. The administration of topical, subconjunctival, and systemic broad-spectrum antibiotics is required until cultures and sensitivity testing have identified the most appropriate drugs for the infecting organism. If the infection is limited to the anterior segment, the purulent material may be irrigated from the anterior chamber with an antibiotic solution and the graft replaced.

The development of a corneal ulcer shortly following keratoplasty may be the result of donor-transmitted infection; however, it is more likely to be caused by host-related organisms, such as staphylococcus. It is often associated with the presence of a persistent epithelial defect or suture abscess (Fig. 1). Treatment consists of debridement, removal of the suture if appropriate, cultures, and sensitivity testing with the administration of appropriate topical and subconjunctival antibiotics. An anterior chamber or vitreous tap should not be performed if the infection appears to be the result of corneal ulceration or suture abscess since the introduction of an organism into the interior of the eye may occur and appropriate cultures may be obtained externally.

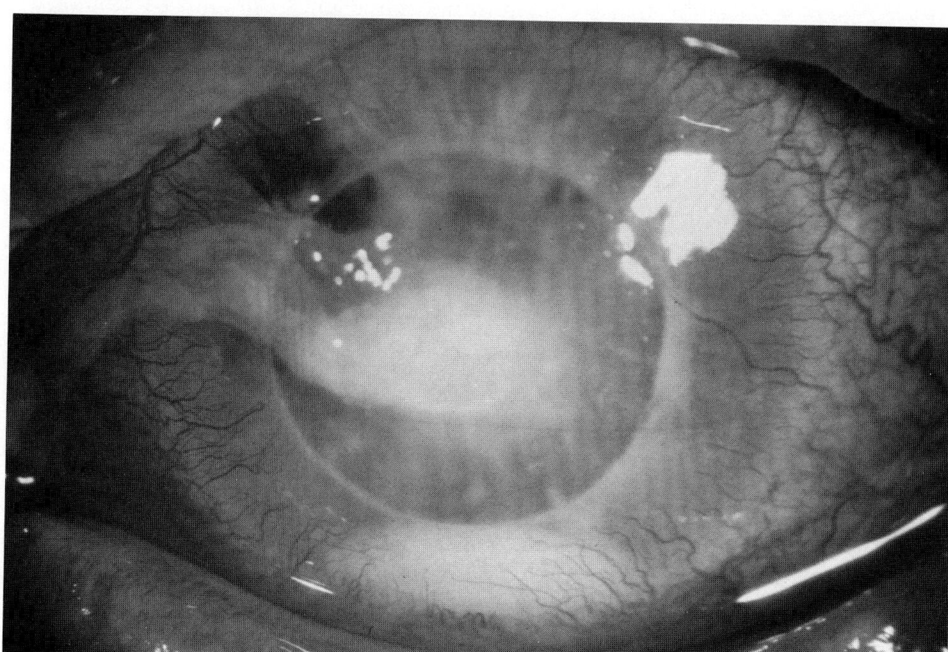

Figure 1 Corneal ulcer in graft due to persistent epithelial defect.

3. Healing Disorders

Re-epithelialization of a corneal graft in a patient with healthy recipient epithelium will normally occur over a denuded donor graft by postoperative day 3. Patients with ocular surface disorders, especially corneal scarring secondary to alkali burns. Stevens-Johnson syndrome, trachoma, ocular pemphagoid, exposure keratitis, and keratitis sicca, will have retarded healing of the epithelium and may develop a persistent epithelial defect of the portion of the donor graft. This disorder, if not successfully treated, results in increased risk of infection, superficial corneal scarring, or melting of the corneal stroma, which could cause perforation within 1 week.

The treatment of an epithelial defect is closure of the eyelid by pressure patching after the application of an antibiotic and the elimination of any possible causes of exposure keratitis or keratitis sicca. If the defect fails to improve over a 48-hr period, a bandage soft contact lens should be utilized to cover the defect in order to protect the regenerating epithelium from trauma or drying. Artificial tears and antibiotic drops are used frequently to prevent drying of the bandage lens. If a bandage lens cannot be tolerated, a temporary central suture tarsorrhaphy should be performed. The applications of topical medications and examination of the cornea are still possible. The suture is removed in approximately 2 weeks if epithelial healing has occurred.

Topical medications that are toxic to the epithelium should not be utilized. Collagenase inhibitors or fibrinonectin have been reported to promote re-epithelialization; however, they have not received widespread acceptance. The patient must be followed closely for recurrence of the defect.

4. Glaucoma

All patients with pre-existing glaucoma will continue to require treatment postoperatively, often additional or stronger antiglaucomatous medications. The measurement of the intraocular pressure postoperatively requires the use of an electronic tonometer since applanation or Schiotz tonometry is difficult or inaccurate on an eye with an irregular corneal surface that recently underwent a penetrating keratoplasty. In eyes that have undergone multiple surgical procedures, the development of a postoperative glaucoma following keratoplasty is not unusual since there may be additional scarring in the area of the trabecular meshwork, inflammatory debris, including blood and fibrin, or the development of peripheral anterior synechiae [6]. A common cause of increased pressure is the use of Healon during the surgical procedure. Fortunately, in most cases this is a transient elevation of the intraocular pressure. The treatment for an early glaucoma is the use of oral Diamox or topical Timoptic. Additional antiglaucomatous medicines may be required. Other surgically induced causes of glaucoma must be identified and corrected as described under the section on surgical complications.

B. Late Medical Complications

1. Corneal Decompensation

Corneal decompensation occurs because of inadequate endothelial cells or endothelial cell dysfunction, which if severe may cause the epithelial edema known as bullous keratopathy. The causes of corneal edema or decompensation after keratoplasty include defective donor tissue, surgical trauma, inflammation, allograft rejection, and glaucoma.

2. Allograft Rejection Reaction

Allograft rejection may involve the epithelium stroma, endothelium, or a combination of any of these cell-containing layers. The incidence varies depending upon the degree of vascularity of the recipient cornea. In nonvascularized recipients, the incidence of the immune reaction has been reported to vary from 10 to 26% [7]. Rejection may occur as early as 2 weeks after corneal transplantation and any time thereafter, although 90% of graft rejections occur within the first year and 50% within 3 months after surgery [8]. The symptoms of decreased vision, photophobia, and redness of the eye may be overlooked by a patient who has not yet gained useful vision in the operated eye. This makes the need for frequent follow-up examinations crucial if such a reaction is to be detected in time for successful treatment.

The identification of an immune allograft rejection is identified by the following criteria: (1) uncomplicated surgery (minimal trauma to endothelium, rapid restoration of anterior chamber, absence of hemorrhage, and so on); (2) absence of postoperative complications that could cause corneal edema (poor wound closure, rupture, severe uveitis, glaucoma, synechiae, vitreous touch, and others); (3) a clear graft for at least 2 weeks postoperatively; (4) rapid onset of graft edema, usually localized, with a relatively mild anterior chamber reaction; and (5) development of an endothelial rejection line.

Alldredge and Krachmer reported three different types of rejection reactions [9]. An epithelial rejection is diagnosed by the present of an epithelial rejection line. This is an elevated line in the epithelium that stains with fluorescein and progresses from the periphery toward the center of the graft over a course of several days to a few weeks. Subepithelial infiltrates found only in the donor tissue are another form of epithelial rejection. They appear as irregular, round, whitish deposits in the anterior stroma approximately 0.2-0.5 mm in diameter [9]. There may be an associated epithelial or endothelial rejection line and keratic precipitates with other signs of inflammation.

The classic endothelial rejection is manifest as a linear accumulation of keratic precipitates on the endothelium that will move over a period of several days from an area of marginal vascularization toward the center of the graft, usually accom-

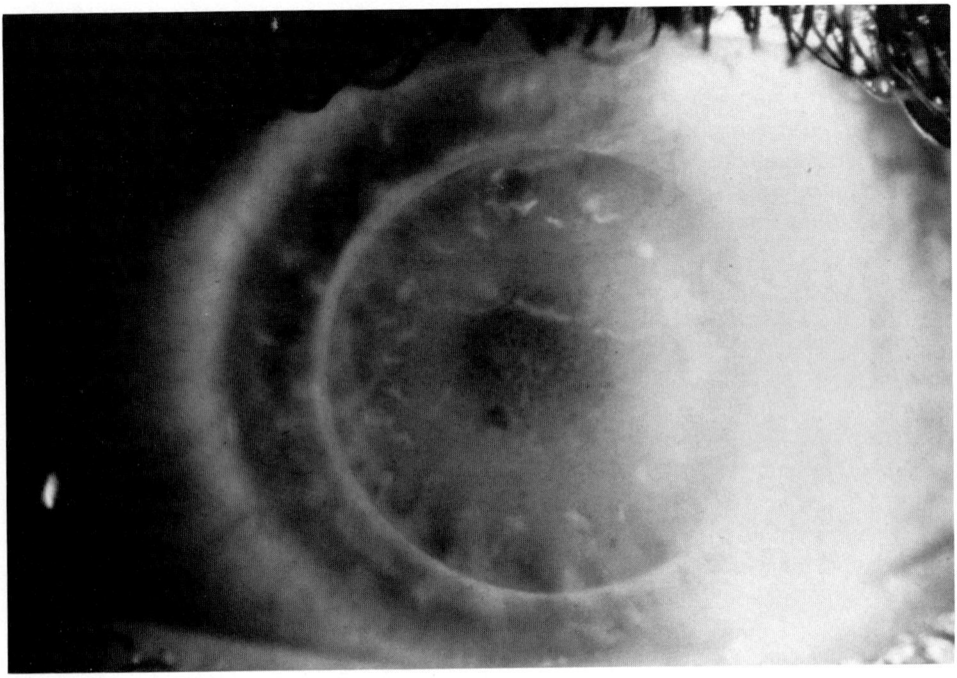

Figure 2 Rejection line in acute allograft rejection reaction.

panied by localized stromal and epithelial edema (Fig. 2) [10]. The line consists of lymphocytes that attack the donor endothelial cells. If the condition is allowed to progress untreated, it will destroy the entire donor endothelium within less than 1 week. Therefore, rapid diagnosis and treatment are essential if the graft is to be salvaged.

The treatment of an immune allograft rejection of any type is the frequency application of concentrated topical steroids, plus sub-Tenon's repository steroids or systemic steroids. Suppression of the reaction is usually achieved within several days. If no response is noted within a 2-week period, the systemic steroids are discontinued and topical steroid drops gradually reduced. (A suggested treatment of graft rejection consists of the immediate instillation, on an hourly basis, of 1% prednisolone acetate drops, and the use of prednisone, 80 mg orally, every morning for 2 weeks. If systemic prednisone is contraindicated, or the patient is not reliable in the administration of topical steroid drops, a sub-Tenon's injection of Depo-Medrol, 80 mg, may be utilized. The administration of topical cycloplegics, such as atropine 1% four times a day, is also indicated.)

A favorable response to treatment will occur within 7-10 days in five-sixths of the cases of graft rejection reactions diagnosed and treated within the first 3 days of onset. Improvement is noted by decrease in corneal thickness, resolution of the rejection line and anterior chamber reaction, and subsequent visual improvement.

Predisposing factors to rejection include pre-existing vascularization of the recipient cornea, postoperative neovascularization, synechiae, inflammation, previous corneal transplant, and especially a history of prior allograft rejection [11]. Rejection rates as high as 60-70% have been reported in these high-risk groups. Although HLA typing in ordinary corneal transplantation has not been shown to be effective in reducing rejection episodes, some studies in patients with vascularized corneas or prior allograft rejection have shown that the absence of preformed circulating lymphocytotoxic antibodies (demonstrated by a negative lymphocyte cross-match), with a relative HLA-A,B antigen matching, improved the corneal allograft survival for these high-risk patients [12,14].

3. Vascularization

The healing of a corneal incision occurs because of the formation of fibroblasts, normally without vascularization of the scar. Vascularization of the graft occurs as a result of a previously vascularized recipient cornea, exposed irritating suture knots, localized inflammation, or edema. The vessels will grow toward the area of irritation or edema; however, once they reach the graft margin, the vessels usually begin to circle around the new cornea unless there is inflammation or edema within the graft. If the vessels pass directly into the stroma, there is a strong liklihood that a severe rejection reaction will occur and the graft may fail. Occasionally a portion of the graft may be vascularized with the deposition of a dense lipid material, which may prevent a good visual result.

The treatment for the development of vascularization in a graft is to immediately remove any sutures that have caused vessels to migrate to the graft margin and treat vigorously with topical and injectable steroids to reduce inflammation.

C. Recurrent Disease

The recurrence of the original disease that resulted in corneal scarring or decompensation requiring a corneal transplant may occur in the new graft. Recurrent herpes simplex keratitis occurs in approximately 10% of corneal transplants done for scarring caused by the herpesvirus (Fig. 3). Special care must be taken, when using topical or systemic steroids, to treat with prophylactic antivirals following a corneal transplant done for this condition.

The hereditary stromal dystrophies will gradually involve the peripheral portion of the corneal grafts and may require a replacement of the graft in 15-20 years in some patients because of the accumulation of new deposits that resulted

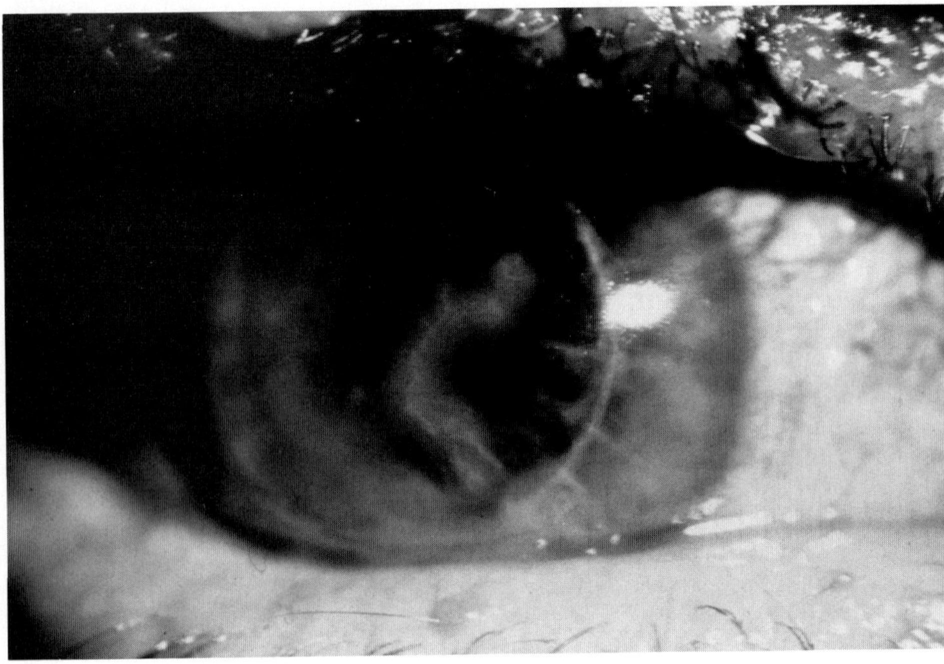

Figure 3 Recurrent dendrite in graft due to herpes simplex virus.

in the original corneal opacification. In mucopolysaccharidosis, especially Hurler's disease, the deposition of the mucopolysaccharide may be seen as early as 3 or 4 years following the corneal transplant.

The development of recurrent keratoconus in a patient who had undergone a corneal transplant previously is usually due to failure to remove the entire area of corneal thinning at the time of the original surgery. If the entire cone was not excised and a small graft was done, the keratoconus may continue with the protrusion of a clear graft at the tip of a new cone [15]. Treatment would require a repeat corneal transplant with a very large diameter.

Recurrent ulceration of the cornea due to keratitis sicca or exposure keratitis is a serious problem that could result in the loss of a graft unless the conditions have been recognized and properly treated in order to prevent ulceration. In some cases of rheumatoid arthritis, a recurrent epithelial defect with stromal melting in the graft occurs that is identical to the original problem the patient experienced (Fig. 4). This melting syndrome is extremely difficult to manage despite frequent lubrication and may require a conjunctival flap or tarsorrhaphy in order to prevent the loss of the eye.

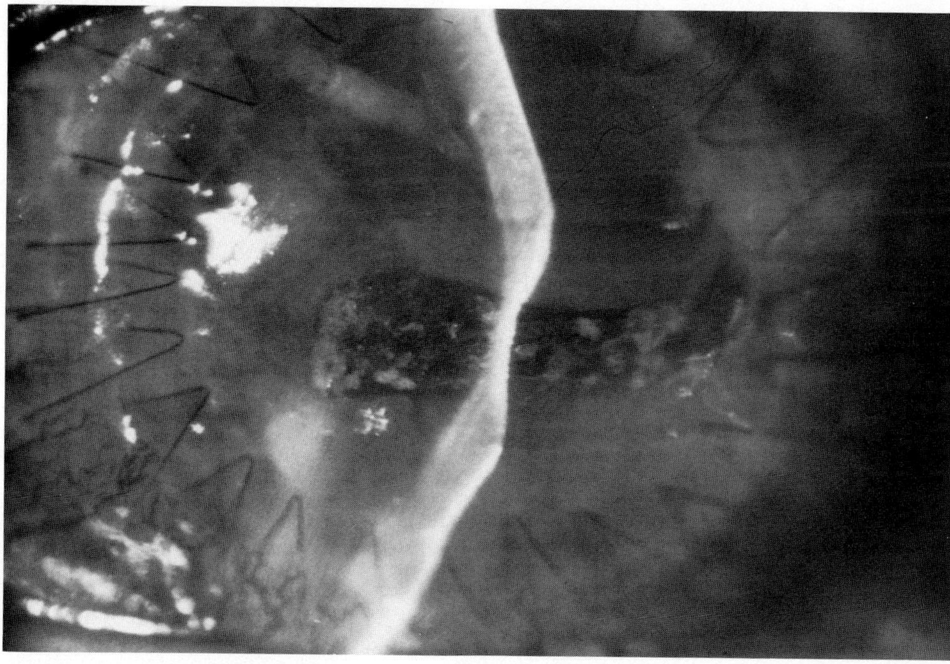

Figure 4 Graft melting in rheumatoid arthritis.

D. Other Medical Complications

Ocular conditions that may not have existed prior to surgery may occur as the result of a corneal transplant. The development of cystoid macular edema in an aphakic eye may prevent a good visual result. This could have existed prior to the corneal surgery and may resolve spontaneously, although 50% of the cases are persistent over a 2-year period.

Diplopia or double vision may be caused by a successful corneal transplant, restoring vision to an eye that had developed a deviation and/or visual suppression. This is treated by realignmant of the eyes with prisms or ocular muscle surgery.

A cataract may develop postoperatively as a rapid progression of a pre-existing cataract, secondary to traumatic surgery or the administration of high doses of topical or systemic steroids. If a visually significant cataract develops post-keratoplasty, it should be removed prior to suture removal in order to prevent corneal graft wound dehiscence at the time of the cataract surgery. Otherwise, a wait of 6-12 months following suture removal will be required before further surgery to assure adequate wound healing. There is a risk of causing corneal decompensation with any intraocular surgical procedure after a corneal transplant.

There are few serious risks to patients' lives resulting from corneal transplantation; however, the very rare transfer of a lethal infection has been reported in rabies, serum hepatitis, and Creutzfeldt-Jakob syndrome. There are no reported cases of malignancy caused by corneal transplantation.

III. SURGICAL COMPLICATIONS

A. Intraoperative Complications

The surgical complications of corneal transplantation include the intraoperative complications of hemorrhage, donor-recipient disparity, surgical trauma to the iris or lens, vitreous loss, and inability to re-form the anterior chamber.

1. Hemorrhage

A retrobulbar hemorrhage may occur at the time of the retrobulbar block and must be recognized prior to the beginning of surgery if disaster is to be avoided. This can be identified by protrusion and firmness of the globe against the eyelids with subconjunctival blood, which gradually creeps forward, appearing around the equator of the eye. Should this be identified the procedure must be canceled. Usually the increased pressure is transient and does not require any specific treatment, although in some cases a lateral canthotomy is performed to relieve the retrobulbar pressure against the globe.

If the patient's cornea is highly vascularized, there may be a significant amount of hemorrhage from the corneal vessels that are cut at the time of the trephination. Bleeding into the anterior chamber interferes with the procedure. Bleeding into the posterior chamber may prevent satisfactory visual recovery due to the vitreous hemorrhage. In order to prevent this, the superficial vessels should be cauterized at the limbus. The removal of a fibrovascular pannus, when present, from the surface of the cornea will also help to reduce bleeding. Deeper corneal vessels may bleed excessively when cut and cannot easily be cauterized because of shrinkage of the corneal incision, which will prevent good wound closure. A topical drop of 1:10,000 epinephrine may help to slow the hemorrhage by vasoconstriction. The best method is to rapidly suture the new cornea into position, tamponading the vessels.

Hemorrhage may occur from the iris or anterior chamber angle because of the presence of rubeosis iridis or abnormal vessels in the anterior chamber angle. Care must be taken to avoid excessive manipulation or pulling on the iris, which could result in an iridodialysis causing a significant hemorrhage from the angle. This is controlled by allowing the iris to flatten against the host cornea for a short period of time until clotting has occurred. In an aphakic eye, if the vitreous face is not intact, this may not be practical and a large amount of blood may enter the posterior chamber. If this occurs, an anterior vitrectomy should be performed with removal of the blood, after adequate clotting has been achieved, from the area of hemorrhage. Residual blood may be gently irrigated from the anterior chamber with balanced salt solution. A blood clot in the pupil should be removed; however, care should be taken not to disturb the clot in the area from which the hemorrhage occurred.

The most serious ocular surgical emergency is the development of an expulsive choroidal hemorrhage. This disaster can be identified prior to its occurrence by progressive vitreous loss with a dark rising mass seen through the pupil. Should this be seen prior to the expulsion of blood, retina, and choroid from the eye, immediate tamponade is required. Place the index finger or other instrument over the trephine opening if the cornea cannot be closed immediately. A posterior sclerotomy is made in the region of the mass with aspiration of the blood in a syringe followed by immediate corneal wound closure. If the expulsive hemorrhage has occurred with loss of intraocular contents, the eye is lost and evisceration or enucleation will be required.

2. Donor-Recipient Disparity

A disparity between the donor corneal diameter and the recipient trephine diameter may be planned to provide a steeper cornea by placing a larger donor in a smaller recipient opening or a flatter cornea by placing a small donor in a larger recipient opening. This is done to reduce an expected refractive error in order to provide the patient with better uncorrected vision. An irregular trephine opening or donor button may produce high degrees of postoperative astigmatism due to the placement of an oval donor in a round hole, or vice versa. Poor technique in preforming the trephination of either the donor or recipient cornea accounts for the majority of the postoperative astigmatism that occurs [16]. Extreme care must be taken in trephining the recipient cornea to assure that the trephine blade is perpendicular to the surface, and even pressure is applied in order to penetrate the cornea in a perpendicular manner without sliding to the side. Care must also be taken to avoid pressing on the globe with the fixation forceps during the trephination, or an oval opening will be made. The corneal scissors must be held perpendicularly when cutting out the recipient corneal button if a posterior lip is to be avoided. If this happens, the lip must be carefully excised in a continuous strip to prevent notching resulting in posterior wound gap and a possible wound leak. The donor button, when supplied in tissue culture media, is usually trephined with the endothelial surface up. Care must be taken to assure a perpendicular cut with a very sharp-edged trephine, or an irregular or oval-shaped button may be produced with a posterior or anterior lip of the button itself.

A disparity in the donor-recipient edge thickenss may develop in cases of keratoconus when the recipient may be thinner than the donor or in cases of bullous keratopathy with a thickened recipient cornea compared with the donor. If the donor is thicker than the recipient, it will be necessary to use an increased number of sutures to close the area with the thinned recipient cornea in order to prevent a wound leak. In cases of a thinned donor with an extremely thick recipient, the endothelial surfaces should be aligned by placing extremely deep sutures on both sides of the wound. This will help to prevent the development of a retrocorneal membrane.

3. Surgical Trauma to the Iris or Lens

Inadvertent trauma to the iris or lens occurs at the time of trephination if the trephine is allowed to penetrate into the eye with the loss of aqueous and flattening of the anterior chamber. A traumatic iridodialysis may be produced by excessive pulling of the iris if it is adherent to the cornea during removal. In complicated keratoplastics with flat anterior chambers, it may be impossible to avoid excising a portion or most of the iris. Care must be taken to avoid a closed chamber angle by separating the iris from the peripheral cornea or performing a large-sector iridectomy. If a lens implant is to be performed in aphakic eyes, large iridectomies or an iridodialysis may require repair.

If the anterior lens capsule is lacerated unintentionally, a lens extraction must be performed since a cataract is inevitable. If a cataract is present at the time of surgery, it should be removed using either the intracapsular or extracapsular technique, with or without an intraocular lens implant. Most corneal surgeons now perform the triple procedure, consisting of the corneal transplantation, extracapsular cataract extraction, and posterior chamber intraocular lens implantation in such cases. Occasionally an anterior chamber lens is placed in an eye that is already aphakic or in which an intracapsular cataract extraction was done. Iris-supported lenses are to be avoided because of the movement of the lens, which may result in damage to the new cornea. Likewise, anterior chamber lenses with anterior movement on compression should also be avoided. A special complication has developed with the advent of intraocular lenses that requires removal at the time of keratoplasty because of partial dislocation or chronic irritation producing an iritis. In these cases the intraocular lens may be fixed in position by fibrosis to the iris or to the anterior chamber angle. Frequently it is necessary to cut the supports loose from the optic portion and remove the lens in pieces to prevent hemorrhage or tearing of the delicate structures.

4. Vitreous Loss

Vitreous may be lost from the eye if there is positive vitreous pressure. This can occur from retrobulbar hemorrhage, inadequate general anesthesia, inadequate lid block, scleral collapse, or choroidal hemorrhage. It is imperative to discover what the difficulty may be and immediately to rectify it. An extensive anterior vitrectomy with the removal of all the vitreous from the anterior chamber and from a central core to the middle of the posterior chamber must be done in order to adequately close the wound and prevent adhesions of vitreous to the wound edge, which could result in cystoid macular edema or an epithelial downgrowth.

5. Inability to Re-Form the Anterior Chamber

Inability to re-form the anterior chamber may be due to an insufficient number of sutures used to close the wound or sutures that are too loosely tied, resulting in wound leak. Identification of this complication may be difficult because of iris blocking the area where the wound leak has occurred. Occasionally, positive vitreous pressure will result in a flattening of the anterior chamber with difficulty in re-formation. In some cases there is pressure against the lens-iris diaphragm, despite the presence of a peripheral iridectomy. This may be the result of an aqueous diversion syndrome and will only be alleviated by a pars plana aspiration of vitreous with re-formation of the anterior chamber using air. A choroidal detachment may also cause a flat anterior chamber. Should the anterior chamber flatten during subconjunctival injections, deficient wound closure must be identified and corrected. Under no circumstances should the patient leave the operating room without a formed anterior chamber. In extremely difficult cases, especially those with flat anterior chamber prior to surgery, Healon or other viscoelastic substances may be helpful in maintaining an open anterior chamber angle after a penetrating keratoplasty.

B. Early Postoperative Complications

Early postoperative surgical complications, which may be found during postoperative day 1 or 2, include a flat anterior chamber and glaucoma.

1. Shallow or Flat Anterior Chamber

As previously mentioned, the presence of a flat anterior chamber is usually due to a wound leak that may or may not be demonstrated by a positive Seidel test using fluorescein to demonstrate the leak. If the Seidel test is negative, a wound leak may have occurred but sealed because of iris plugging the wound internally. Light pressure on the peripheral portion of the cornea may produce a positive Seidel test that was otherwise negative. If this is the case the leak must be resutured. This usually can be done under topical anesthesia without returning to the operating room.

A chorodial detachment may also be the cause of a flat anterior chamber. If a choroidal detachment can be seen or diagnosed by ultrasound, cycloplegics and mannitol or carbonic anhydrase inhibitors may be successful in re-establishing the anterior chamber. If there is no improvement over a 2- to 3-day period or if the lens is up against the back of the new cornea, surgical intervention consisting of drainage of the choroidal detachment and air injection of the anterior chamber will be required in order to minimize damage to the corneal graft.

2. Aqueous Diversion Syndrome

An acute glaucoma may be caused by the aqueous diversion syndrome. In pupillary or lens block glaucoma there is a flat anterior chamber due to the posterior diversion of aqueous, which pushes vitreous and the lens iris diaphragm forward, blocking the anterior chamber angle. In such cases a pars plana vitreous aspiration, re-formation of the anterior chamber with air, and rupture of the vitreous face are usually required. In some cases of secondary glaucoma the removal of the lens, if present, may be necessary.

A peripheral iridectomy may become blocked by vitreous or blood, resulting in high intraocular pressure. Blood, Healon, or other material in the angle will gradually disappear if the pressure can be temporarily controlled with oral or topical glaucoma medications. An open-angle glaucoma may develop in aphakic eyes from placement of a small-diameter graft in a larger recipient opening because of anatomic pressure on the trabecular meshwork. If this cannot be controlled medically, a larger corneal graft may be necessary rather than resorting to a glaucoma surgical procedure.

C. Late Postoperative Complications

Late postoperative surgical complications are related to poor surgical technique or to healing problems. Excessive scarring, inadequate wound healing, astigmatism, cataract formation, or secondary glaucoma may develop, resulting in poor vision.

1. Subepithelial Fibrosis

Subepithelial fibrosis is a benign proliferation of fibrous tissue that results in a superficial corneal scar. This is often seen in the peripheral portion of the graft because of unburied or excessively tightened sutures. It is also associated with prolonged epithelial defects from a tear film deficiency or graft inflammation (Fig. 5). If opacification occurs in the visual axis, poor vision will result. Usually this will require a repeat keratoplasty if a contact lens does not provide adequate visual improvement. A superficial keratectomy can be done to remove the scar in certain cases to improve the vision.

2. Epithelial Downgrowth

The development of an epithelial downgrowth is catastrophic for the eye. This progressive spread of epithelium inside the anterior chamber may result from inadequate closure of a penetrating or surgical wound. The epithelial layer grows across the back of the cornea, over the trabecular meshwork and anterior iris surface, through the pupil, across the posterior iris, and over the ciliary body

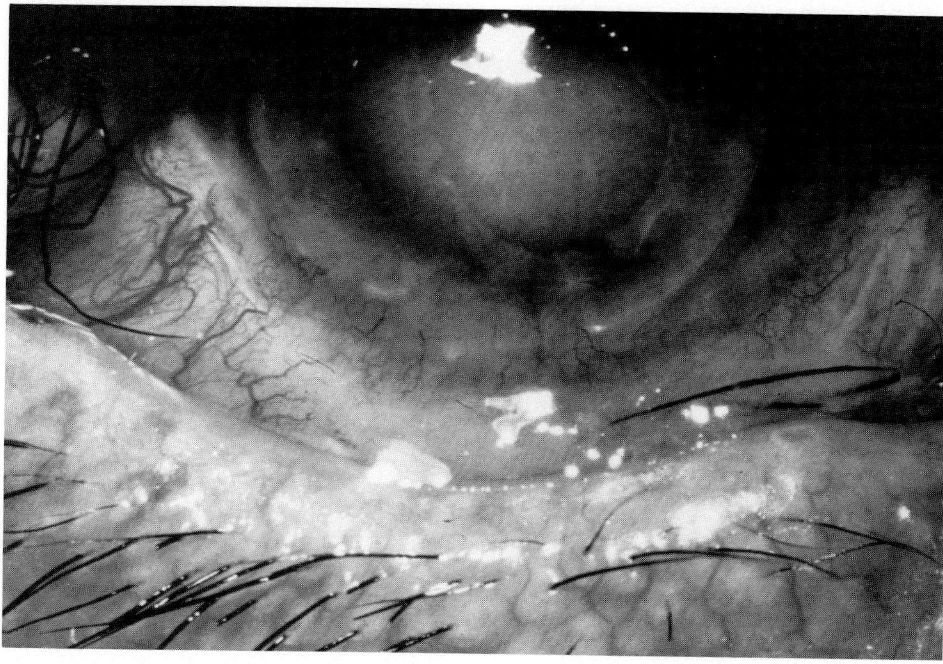

Figure 5 Subepithelial fibrosis in area of persistent epithelial defect.

and processes, eventually destroying the entire eye because of uncontrollable secondary glaucoma (Fig. 6). Photocoagulation of an abnormal-appearing area of the anterior surface of the iris produces a small snowball-appearing burn of contracted epithelium, which is diagnostic. This does not occur in areas of normal iris. The only successful treatment is the heroic surgical intervention to excise the retrocorneal membrane and all areas of involved iris and to apply cryotherapy to the area of involved iris, ciliary body, and the corneal endothelial surface to completely kill all remaining epithelial tissue. If the glaucoma can be controlled, the eye may be salvaged; however, the cornea is usually markedly edematous and a penetrating keratoplasty is required if any vision is to be obtained.

A fibrous downgrowth may occur from a poorly closed corneal incision without the development of epithelial invasion. This extends across the back of the cornea, forming a retrocorneal membrane, resulting in destruction of endothelium and corneal decompensation. Or it can involve the anterior chamber angle, resulting in a secondary glaucoma.

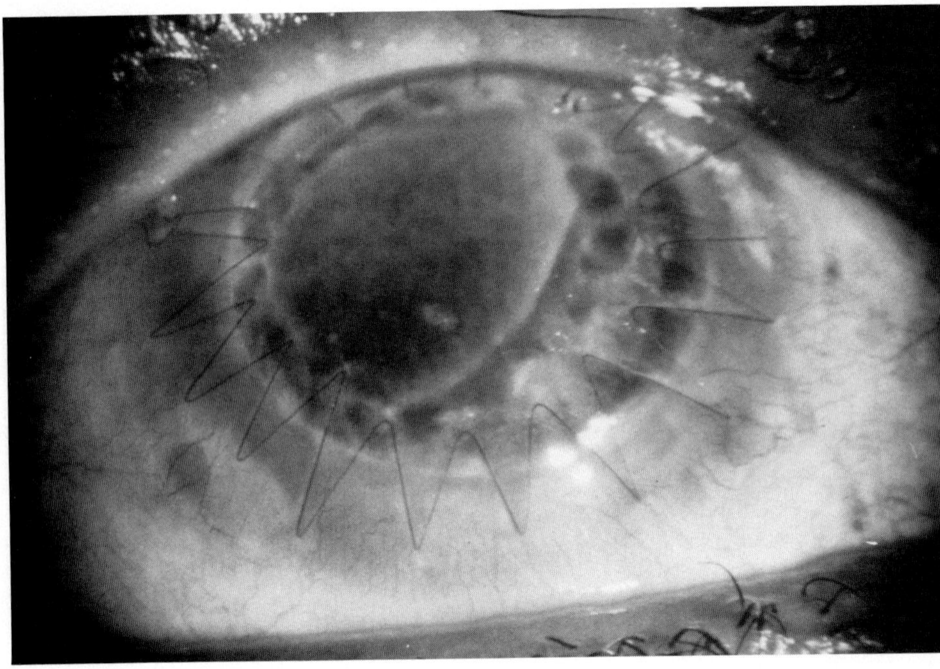

Figure 6 Epithelial downgrowth covering iris and pupillary membrane.

3. Wound Dehiscence

A traumatic wound dehiscence due to a direct blow to the globe may accidentally occur at any time following surgery. Several reports have indicated a Predominance of young males, particularly those with keratoconus, who sustained a ruptured corneal graft wound while the sutures were still present [17,18]. Immediate primary repair of the wound dehiscence was performed whenever possible, with most cases resulting in a clear graft. In the majority of the cases, the injury was caused by the patient either accidently poking the eye or falling; however, several patients reported injury from a flying object or being struck by another individual. Iris prolapse, extrusion of the lens, vitreous loss, retinal detachment, and choroidal hemorrhage secondary to the injury may result in the loss of vision or the eye (Fig. 7).

A special type of wound dehiscence may occur at the time of suture removal following a penetrating keratoplasty, if the intraocular pressure is elevated, in older patients or diabetics who heal slower. This is an anterior lip dehiscence in which the donor cornea protrudes forward after removal of the sutures; however,

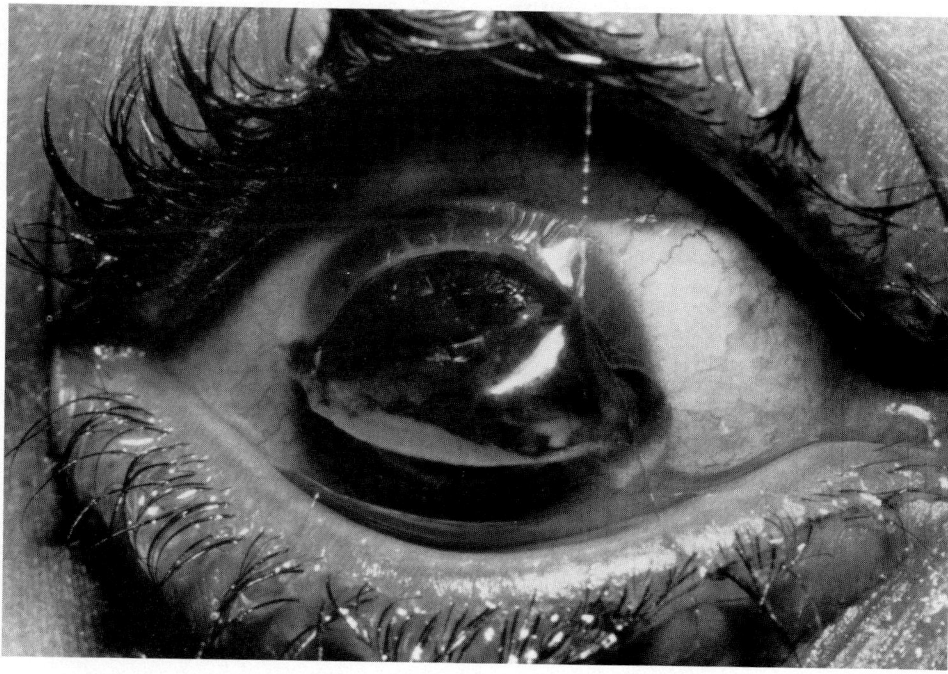

Figure 7 Traumatic graft wound dehiscence 1½ years after PKP.

no wound leak is present (Fig. 8). If small, a bandage contact lens can be used for several months, although high corneal astigmatism may remain. If this is anticipated, resuturing of the corneal wound is advisable. A posterior wound dehiscence may result in the acute onset of stromal edema due to the sudden swelling of the stroma with aqueous fluid.

It is mandatory to examine the patient the day after all sutures have been removed in order to check for a wound leak or flat anterior chamber. If one of these conditions is present, resuturing of the corneal incision is required with reformation of the anterior chamber.

4. Astigmatism

Many corneal transplants will have a significant amount of postoperative astigmatism, especially in cases of keratoconus. High irregular astigmatism may be caused by a donor-recipient size or shape disparity, improper suturing technique, partial wound dehiscence, vitreous loss, or postoperative anterior synechiae [13]. Irregular corneal astigmatism due to the healed incision scar, subepithelial fibrosis, or thinning may also occur and cannot be corrected satisfactorily with spectacles.

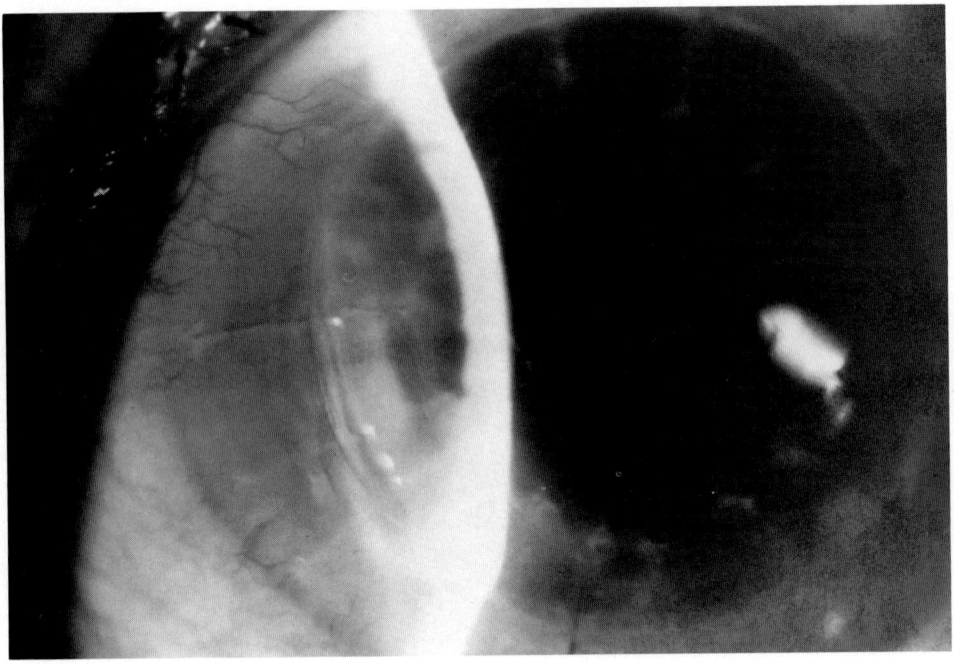

Figure 8 Anterior lip elevation 1 day after suture removal.

The treatment for high or irregular astigmatism is the use of a contact lens. Either a soft contact lens with spectacle overrefraction or a hard contact lens for a very high astigmatism will be required. If a contact lens cannot be fit because of a high astigmatism, a refractive surgical procedure is necessary. This consists of a wedge resection or relaxing incisions in order to reduce the astigmatism by changing the corneal curvature [19].

5. Conclusion

The successful corneal surgeon must anticipate complications and be prepared to manage them as soon as they arise. Frequent observation postoperatively and rapid intervention to correct any problems that occur will be rewarded by a higher long-term success rate in patients who can see again.

REFERENCES

1. Barraquer, J., and Rutllan, J.: Microsurgery of the Cornea: An Atlas and Textbook (Thoft, R. A., and Luther, E., Translators), Barcelona: Edicoones S.A., 1984, Chap. 17, pp. 313-328; Chap. 18, pp. 329-390.

2. Leveille, A. S., McMullan, F. D., and Cavanagh, H. D.: Endophthalmitis following penetrating keratoplasty. Ophthalmology, 90:38-39, 1983.
3. Clark, W. M., Heaton, K. T., Snider, G. R., Reeve, R. B., Caskey, P. J., and Olson, R. J.: Donor eye contamination. Am. J. Ophthalmol. 94:395-397, September 1982.
4. Levenson, J. E., Duffin, R. M., Gardner, S. K., and Pettit, T. H.: Dematiaceous fungal keratitis following penetrating keratoplasty. Ophthalmic Surg. 15(7):578-582, 1984.
5. Beyt, B. E., and Waltman, S. R.: Cryptococcal endophthalmitis after corneal transplantations. N. Engl. J. Med. 298:826-836, April 1978.
6. Karesh, J. W., and Nirankari, V. S.: Factors associated with glaucoma after penetrating keratoplasty. Am. J. Ophthalmol. 96:160-164, 1983.
7. Pollak, F. M.: Flinical and pathological aspects of the corneal graft reaction. Trans. Am. Acad. Ophthalmol. Otolaryngol. 77:418, 1973.
8. Manumence, A. E.: Clinical patterns of corneal graft failure: Corneal graft failures. Ciba Symposium, London, 1972.
9. Alldredge, O. C., and Krachmer, J. H.: Clinical types of corneal transplant rejection: Their manifestations, frequency, preoperative correlates and treatment. Arch. Ophthalmol. 99:599-604, April 1981.
10. Paque, J., and Poirier, R. H.: Corneal allograft reaction and its relationship to suture site neovascularization. Ophthalmic Surg. 8(4);71-74, August 1977.
11. Arentsen, J. J.: Corneal transplant allograft reaction: Possible predisposing factors. Trans. Am. Ophthalmol. Soc. 81:361-402, 1983.
12. Foulks, G. N., Sanfilippo, F. P., Locascido, J. A., MacQueen, J. M., and Dawson, D. V.: Histocompatibility testing for keratoplasty in high-risk patients. Am. Acad. Ophthalmol. 90(3):239-244, March 1983.
13. Braude, L. S., and Chandler, J. W.: Corneal allograft rejection. The role of the major histocompatibility complex. Surv. Ophthalmol. 27(5):290-305, March-April 1983.
14. Stark, W. J., Taylor, H. R., Datiles, M., Young, E., and Klein, P.: Transplantation antigens and keratoplasty. Aust. J. Ophthalmol. 11:333-339, 1983.
15. Nirankari, V. S., Kresh, J., Bastion, F., Lakhanpal, V., and Billings, E.: Recurrence of keratoconus in donor cornea 22 years after successful keratoplasty. Br. J. Ophthalmol. 67:23-28, 1983.
16. Cherry, P. M. H., Pashby, R. C., Tadros, M. L., Wolf, A., Chipman, M. L., Basu, P. K., Dixon, W. S., Hunter, W. S., and Thompson, G. A.: An analysis of corneal transplantation. II. Postoperative astigmatism. Ann. Ophthalmol. 669-672, April 1979.
17. Raber, I. M., Arentsen, J. J., and Laibson, P. R.: Traumatic wound dehiscence after penetrating keratoplasty. Arch. Ophthalmol. 98:1407-1409, 1980.
18. Topping, T. M., Stark, W. J., Maumenee, E., and Kenyon, K. R.: Traumatic wound dehiscence following penetrating keratoplasty. Br. J. Ophthalmol. 66: 174-178, 1982.
19. Paton, D.: The principal problems of penetrating keratoplasty: Graft failure and graft astigmatism. Symposium in Medical and Surgical Diseases of the Cornea. Trans. New Orleans Acad. Ophthalmol, 1980.

22

Bone Marrow Transplant Complications

OLIVER W. PRESS, ROBERT T. SCHALLER, JR., and
E. DONNALL THOMAS
Fred Hutchinson Cancer Research Center and University of Washington, Seattle, Washington

I. INTRODUCTION

Recent advances in transplant immunobiology, supportive care, and graft-versus-host disease (GVHD) prevention and treatment have resulted in dramatic progress in curing hematologic diseases with bone marrow transplantation (BMT) since the beginning of the "modern" era [1]. Long-term disease-free survival for HLA-matched, allogeneic transplant recipients is now achievable in 80% of untransfused patients with aplastic anemia (AA) [2,3], 50-60% of patients with acute nonlymphocytic leukemia (ANL) in first remission [4,5], 50-60% of patients with chronic myelogenous leukemia (CML) in chronic phase [6,7,85], 30% of patients with acute lymphoblastic leukemia (ALL) in second remission [8, 9], and 15% of patients with acute leukemia in relapse [10]. Prospective comparative analyses have demonstrated unequivocal survival advantages favoring bone marrow transplantation over conventional management for AA [11], ANL in first remission [12-14], and ALL in second or subsequent remission [15]. Furthermore, preliminary evidence is encouraging for the future application of allogeneic or autologous BMT for patients with preleukemia [16], non-Hodgkin's lymphomas [17,18], solid tumors [19], and genetic diseases [20]. Despite these extremely encouraging developments, marrow grafting remains a hazardous undertaking with sobering morbidity and mortality rates. For details of the transplantation procedure, conditioning regimens, and pretransplant complications, the reader is referred to other reviews [1,21]. In this chapter we summarize the most important medical and surgical complications occurring following bone marrow transplantation (Fig. 1).

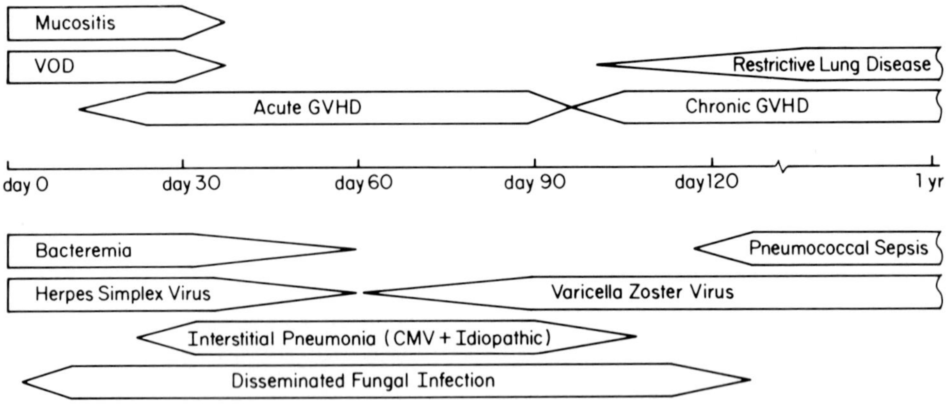

Figure 1 Temporal sequence of major complications following allogeneic bone marrow transplantation on day 0.

II. GRAFT FAILURE

Failure of infused histocompatible marrow to result in sustained hematologic reconstitution following BMT is of primary importance in multiply transfused patients with aplastic anemia. Early transplant experience demonstrated that 30-60% of transfused aplastics conditioned with cyclophosphamide alone experienced graft failure that ultimately proved fatal [2,21]. Sensitization of host lymphocytes to minor transplantation antigens as a result of prior blood transfusions is believed to be responsible for the immunologic rejection of marrow grafts observed in these patients. Three factors have been shown to correlate with graft rejection: (1) positive in vitro reactivity of host lymphocytes against donor cells prior to transplantation, (2) low numbers of transplanted marrow cells ($<3 \times 10^8$ cells per kg), and (3) marrow grafting from male donors. Administration of total-body irradiation (TBI) in addition to cyclophosphamide has been successful in decreasing graft rejection rates by increasing host immunosuppression (reviewed in Ref. 21). However, survival rates are generally not improved because of increased incidences of interstitial pneumonia and GVHD. In Seattle, donor buffy coat infusions are employed for 5 days following allografting to serve as a source of additional stem cells and donor lymphocytes capable of overcoming host rejection. Using this approach, the rejection rate for multiply transfused AA patients has plummeted to 14%, and the long-term survival rate has improved to 70% [22]. Clearly the optimal approach, however, is avoidance of transfusions (especially from family members) prior to transplantation. Untransfused aplastics have a rejection rate less than 10% and a "cure" rate following BMT of over 80% [2].

Graft failure had been a rare event in patients transplanted for leukemia until recent years, when T-cell depletion of marrow grafts with monoclonal antibodies and complement gained popularity as a means of preventing GVHD [23,24]. Although GVHD has been successfully prevented by these maneuvers, a striking increase in graft failure rates has been observed (6 of 20 patients with hematologic malignancies receiving T-cell-depleted marrow in Seattle and 5 of 20 at UCLA) [23,25].

III. RELAPSE OF HEMATOLOGIC MALIGNANCY

Early clinical trials of BMT in 100 patients with end-stage, refractory leukemia resulted in an actuarial 75% relapse rate in the first 2 years. No recurrences were observed after this time, however, and 12% of these patients are alive and well between 7 and 12 years later without further therapy [26]. Because recurrence was assumed to be due to incomplete eradication of tumor in patients with heavy tumor burdens and resistance to conventional chemotherapy, higher doses of TBI were employed as a means of decreasing the relapse rate. This approach has doubled the survival rate for ANL in relapse (to 25%) but has not improved the results for ALL [21].

Relapse has been much less of a problem in patients transplanted earlier in the course of their disease. Leukemic recurrence occurs in only 10-20% of patients with ANL in first remission [4] and 4-25% of patients with CML in chronic phase [7,85]. Presumably, eradication of leukemia is more successful in these patients because of lower tumor burdens and absence of therapy-resistant cells. Cytogenetic and enzyme marker analyses have documented the occurrence of leukemic relapse in donor cells in a minority of cases transplanted for ANL, ALL, and CML (reviewed in Ref. 27). Current estimates suggest that 5% of all leukemic relapses occur in donor-type cells [28]. It is speculated that these "new" leukemias may result from transfection of viral oncogenes from dying tumor cells to transplanted donor cells.

Considerable evidence has been accumulated to support the existence of a graft-versus-leukemia (GVL) effect occurring in patients following allogeneic BMT. Patients acquiring acute or chronic GVHD have been shown to have roughly one-third the risk of leukemic relapse of patients who do not develop GVHD [29,30]. A survival advantage is also observed for patients developing GVHD; however, this trend reaches statistical significance only for chronic GVHD because of offsetting mortality from nonleukemic causes in patients with acute GVHD. This beneficial GVL effect is most apparent in patients at high risk for relapse, especially for patients with ALL and for patients transplanted in relapse rather than remission. Unfortunately, attempts to improve survival of patients with poor prognoses by manipulating GVHD prophylaxis and exploiting the GVL effect have not yet proven beneficial.

IV. IMMUNODEFICIENCY

Bone marrow transplantation results in profound deficiencies of both humoral and cellular immunity that gradually become reconstituted over 1-2 years after transplantation unless chronic GVHD ensues [31,32]. Within the first month after marrow grafting most patients acquire normal numbers of T and B lymphocytes, and in vitro tests of antibody-dependent cellular cytotoxicity and natural killer activity return to normal. A reversal of the normal T4/T8 T-cell ratio is observed for 3 months after BMT due to decreased numbers of OKT4+ helper cells and normal or increased numbers of OKT8+ suppressor cells. Mitogen reactivity and mixed lymphocyte culture responsiveness return in 1-2 months. Host immunoglobulins, including isohemagglutinins, persist for up to 3 months following BMT, at which time donor antibody production begins. Normal IgG and IgM levels are reached in the first year after transplantation, but IgA levels remain subnormal for longer periods. Specific antibody production to T-dependent antigens (e.g., ΦX 174) is generally depressed for at least 3 months, and responsiveness to pneumococcal vaccine is minimal for 7 months after BMT. Cellular immunity appears to recover later than humoral immunity, and skin test anergy to DNCB, mumps, *Candida,* and tuberculin is often demonstrable for up to 4 years.

Patients who develop chronic GVHD have persistent severe immunodeficiencies with impaired humoral responses to T-dependent and T-independent antigens, inability to switch isotypes from IgM to IgG, diminished T-cell helper activity, augmented nonspecific T-cell suppressor activity, and recurrent infectious episodes.

V. INFECTIONS

As a result of disruption of mucosal barriers, profound neutropenia, complete abrogation of humoral and cellular immunity, and posttransplantation immunosuppression with methotrexate or cyclosporine, severe infections commonly occur after BMT. Attempts at infection prophylaxis with laminar airflow (LAF) isolation, gut decontamination with oral nonabsorbable antibiotics, prophylactic granulocyte transfusions, and prophylactic systemic antibiotics have been moderately successful at decreasing the incidence of septicemia and local major infections [33-35]. Trends suggesting improved survival for patients treated with these prophylactic measures have been repeatedly observed, but statistical significance has only been demonstrable for patients with aplastic anemia in whom the enhanced survival for patients in LAF isolation was mainly attributable to a diminished risk of fatal GVHD [35,36]. The posttransplant course can be conveniently divided into three separate phases characterized by unique constellations of infectious complications [37].

A. Phase I (Days 0-30)

Profound granulocytopenia dominates the clinical picture in the first 3-4 weeks following transplantation. Virtually all patients develop fever during this period and are placed on empiric broad-spectrum antibiotics. If fever does not defervesce in 4-5 days, empiric amphotericin is generally instituted. A demonstrable pathogen will be isolated in roughly one-third of febrile episodes. Bacteremia emanating from denuded oropharyngeal and gastrointestinal sites or from infected Hickman catheters constitutes a majority of these episodes. Early studies emphasized the importance of gram-negative rods (*Escherichia coli, Klebsiella,* and *Pseudomonas*) and *Candida* in septicemic BMT patients [38,39]. However, in more recent years, gram-positive organisms, particularly *Staphylococcus epidermidis,* have arisen as the predominant pathogens (Table 1) [40].

Table 1 Pathogens Isolated from 111 Septicemic Episodes in 95 Bone Marrow Transplant Patients (1980-1983)

Organism	No. isolates[a] (%)
Staphylococcus epidermidis	46 (35.9)
Candida sp.	14 (10.9)
Klebsiella sp.	11 (8.6)
Staphylococcus aureus	10 (7.8)
Streptococcus sp.	8 (6.3)
Escherichia coli	7 (5.5)
Pseudomonas aeruginosa	6 (4.7)
Enterobacter cloacae	6 (4.7)
Enterococcus	4 (3.1)
Propionebacter sp.	4 (3.1)
Serratia liquifaciens	3 (2.3)
Diphtheroids	2 (1.6)
Other	7 (5.5)
Total	128

[a]Some patients had polymicrobial bacteremia.
Source: Modified from F. Peterson et al. [39].

Silicone elastomer right atrial Hickman catheters have proven indispensable in the supportive care of BMT patients. However, their use is associated with risks of catheter infection, thrombosis, and dislodgement [40,41]. A recent review at our institution disclosed that there were 111 episodes of septicemia and 25 episodes of local catheter infection associated with 407 catheters in 357 consecutive BMT patients [40]. In this group, 39 catheters (9.6%) were removed for infections and 24 (5.9%) for mechanical complications. Exit site infections and bacteremia alone generally resolved with antibiotic therapy, but infections of the subcutaneous catheter tunnel and cases of septic thrombophlebitis required catheter removal [41].

Despite the frequency of bacteremia in the first 30 days after transplantation and the attendant risks of septic shock, disseminated intravascular coagulation, acute respiratory distress syndrome, and renal failure, the vast majority of these episodes are successfully managed without significant sequelae. Infections associated with Hickman catheters and those in which *S. epidermidis* is the pathogen are particularly benign in outcome [41]. Currently, early bacterial infections are responsible for less than 10% of transplant deaths in Seattle.

Unlike bacterial infections, which are concentrated in the first month after BMT, fungal infections are prone to arise at any time after marrow grafting. Disseminated fungal disease, usually due to *Candida* or *Aspergillus* species, tends to arise in the setting of prolonged granulocytopenia [42], graft failure, leukemic relapse, CMV infection, or GVHD. Diagnosis is difficult, with fungemia demonstrable in less than 50% of cases of fulminant candidiasis; blood cultures are virtually never positive with aspergillosis. Unfortunately, serological tests are not yet reliable enough to be useful clinically. Colonization of multiple surveillance sites (sputum, oropharynx, urine, and stool) with a single fungal species often furnishes a useful diagnostic clue. Cutaneous and ocular candidal lesions help in confirming disseminated candidiasis when they are present. However, most patients with fungal infections are initially treated with amphotericin B empirically because of persistent fever despite antibiotic therapy. Unfortunately, 90% of affected patients with aspergillosis and 50% of patients with disseminated candidiasis die of progressive disease.

Reactivation of endogenous herpes simplex virus (HSV) infection occurs in 80% of seropositive patients following BMT and generally is manifest as an acute exacerbation of oropharyngeal mucositis [37]. Isolation of HSV peaks in the third week following BMT, and in the absence of specific antiviral therapy, lesions heal slowly and rarely resolve until granulocyte levels rise above $500/mm^3$. Extension of HSV infection can result in painful esophagitis, and in rare instances, viremia or aspiration of oropharyngeal secretions can lead to fatal HSV pneumonia [43]. Prophylactic intravenous acyclovir is virtually 100% effective in controlling HSV reactivation following BMT and is indicated for all seropositive patients [44,45].

B. Phase II (Days 30-100)

In the second and third months following marrow transplantation, nonbacterial interstitial pneumonia and viral and protozoal infections assume primary importance as infectious sequelae. During this period, persistent defects of cellular and humoral immunity predispose to infectious episodes, but granulocytopenia usually has resolved. Of 952 allogeneic transplant recipients in Seattle between 1969 and 1982, 332 (35%) developed diffuse interstitial pneumonitis (IP) [46]. As shown in Table 2, cytomegalovirus infections were responsible for 44% of the cases of IP, and 88% of these cases ended fatally, "Idiopathic" IP, which presumably represents chemoradiation pulmonary toxicity, caused 27% of the cases of IP, and of these 64% were lethal. A minority of cases were caused by other viruses (herpes simplex virus, varicella zoster, and adenovirus) or by *Pneumocystis carinii.* The latter pathogen has virtually disappeared since the institution of cotrimoxazole prophylaxis in the peritransplant period. Multivariate proportional hazards regression analysis has revealed the following risk factors for acquisition of CMV pneumonia: age > 20 years, moderate or severe acute GVHD, CMF seropositivity prior to BMT, conditioning with agents in addition to cyclophosphamide prior to BMT, and antithymocyte globulin therapy for GVHD. The

Table 2 Etiology of 332 Cases of Nonbacterial Interstitial Pneumonia Occurring in 952 Bone Marrow Transplant Patients (1969-1982)

Etiology	No cases (% of affected patients)[a]
Cytomegalovirus	147 (44)
Idiopathic	90 (27)
Pneumocystis carinii	39 (12)
Herpes simplex virus	12 (4)
Varicella zoster virus	10 (3)
Adenovirus	4 (1)
Unknown	49 (15)
	351

[a]More than one pathogen was isolated in some patients.
Source: Modified from J. Meyers et al., in *Recent Advances in Bone Marrow Transplantation,* 1983, pp. 405-423, New York: Alan R. Liss, Inc. [44].

only clearly defined risk factor for idiopathic IP is the pretransplant conditioning regimen, with fractionated TBI associated with a lower IP incidence than single-dose irradiation [46]. Similarly, low-dose-rate irradiation is seemingly safer than high-dose-rate TBI [47]. Patients receiving allogeneic transplants for end-stage leukemia have higher risks of IP (48%) than patients with leukemia in remission (20-25%) or aplastic anemia (27%) or patients receiving syngeneic (twin) transplants (7.5%) [48]. The onset of IP typically occurs between weeks 5 and 12 after BMT and is manifested by dyspnea, tachypnea, rales, hypoxemia, and diffuse radiographic infiltrates. Noninvasive diagnostic techniques are generally unsuccessful. Several prospective trials have shown open lung biopsy to be superior to other diagnostic methods, with a sensitivity of 83-100% [49-51]. Unfortunately, knowledge of a specific diagnosis does not improve the outcome of most cases of IP [48], and consequently many physicians prefer reliance on transbronchial biopsy, washings, and brushings (sensitivity, 59-84%) in cases with adequate platelet levels (50,000 mm^{-3} after transfusion) and tolerable hypoxemia ($PaO_2 \geqslant 60$ on mask oxygen). Cases with nondiagnostic bronchoscopy or in whom bronchoscopy is contraindicated are either referred for open lung biopsy or treated empirically with broad-spectrum antibiotics, high-dose cotrimoxazole (for *Pneumocystis*), amphotericin (for fungi), and acyclovir (for herpes viruses). Unfortunately, there are no effective known forms of therapy for the two major groups of IP, namely, CMV and idiopathic pneumonitis, despite trials of acyclovir, interferon, and vidarabine for the former and steroids for the latter [37].

Recent studies suggest that 62% of seropositive patients and 33% of seronegative patients acquire some form of CMV infection posttransplant [52]. The risk of CMV infection occurring in seronegative patients is dramatically increased to 75% if granulocyte transfusions from seropositive donors are administered [52,53]. Manifestations of CMV infection besides CMV pneumonia include fever, myelosuppression (which can result in graft failure), hepatitis, atypical lymphocytosis, arthralgias, esophagitis, enteritis, and predisposition to bacterial and fungal superinfections. CMV infections (particularly CMV pneumonia) are associated with more deaths following BMT than any other single infectious agent. In the absence of effective therapy of established infections, efforts at CMV prophylaxis have been stressed. Administration of CMV hyperimmune globulin in three controlled trials has dramatically decreased the incidence of CMV infection and interstitial pneumonia [54-56]. This improvement is primarily due to prevention of exogenous acquisition of infection in seronegative patients. Pre-existent antibody and administered immune globulin does not appear to be effective in preventing endogenous reactivation in seropositive patients [54]. Careful screening of blood products and transfusion of only seronegative blood components to seronegative recipients may be an alternate strategy for preventing CMV infections. It has proven beneficial in a prospective randomized study [87].

C. Phase III (After Day 100)

Following the first 3 months posttransplant, the incidence of severe infections declines markedly (except in patients with chronic GVHD). Late reactivation of varicella zoster virus (VZV) is the most frequent infection in this time period, occurring in 17% of all patients transplanted in Seattle between 1969 and 1982 and in 50% of patients surviving for longer than 6 months. The median time of onset was 5 months after BMT; 45% of cases disseminated, and 12% of cases ended fatally (all deaths occurred in the first 9 months). Acute GVHD was the major risk factor predisposing to dissemination or death. Considerable neurological morbidity (blindness and deafness) was incurred in surviving cases, particularly those with cranial nerve involvement. Antiviral therapy resulted in less scarring, neurological morbidity, and bacterial superinfection but did not significantly alter the rates of mortality (10%), postherpetic neuralgia, or recurrence. Acyclovir therapy is currently recommended for all patients who develop VZV infection in the first 9 months after BMT and for all patients with cranial nerve involvement. When VZV occurs more than 9 months after BMT, antiviral therapy is instituted only if there is evidence of visceral or cutaneous dissemination [86].

Patients who develop chronic GVHD remain immunologically crippled by their disease and by continued immunosuppressive therapy and consequently have persistently high rates of infection. Sinopulmonary infections and septicemia with pneumococci have been particularly common in this population [37,57]. In accordance with these findings, patients with chronic GVHD should be maintained indefinitely on prophylactic cotrimoxazole or penicillin, and attempts at pneumococcal vaccination are advocated. Unfortunately, antibody responses to pneumococcal vaccine are poor in patients on corticosteroids and those vaccinated less than 7 months after BMT [58].

VI. ACUTE GRAFT-VERSUS-HOST DISEASE

Despite postgrafting immunosuppression, 35-50% of HLA-matched, MLR-unresponsive, allogeneic sibling marrow transplant recipients develop moderate to severe acute GVHD. Although the pathophysiology of this phenomenon remains controversial, it is assumed that grafted donor T lymphocytes recognize polymorphic non-HLA host antigens and initiate cytotoxic injury directed against the foreign host environment. The major target organs for this immune attack are the skin, liver, and gut, with resultant development in severe cases of maculopapular rashes, skin desquamation, nausea, voluminous watery diarrhea, abdominal pain, jaundice, and immunodeficiency. The severity of this complication varies markedly, and a clinical staging and grading system has proven useful [1,59]. The median onset of acute GVHD is day 25 (range, days 10-70). The only clearly defined risk factors for acute GVHD are age and transplantation out of LAF isolation. (The latter has been proven only for patients with aplastic anemia [21]).

Conventional attempts to prevent this immunologic reaction have employed prophylactic immunosuppressive therapy with methotrexate or cyclosporine [59,60]. Controlled studies have demonstrated a slight decrease in acute GVHD in patients treated prophylactically with cyclosporine, but there has been no significant survival advantage compared with methotrexate. Advantages of cyclosporine include faster engraftment, less mucositis, a decrease in platelet transfusion requirements, and a shorter hospital stay. However, an increased incidence of nephrotoxicity is seen with cyclosporine. Newer preventive measures include T-cell depletion of donor marrow prior to transplantation with monoclonal antibodies plus complement [23-25], soybean agglutinin, and sheep red cells [61], or T-cell immunotoxins [62]. These studies show convincing abrogation of GVHD, but unfortunately increased incidences of late graft failure and leukemic relapse have been observed [23,25]. Therapeutic attempts to control established acute GVHD with cyclosporine, antithymocyte globulin, or corticosteroids are successful in roughly half the affected patients, but the remainder die of this complication, generally from intercurrent infection [21]. Recent attempts at salvage therapy employing intravenous infusion of anti-T-cell monoclonal antibodies have resulted in improvement in some patients treated with intermediate or high doses of antibody [63,64]. The exact role of this modality in GVHD therapy remains to be defined.

VII. CHRONIC GRAFT-VERSUS-HOST DISEASE

Approximately 35% of allogeneic transplant recipients experience the onset of chronic GVHD (C-GVHD) between 70 and 400 days after BMT. The protean manifestations of this multisystem autoimmune disease include cutaneous dyspigmentation, sclerodermatous skin changes, joint contractures, xerostomia, keratoconjunctivitis sicca, esophageal and vaginal strictures, pulmonary insufficiency, chronic liver disease, diarrhea, a wasting syndrome, and profound humoral and cellular immunodeficiencies [60,65]. The three risk factors that have been identified as predisposing to C-GVHD are (1) grade II-IV acute GVHD, (2) age over 30, and (3) administration of donor buffy coat transfusions to recipients with aplastic anemia [66]. There are three patterns of onset: (1) "progressive" (a direct extension of acute GVHD–62% mortality), (2) "quiescent" (beginning after resolution of acute GVHD–33% mortality), and (3) "de novo" (no antecedent acute GVHD–20% mortality) [65]. "Limited" C-GVHD involves only the skin and liver without associated sicca, mucositis, weight loss, or recurrent infections. Patients with limited C-GVHD have an excellent prognosis without therapy, and fatalities are rare in this group. Patients with "extensive" C-GVHD have involvement of organs other than liver and skin and have a poor prognosis without treatment, developing progressive wasting, joint contractures, debility, and recurrent infections. Only 2 of 13 untreated patients with extensive C-GVHD survived with Karnofsky performance scores >70%. In contrast, treatment of extensive C-GVHD with prednisone and/or azathioprine results in Karnofsky scores of 90-100 in 75-80% of patients [65,66]. Patients with C-GVHD and persistent thrombocytopenia (<100,000 mm^{-3} after day 100) have been identified as a subgroup with a particularly unfavorable prognosis despite current therapy.

VIII. GASTROINTESTINAL TOXICITY

A. Mucositis

As a consequence of high-dose cyclophosphamide, TBI, methotrexate GVHD prophylaxis, and coexistent herpes simplex virus infection, many patients experience severe, painful denudation of the oropharyngeal mucosa in the first 3-4 weeks following transplantation. Because of concomitant thrombocytopenia, oral and pharyngeal bleeding often ensues and may lead to aspiration pneumonia unless platelet transfusion therapy is promptly instituted. In a prospective trial, patients treated with cyclosporine for GVHD prophylaxis experienced only 7.6 days of mucositis, whereas methotrexate-treated patients incurred 27.7 days of moderate to severe mucositis [67]. Maintenance of good oral hygiene with saline mouthwashes, prompt institution of acyclovir in cases with superimposed herpes infections, and application of topical anesthetics (such as Xylocaine or Dyclone) prove to be beneficial for many patients. However, the majority of patients with severe mucositis require temporary intravenous morphine infusions to palliate their severe pain. Fortunately, mucositis generally heals promptly once engraftment ensues and granulocytopenia resolves. Serious long-term sequelae are rare, provided aspiration pneumonia or bacteremic seeding of the bloodstream have not transpired.

B. Protracted Nausea and Esophagitis

During conditioning for BMT with cyclophosphamide and TBI, most patients experience nausea and vomiting, which generally is well controlled with prophylactic antiemetics. In a significant minority of patients, however, nausea and vomiting persist long into the posttransplant period. Spencer et al. have recently analyzed 50 patients with protracted nausea lasting >4 days and occurring after day 15 following BMT (Spencer, G., and McDonald, G., unpublished data). Upper gastrointestinal endoscopy with duodenal biopsy was performed in all patients. Presumptive causes of nausea were eventually identified in 39 of 50 patients (78%), including 15 with gastrointestinal infections alone, 13 with acute GVHD alone, 8 with GVHD and infection, 1 with sepsis, 1 with a subdural hematoma, and 1 with encephalopathy. CMV (17 isolates) and HSV (5 isolates) were the most common infectious pathogens. Surprisingly, there was no evidence for an increased risk of CMV pneumonia among patients with CMV esophagitis compared with the pneumonia risk in cases of GVHD esophagitis. Nausea and vomiting were slow to resolve in all patients, particularly those with CMV, and often persisted for weeks.

C. Veno-Occlusive Disease of the Liver (VOD)

A prospective evaluation of 255 BMT patients between 1978 and 1980 disclosed 53 (21%) who developed the clinicopathologic picture of VOD. This entity is characterized by fibrous obliteration of the small centrilobular hepatic venules, presumably as a result of chemoradiation toxicity to the liver [68]. Risk factors for VOD determined by multivariate analysis include age > 15 years, antecedent hepatitis prior to BMT (relative risk = 3.4), and transplantation for malignancy other than ALL (ANL > ALL > AA). The clinical diagnosis of VOD can be established with 89% accuracy if a patient develops two of the following three characteristics before day 30 after BMT: (1) jaundice, (2) hepatomegaly or right upper quadrant pain, or (3) ascites or unexplained weight gain. The differential diagnosis of liver disease in BMT patients is often difficult and must include such entities as VOD, GVHD, congestive hepatomegaly from cardiomyopathy, shock liver, hepatic vein thrombosis, pyogenic liver abscesses, pancreatitis, viral hepatitis, drug toxicity, malignant infiltration, and hyperalimentation-induced liver injury. Clinically, the most difficult distinction is generally between VOD and GVHD. Clinical criteria permitting distinction of these two entities are summarized in Table 3. Percutaneous liver biopsy is generally precluded in these patients because of severe thrombocytopenia. VOD attains serious magnitude in 45% of afflicted patients and is fatal in 32% (6% of BMT patients overall). Features signifying a poor prognosis include a bilirubin > 20, weight gain > 12%, SGOT > 400, or development of encephalopathy. There is no effective specific therapy. Supportive care measures consist of saline restriction, maintenance of intravascular volume with red cells and albumin, spironolactone, and maintenance of renal perfusion with low-dose dopamine. Patients generally either recover or die by day 35 after BMT.

D. Acute Abdominal Crises

The occurrence of acute catastrophic intra-abdominal events in patients following BMT poses difficult diagnostic and therapeutic problems. Symptoms and signs of viscus perforation and peritonitis are frequently obscured by corticosteroid therapy, and complaints are often erroneously ascribed to coexistent GVHD or VOD.

Table 3 Distinguishing Features of Hepatic Veno-occlusive Disease and Graft-Versus-Host Disease

Feature	VOD	GVHD
Typical onset	Before day 14	After day 20
Enzyme pattern	Hepatitic (variable cholestasis)	Cholestatic (variable hepatitis)
Diarrhea and rash	No	Frequent
Ascites	Frequent	Rare
Liver failure	Frequent	Rare
Therapy	Supportive	Immunosuppression

Source: From G. Spencer and G. McDonald (unpublished data).

When the true nature of the abdominal event is recognized, emergency surgical intervention is often hampered by refractory thrombocytopenia, septic shock, and hepatic and renal dysfunction. Nevertheless, an aggressive surgical approach has been shown to salvage a significant proportion of BMT patients (4 of 16) afflicted with otherwise fatal complications, including massive gastrointestinal hemorrhage, biliary tract obstruction, and typhlitis [69]. Careful serial physical examinations are most useful in determining the need for operative intervention. Postoperative wound healing is often impaired because of the presence of GVHD and immunosuppressive therapy.

Surgical procedures, even minor ones, must be carried out with meticulous technique because of the increased risk of bleeding and infection. Minor procedures, such as skin biopsy and marrow aspiration, can be performed regardless of platelet count. For major operative procedures, bleeding has usually not been excessive if platelet transfusions can keep the platelet count at or above 50,000 mm^{-3}. If the patient is refractory to platelets from family members or HLA-matched unrelated donors, surgery should not be undertaken except in life-threatening situations.

IX. INVASIVE PROCEDURES

A variety of invasive diagnostic and therapeutic maneuvers are frequently required for the optimal management of complications following marrow transplantation. Table 4 depicts the frequency with which such interventions were necessary in a series of 840 consecutive, allogeneic, HLA-matched BMT patients treated in Seattle for aplastic anemia or leukemia between January 1978 and June 1984. Virtually all patients had elective placement of Hickman right atrial catheters

Table 4 Invasive Procedures Performed in 840 Bone Marrow Transplant Patients[a]

Procedure	No. patients undergoing procedure (%)
Skin biopsy	649 (77.3)
Hickman catheter placement	627 (74.6)
Endotracheal tube placement	149 (17.7)
Gastrointestinal endoscopy	137 (16.3)
Artificial ventilation	136 (16.2)
Chest tube placement	123 (14.6)
Open lung biopsy	122 (14.5)
Arteriovenous shunt insertion	86 (10.2)
Bowel biopsy	65 (7.7)
Rectal biopsy	50 (6.0)
Liver biopsy	48 (5.7)
Bronchoscopy	40 (4.8)
Cystoscopy	8 (1.0)

[a]Includes consecutive patients receiving HLA-matched allogeneic transplants at Fred Hutchinson Cancer Research Center from January 1978 through June 1984.

either at the referring institution or after arrival in Seattle (only the latter are depicted in Table 4). Skin biopsies were done as clinically indicated by the appearance of skin rashes and were also performed according to protocol 100 days following BMT to screen for C-GVHD. Respiratory failure, generally due to interstitial pneumonitis, was responsible for the greatest number of nonprotocol procedures. Endotracheal intubation was necessary in 149 of 840 patients, and 136 of these patients required mechanically assisted ventilation. Open lung biopsies were performed in 122 patients and were responsible for the high frequency of chest tube insertion observed in this series. Renal failure required the insertion of arteriovenous shunts for hemodialysis in 86 patients (10.2%). Gastrointestinal complaints led to endoscopic examination of the alimentary canal in 137 patients, sigmoidoscopy in 32, and proctoscopy in 3. Biopsies of the bowel, rectum, and liver were each done in 5-8% of patients, primarily to assist in the diagnosis of GVHD.

X. CARDIOMYOPATHY

Congestive cardiomyopathy develops in a small minority of patients as a result of high-dose cyclophosphamide given in preparation for BMT. Even young patients can develop sudden cardiomegaly, congestive heart failure, and fluid retention within days after cyclophosphamide administration. Careful regulation of fluid balance is essential in these patients to avoid iatrogenic pulmonary edema. Fortunately, the majority of cases are easily managed with diuretics and cardiac glycosides, and serial radionuclide ventriculograms generally document gradual improvement of cardiac ejection fraction during the first 100 days after BMT. In a few unfortunate individuals, however, permanent cardiomyopathy occurs and occasionally is fatal ($<1\%$ of BMT patients, unpublished data).

XI. CHRONIC LUNG DISEASE

Prospective serial spirometric evaluation of transplant recipients has documented the development of transient mild restrictive lung disease in 21% of patients [70]. Affected patients demonstrate a mean maximal decrement in total lung capacity of 0.81 L, in vital capacity of 0.54 L, and in carbon monoxide diffusing capacity of 4.4 mL/min. These changes are maximal 1 year after BMT and subsequently improve to normal within 4 years. Patients with previous IP demonstrate the greatest abnormalities, but there is no association with C-GVHD or TBI.

A separate, distinct, progressive syndrome of severe obstructive lung disease (forced expiratory volume in 1 min divided by vital capacity $< 50\%$ predicted) associated with obliterative bronchiolitis is observed in 10% of BMT patients examined 4 years after grafting. This syndrome has been considered a manifestation of C-GVHD by many workers [71], but such an association could not be demonstrated in an analysis of the Seattle patients [70].

XII. RENAL DYSFUNCTION

Renal function deteriorates in a majority of BMT recipients as a result of exposure to nephrotoxins (amphotericin B, cyclosporine, methotrexate, and aminoglycosides) superimposed on such untoward events as septic and cardiogenic shock, volume depletion due to diarrhea, and hepatorenal syndrome associated with VOD. In most patients the magnitude of dysfunction is mild, and patients can be managed by medication dose adjustments and careful fluid management. However, approximately 5-10% of BMT patients require dialysis at least transiently.

Cyclosporine, often in concert with other nephrotoxins, is frequently associated with renal failure. The three distinct syndromes of cyclosporine-induced nephropathy that have been identified are (1) asymptomatic azotemia, proteinuria, and hypertension; (2) acute reversible renal failure requiring dialysis; and (3) a rapidly fatal progressive syndrome resembling thrombotic thrombocytopenic purpura [72]. Pathologically, cyclosporine appears to induce a tubulointerstitial injury with focal glomerular thrombosis and sclerosis, which in some cases is irreversible [72,73]. Careful monitoring for rises in creatinine along with measurement of cyclosporine trough levels and appropriate dose modifications will prevent most cases of serious cyclosporin nephropathy.

XIII. NEUROLOGICAL SEQUELAE

A small proportion of marrow transplant recipients will develop leukoencephalopathy days to months after BMT. This complication is generally restricted to patients who have received previous cranial irradiation and intrathecal methotrexate and appears to be no more frequent following BMT than when such patients are treated conventionally.

Approximately 8% of patients treated with cyclosporine will develop neurotoxicity manifest by grand mal seizures, cerebellar ataxia, tremor, depression, expressive aphasia, or quadriparesis [75,76]. Recent studies in Seattle implicate hypomagnesemia due to cyclosporine-induced renal magnesium wasting as the cause of these symptoms. Magnesium replacement has been shown to be effective in the prevention and treatment of such neurological sequelae [76].

XIV. ENDOCRINE SEQUELAE

Subclinical thyroid dysfunction manifest by elevated thyroid stimulating hormone levels are evident in 10-43% of patients receiving TBI (J. Sanders, unpublished results) [77]. However, only 5-10% have clinically significant hypothyroidism associated with depressed thyroxine levels. Thyroid supplementation is indicated for such patients.

Gonadal function was evaluated in 94 patients with aplastic anemia conditioned with cyclophosphamide alone prior to BMT [78]. Prepubertal males subsequently underwent puberty normally with development of adult gonadotrophin levels and normal development of secondary sex characteristics. Similarly, 9 of 12 evaluable girls experienced menarche and secondary sex characteristic development at an appropriate age; in the remaining 3 girls menarche was delayed. Postpubertal women younger than age 26 treated with cyclophosphamide conditioning alone experienced return of menses 3-4 months following BMT. Their gonadotrophin levels were all normal. In contrast, 6 of 9 postpubertal women older than age 26 developed early menopause with elevated luteinizing hormone (LH) and follicle stimulating hormone (FSH) levels. Of 31 postpubertal males, 20 experienced return of normal gonadal function with normal LH and FSH levels and normal to low sperm counts. In contrast, 11 of these 31 developed azoospermia and elevated FSH levels. Leydig cell function was present in all patients, however, as manifest by normal testosterone levels. A total of eight normal children have been born to four men and three women undergoing BMT with cyclophosphamide conditioning alone.

The effects of conditioning regimens employing both cyclophosphamide and TBI on gonadal function were examined in a parallel fashion in 123 patients with ANL [78]. All prepubertal girls subsequently experienced primary ovarian failure with amenorrhea, elevated gonadotrophin levels, and failure of secondary sex characteristics to develop. Of 16 evaluable boys, 5 developed secondary sex characteristics at an appropriate age, but 11 experienced delayed onset of puberty. All 38 postpubertal women in this series developed primary ovarian failure after BMT with cyclophosphamide and TBI, although 2 subsequently had return of menses and became pregnant. All 41 postpubertal males receiving the combined conditioning regimen had primary gonadal failure with elevated FSH levels and azoospermia. Of these, 2 men had delayed recovery 6 years later, and 1 of these men has fathered two normal children. In general, however, gonadal failure should be expected following TBI. Women should be given cyclic hormonal replacement therapy to prevent menopausal symptoms, and young men should have sperm stored prior to BMT.

Additional hormonal abnormalities observed in patients conditioned with TBI include impaired adrenocortical function in 30-40% and subnormal growth hormone levels in 25%. Children who received cranial irradiation prior to conditioning with TBI routinely experienced growth impairment, whereas normal growth velocity curves were observed in 39 children treated with cyclophosphamide alone (Sanders, J., unpublished data).

XV. CATARACTS

Deeg et al. studied cataract development in 277 patients following allogeneic BMT [79]. Of patients receiving single-dose TBI, 80% developed cataracts by 6 years posttransplant and half of the affected patients required cataract extraction. Recipients conditioned with fractionated TBI fared much better; only 19% developed cataracts, and only 20% of affected patients required surgical intervention. Among patients transplanted for aplastic anemia who received no TBI at all, 18% developed cataracts (presumably due to corticosteroid therapy) but none required extraction.

XVI. HEMORRHAGE

Prior to the availability of platelet transfusions, exsanguinating hemorrhage during the period of marrow aplasia preceding engraftment was a major impediment to successful marrow transplantation. However, with the evolution of modern transfusional support services the specter of hemorrhage has diminished greatly. Patients who become refractory to random platelet transfusions can be supplied with HLA-matched platelets garnered by plateletphoresis from compatible family members. Transplant recipients with coexistent liver disease (VOD or GVHD) may also require supplemental coagulation factor replacement in the form of whole blood, fresh-frozen plasma, or cryoprecipitate. These measures are effective in staunching most posttransplant bleeding episodes, such as epistaxis, oropharyngeal bleeding from mucositis, stress gastritis, and hemorrhagic cystitis. Catastrophic intracranial hemorrhage and fulminant gastrointestinal bleeding still prove fatal in 1% of BMT patients, however (unpublished data).

XVII. HEMOLYSIS

Patients receiving marrow grafts from ABO-incompatible donors are at risk of major hemolytic transfusion reactions at the time of marrow infusion. In practice, however, this theoretical obstacle has not been a major clinical concern. Depletion of host isohemagglutinin levels by exchange transfusions, plasmapheresis, or extracorporeal immunoabsorption has proven effective in preventing acute hemolysis [80-82]. An alternate approach is red cell depletion of the marrow graft by differential centrifugation prior to infusion. There is no evidence that engraftment, graft rejection, graft-versus-host disease, or patient survival is adversely influenced by transplantation across major or minor ABO or Rh barriers [82].

XVIII. SECOND MALIGNANCIES

Since both alkylating agents and irradiation are known carcinogens, it can be anticipated that patients surviving marrow transplantation will be at increased risk for the development of second neoplasms. Such an increased risk has been clearly shown in dogs, in which a fivefold increased risk of second malignancies was seen in radiation chimeras compared with control animals [60]. So far, 17 second tumors have been observed in patients following BMT: 5 patients with recurrent leukemia in donor cells, 7 patients with lymphomas (3 of which have been Epstein-Barr virus associated), and 5 cases with solid tumors (2 glioblastomas, 2 rectal adenocarcinomas, and 1 undifferentiated sarcoma) [60].

XIX. CONCLUSION

This brief review has summarized the numerous complications that can ensue following allogeneic marrow transplantation. In spite of the formidable array of obstacles delineated in the foregoing paragraphs, one must not lose sight of the dramatic progress that has been made in this field. We are now able to provide long-term disease-free survival for the majority of patients with aplastic anemia, thalassemia, ANL in first remission and CML in chronic phase, and a minority of patients with end-stage leukemia or lymphoma. Nevertheless, much work still needs to be done. Better conditioning regimens need to be developed to decrease the incidence of leukemic relapse. New approaches for the prophylaxis and treatment of GVHD, interstitial pneumonia, and CMV infections need to be developed. Further clinical trials investigating the utility of bone marrow transplantation in the management of lymphomas, solid tumors, and inborn errors of metabolism need to be undertaken. Methods for expanding the potential pool of transplant candidates by employing partially matched marrow donors and unrelated phenotypically matched donors must be refined [83,84]. Although these goals all represent challenging hurdles to overcome, the progress in marrow transplantation in the past decade engenders optimism for future advances in the field.

ACKNOWLEDGMENTS

The authors gratefully acknowledge the expert assistance of Jan Freedle and Lynn Richardson in manuscript preparation and that of Deborah Amos in data analysis. This investigation was supported by Grants CA 15704, CA 18029, and CA 30924 awarded by the National Cancer Institute, DHHS. Dr. Thomas is a recipient of a Research Career Award (AI 02425) from the National Institute of Allergy and Infectious Diseases. Dr. Press is a recipient of a Young Investigator Award from the American Society of Clinical Oncology and Stuart Pharmaceuticals and of a Clinical Oncology Career Development Award from the American Cancer Society.

REFERENCES

1. Thomas, E. D., Storb, R., Clift, R. A., Fefer, A., Johnson, F. L., Neiman, P. E., Lerner, K. G., Glucksberg, H., and Buckner, C. D.: Bone-marrow transplantation. N. Engl. J. Med. 292:832-843; 895-902, 1975.
2. Storb, R., Thomas, E. D., Buckner, C. D., Clift, R. A., Deeg, H. J., Fefer, A., Goodell, B. W., Sale, G. E., Sanders, J. E., Singer, J., Stewart, P., and Weiden, P. L.: Marrow transplantation in thirty "untransfused" patients with severe aplastic anemia. Ann. Intern. Med. 92:30-36, 1980.
3. Feig, S. A., Champlin, R., Arenson, E., Yak, C., Ho, W., Tesler, A., and Gale, R. P.: Improved survival following bone marrow transplantation for aplastic anaemia. Br. J. Haematol. 54:509-517, 1983.
4. Thomas, E. D., Buckner, C. D., Clift, R. A., Fefer, A., Johnson, F. L., Neiman, P. E., Sale, G. E., Sanders, J. E., Singer, J. W., Shulman, H., Storb, R., and Weiden, P. L.: Marrow transplantation for acute nonlymphoblastic leukemia in first remission. N. Engl. J. Med. 301:597-599, 1979.
5. Gale, R. P., Kay, H. E. M., Rimm, A. A., and Bortin, M. M.: Bone-marrow transplantation for acute leukaemia in first remission. Lancet 2:1006-1009, 1982.
6. Speck, B., Gratwohl, A., Osterwalder, B., and Nissen, C.: Bone marrow transplantation for chronic myeloid leukemia. Semin. Hematol. 21:48-52, 1984.

7. Goldman, J. M., Wyatt, S. E., Baughan, A. S. J., Cranfield, T., McCarthy, D. M., Worsley, A. M., Yin, J., Hows, J. M., Reid, C. D., Catovsky, D., Gordon-Smith, E. C., and Galton, D. A. G.: Allogeneic bone marrow transplantation (BMT) for chronic granulocytic leukaemia (CGL). Exp. Hematol. 12(Suppl. 15):34-35, 1984.
8. Thomas, E. D., Sanders, J. E., Flournoy, N., Johnson, F. L., Buckner, C. D., Clift, R. A., Fefer, A., Goodell, B. W., Storb, R., and Weiden, P. L.: Marrow transplantation for patients with acute lymphoblastic leukemia: A long-term follow-up. Blood 62:1139-1141, 1983.
9. Gale, R. P., Kersey, J. H., Bortin, M. M., Dicke, K. A., Good, R. A., Zwaan, F. E., and Rimm, A. A.: Bone-marrow transplantation for acute lymphoblastic leukaemia. Lancet 2:663-667, 1983.
10. Badger, C., Buckner, C. D., Thomas, E. D., Clift, R. A., Sanders, J. E., Stewart, P. S., Storb, R., Sullivan, K. M., Shulman, H., and Flournoy, N.: Allogeneic marrow transplantation for acute leukemia in relapse. Leuk. Res. 6:383-387, 1982.
11. Camitta, B. M., Thomas, E. D., Nathan, D. G., Gale, R. P., Kopecky, K. J., Rappeport, J. M., Santos, G., Gordon-Smith, E. C., and Storb, R.: A prospective study of androgens and bone marrow transplantation for treatment of severe aplastic anemia. Blood 53:504-514, 1979.
12. Appelbaum, F. R., Dahlberg, S., Thomas, E. D., Buckner, C. D., Cheever, M. A., Clift, R. A., Crowley, J., Deeg, H. J., Fefer, A., Greenberg, P., Kadin, M., Smith, W., Stewart, P., Sullivan, K., Storb, R., and Weiden, P.: Bone marrow transplantation or chemotherapy after remission induction for adults with acute nonlymphoblastic leukemia—a prospective comparison. Ann. Intern. Med. 101:581-588, 1984.
13. Begg, C. B., McGlave, P. B., Bennett, J. M., Cassileth, P. A., and Oken, M. M.: A critical comparison of allogeneic bone marrow transplantation and conventional chemotherapy as treatment for acute nonlymphocytic leukemia. J. Clin. Oncol. 2:369-378, 1984.
14. Powles, R. L., Morgenstern, G., Clink, H. M., Hedley, D., Bandini, G., Lumley, H., Watson, J. G., Lawson, D., Spence, D., Barrett, A., Jameson, B., Lawler, S., Kay, H. E., and McElwain, T. J.: The place of bone marrow transplantation in acute myelogenous leukaemia. Lancet 1:1047-1050, 1980.
15. Johnson, F. L., Thomas, E. D., Clark, B. S., Chard, R. L., Hartmann, J. R., and Storb, R.: A comparison of marrow transplantation with chemotherapy for children with acute lymphoblastic leukemia in second or subsequent remission. N. Engl. J. Med. 305:846-851, 1981.
16. Appelbaum, F. R., Storb, R., Ramberg, R. E., Shulman, H. M., Buckner, C. D., Clift, R. A., Deeg, H. J., Fefer, A., Sanders, J., Stewart, P., Sullivan, K., Witherspoon, R., and Thomas, E. D.: Allogeneic marrow transplantation in the treatment of preleukemia. Ann. Intern. Med. 100:689-693, 1984.
17. Appelbaum, F. R., and Thomas, E. D.: Review of the use of marrow transplantation in the treatment of non-Hodgkin's lymphoma. J. Clin. Oncol. 7:440-447, 1983.

18. Phillips, G. L., Herzig, R. H., Lazarus, H. M., Fay, J. W., Wolff, Sn. N., Mill, W. B., Lin, H.-S., Thomas, P. R. M., Glasgow, G. P., Shina, D. C., and Herzig, G. P.: Treatment of resistant malignant lymphoma with cyclophosphamide, total body irradiation, and transplantation of cryopreserved autologous marrow. N. Engl. J. Med. 310:1557-1561, 1984.
19. Phillips, G. L., Fay, J. W., Herzig, G. P., Herzig, R. H., Weiner, R. S., Wolff, S. N., Lazarus, H. M., Karanes, C., Ross, W. E., Kramer, B. S., and the Southeastern Cancer Study Group: Intensive 1,3-bis(2-chloroethyl)-1-nitrosourea (BCNU) NSC #4366650 and cryopreserved autologous marrow transplantation for refractory cancer. Cancer 52:1792-1802, 1983.
20. Thomas, E. D.: Marrow transplantation for nonmalignant disorders: A retrospective (Editorial Retrospective). N. Engl. J. Med. 312:46-47, 1985.
21. Storb, R., and Thomas, E. D.: Allogeneic bone-marrow transplantation. Immunol. Rev. 71:77-102, 1983.
22. Storb, R., Doney, K. C., Thomas, E. D., Appelbaum, F., Buckner, C. D., Clift, R. A., Deeg, H. J., Goodell, B. W., Hackman, R., Hansen, J. A., Sanders, J., Sullivan, K., Weiden, P. L., and Witherspoon, R. P.: Marrow transplantation with or without donor buffy coat cells for 65 transfused aplastic anemia patients. Blood 59:236-246, 1982.
23. Martin, P. J., Hansen, J. A., Buckner, C. D., Sanders, J. E., Deeg, H. L., Stewart, P., Appelbaum, F. R., Clift, R., Fefer, A., Witherspoon, R. P., Kennedy, M. S., Sullivan, K. M., Flournoy, N., Storb, R., and Thomas, E. D.: Effects of in vitro depletion of T cells in HLA-identical allogeneic marrow grafts. Blood 66:664-672, 1985.
24. Prentice, H. G., Janossy, G., Price-Jones, L., Trejdosiewicz, L. K., Panjwani, D., Graphakos, S., Ivory, K., Blacklock, H. A., Gilmore, M. J. M. L., Tidman, N., Skeggs, D. B. L., Ball, S., Patterson, J., and Hoffbrand, A. V.: Depletion of T lymphocytes in donor marrow prevents significant graft-versus-host disease in matched allogeneic leukaemic marrow transplant recipients. Lancet 1:472-476, 1984.
25. Mitsuyasu, R., Champlin, R., Wells, J., Billing, R., Royston, I., and Gale, R. P.: Bone marrow transplantation after in vitro marrow treatment with monoclonal anti-T cell antibody and complement. Blood 62(Suppl. 1):226a, abstract 807, 1984.
26. Thomas, E. D., Buckner, C. D., Banaji, M., Clift, R. A., Fefer, A., Flournoy, N., Goodell, B. W., Hickman, R. O., Lerner, K. G., Neiman, P. E., Sale, G. E., Sanders, J. E., Singer, J., Stevens, M., Storb, R., and Weiden, P. L.: One hundred patients with acute leukemia treated by chemotherapy, total body irradiation, and allogeneic marrow transplantation. Blood 49:511-533, 1977.
27. Schubach, W. H., Hackman, R., Neiman, P. E., Miller, G., and Thomas, E. D.: A monoclonal immunoblastic sarcoma in donor cells bearing Epstein-Barr virus genomes following allogeneic marrow grafting for acute lymphoblastic leukemia. Blood 60:180-187, 1982.
28. Boyd, C. N., Ramberg, R. C., and Thomas, E. D.: The incidence of recurrence of leukemia in donor cells after allogeneic bone marrow transplantation. Leuk. Res. 6:833-837, 1982.

29. Weiden, P. L., Flournoy, N., Thomas, E. D., Prentice, R., Fefer, A., Buckner, C. D., and Storb, R.: Antileukemic effect of graft-versus-host disease in human recipients of allogeneic-marrow grafts. N. Engl. J. Med. 300: 1068-1073, 1979.
30. Weiden, P. L., Sullivan, K. M., Flournoy, N., Storb, R., Thomas, E. D., and the Seattle Marrow Transplant Team: Antileukemic effect of chronic graft-versus-host disease. Controbution to improved survival after allogeneic marrow transplantation. N. Engl. J. Med. 304:1529-1533, 1981.
31. Witherspoon, R., Lum, L., Storb, R., and Thomas, E. D.: Transplant-related immune deficiency in man. In R. P. Gale, ed., Recent Advances in Bone Marrow Transplantation, New York: Alan R. Liss, Inc., 1983, pp. 473-482.
32. Witherspoon, R. P., Lum, L. G., and Storb, R.: Immunologic reconstitution after human marrow grafting. Semin. Hematol. 21:2-10, 1984.
33. Buckner, C. D., Clift, R. A., Sanders, J. E., Meyers, J. D., Counts, G. W., Farewell, V. T., Thomas, E. D., and the Seattle Marrow Transplant Team: Protective environment for marrow transplant recipients. A prospective study. Ann. Intern. Med. 89:893-901, 1978.
34. Buckner, C. D., Clift, R. A., Thomas, E. D., Hersman, J., Sanders, J. E., Stewart, P. S., Wade, J. C., Murphy, M., Counts, G., and Meyers, J. D.: Early infectious complications in allogeneic marrow transplant recipients with acute leukemia: Effects of prophylactic measures. Infection 11:243-250, 1983.
35. Navari, R. M., Buckner, C. D., Clift, R. A., Storb, R., Sanders, J. E., Stewart, P., Sullivan, K. M., Williams, B., Counts, G. W., Meyers, J. D., and Thomas, E. D.: Prophylaxis of infection in patients with aplastic anemia receiving allogeneic marrow transplants. Am. J. Med. 76:564-572, 1984.
36. Storb, R., Prentice, R. L., Buckner, C. D., Clift, R. A., Appelbaum, F., Deeg, J., Doney, K., Hansen, J. A., Mason, M., Sanders, J. E., Singer, J., Sullivan, K. M., Witherspoon, R. P., and Thomas, E. D.: Graft-versus-host disease and survival in patients with aplastic anemia treated by marrow grafts from HLA-identical siblings. Beneficial effect of a protective environment. N. Engl. J. Med. 308:302-307, 1983.
37. Meyers, J. D., and Thomas, E. D.: Infection complicating bone marrow transplantation. In: Rubin, R. H., and Young, L. S., eds., Clinical Approach to Infection in the Immunocompromised Host, New York: Plenum Press, 1981, Chap. 15, pp. 507-551.
38. Clift, R. A., Buckner, C. D., Fefer, A., Lerner, K. G., Neiman, P. E., Storb, R., Murphy, M., and Thomas, E. D.: Infectious complications of marrow transplantation. Transplant. Proc. 6:389-393, 1974.
39. Winston, D. J., Gale, R. P., Meyer, D. V., and Young, L. S.: Infectious complications of human bone marrow transplantation. Medicine (Baltimore) 58:1-31, 1979.
40. Peterson, F. B., Clift, R. A., Hickman, R. O., Sanders, J. E., Meyers, J. D., Kelleher, J., and Buckner, C. D.: Hickman catheter complications in marrow transplant recipients. J. Parent. Ent. Nutr. 10:58-62, 1986.
41. Press, O. W., Ramsey, P. G., Larson, E., Fefer, A., and Hickman, R. O.: Hick-

man catheter infections in patients with malignancies. Medicine (Baltimore) 63:189-200, 1984.

42. Gerson, S. L., Talbot, G. H., Hurwitz, S., Strom, B. L., Luck, E. J., and Cassileth, P. A.: Prolonged granulocytopenia: The major risk factor for invasive pulmonary aspergillosis in patients with acute leukemia. Ann. Intern. Med. 100:345-351, 1984.
43. Ramsey, P. G., Fife, K. H., Hackman, R. C., Meyers, J. D., and Corey, L.: Herpes simplex virus pneumonia: Clinical, virologic, and pathologic features in 20 patients. Ann. Intern. Med. 97:813-820, 1982.
44. Saral, R., Burns, W. H., Laskin, O. L., Santos, G. W., and Lietman, P. S.: Acyclovir prophylaxis of herpes-simplex-virus infections. N. Engl. J. Med. 305: 63-67, 1981.
45. Meyers, J. D., Wade, J. C., Mitchell, C. D., Saral, R., Leitman, P. S., Durack, D. T., Levin, M. J., Segreti, A. C., and Balfour, H. H., Jr.: Multicenter collaborative herpes simplex virus infection in the immunosompromised host. Am. J. Med. 73:229-235, 1982.
46. Meyers, J. D., Flournoy, N., Wade, J. C., Hackman, R. C., McDougall, J. K., Neiman, P. E., and Thomas, E. D.: Biology of interstitial pneumonia after marrow transplantation. In: Gale, R. P., ed., Recent Advances in Bone Marrow Transplantation, New York: Alan R. Liss, Inc., 1983, pp. 405-423.
47. Barrett, A., Depledge, M. H., and Powles, R. L.: Interstitial pneumonitis following bone marrow transplantation after low dose rate total body irradiation. Int. J. Radiat. Oncol. 9:1029-1033, 1983.
48. Neiman, P. E., Meyers, J. D., Medeiros, E., McDougall, J. K., and Thomas, E. D.: Interstitial pneumonia following marrow transplantation for leukemia and aplastic anemia. In: Gale, R. P., and Fox, C. F., eds., Biology of Bone Marrow Transplantation, New York: Academic Press, 1980, pp. 75-81.
49. Burt, M. E., Flye, M. W., Webber, B. L., and Wesley, R. A.: Prospective evaluation of aspiration needle, cutting needle, transbronchial, and open lung biopsy in patients with pulmonary infiltrates. Ann. Thorac. Surg. 32:146-153, 1981.
50. Haverkos, H. W., Dowling, J. N., Pasculle, A. W., Myerowitz, R. L., Lerberg, D. B., and Hakala, T. R.: Diagnosis of pneumonitis in immunocompromised patients by open lung biopsy. Cancer 52:1093-1097, 1983.
51. Springmeyer, S. C., Silvestri, R. C., Sale, G. E., Peterson, D. L., Weems, C. E., Huseby, J. S., Hudson, L. D., and Thomas, E. D.: The role of transbronchial biopsy for the diagnosis of diffuse pneumonias in immunocompromised marrow transplant recipients. Am. Rev. Respir. Dis. 126:763-765, 1982.
52. Meyers, J. D.: Cytomegalovirus infection following marrow transplantation: risk, treatment, and prevention. In: Plotkin, S. A., Michelson, S., Pagano, J. S., and Rapp, F., eds., CMV: Pathogenesis and Prevention of Human Infection, New York: Alan R. Liss, Inc., 1984, pp. 101-117.
53. Hersman, J., Meyers, J. D., Thomas, E. D., Buckner, C. D., and Clift, R.: The effect of granulocyte transfusions upon the incidence of cytomegalovirus infection after allogeneic marrow transplantation. Ann. Intern. Med. 96: 149-152, 1982.

54. Meyers, J. D., Leszczynski, J., Zaia, J. A., Flournoy, N., Newton, B., Snydman, D. R., Wright, G. G., Levin, M. J., and Thomas, E. D.: Prevention of cytomegalovirus infection by cytomegalovirus immune globulin after marrow transplantation. Ann. Intern. Med. 98:442-446, 1983.
55. Condie, R. M., and O'Reilly, R. J.: Prevention of cytomegalovirus infection in bone marrow transplant recipients by prophylaxis with an intravenous, hyperimmune cytomegalovirus globulin. In: Plotkin, S. A., Michelson, S., Pagano, J. S., and Rapp, F., eds., CMV: Pathogenesis and Prevention of Human Infection, New York: Alan R. Liss, Inc., 1984, pp. 327-344.
56. Kubanek, B., Ernst, P., Schafer, U., Ostendorf, P., and Wolf, H.: A controlled trial of intravenous hyperimmunoglobulin in the prevention of cytomegalovirus infection in bone marrow transplant recipients. Exp. Hematol. 12(Suppl. 15):111-112, 1984.
57. Winston, D. J., Schiffman, G., Wang, D. C., Feig, S. A., Lin, C. H., Marso, E. L., Ho, W. G., Young, L. S., and Gale, R. P.: Pneumococcal infections after human bone-marrow transplantation. Ann. Intern. Med. 91:835-841, 1979.
58. Winston, D. J., Ho, W. G., Schiffman, G., Champlin, R. E., Feig, S. A., and Gale, R. P.: Pneumococcal vaccination of recipients of bone marrow transplants. Arch. Intern. Med. 143:1735-1737, 1983.
59. Deeg, H. J., Storb, R., Thomas, E. D., Flournoy, N., Kennedy, M. S., Banaji, M., Appelbaum, F. R., Bensinger, W. I., Buckner, C. D., Clift, R. A., Doney, K., Fefer, A., McGuffin, R., Sanders, J. E., Singer, J., Stewart, P., Sullivan, K. M., and Witherspoon, R. P.: Cyclosporine as prophylaxis for graft-versus-host disease: A randomized study in patients undergoing marrow transplantation for acute nonlymphoblastic leukemia. Blood 65:1325-1334, 1985.
60. Deeg, H. J., Storb, R., and Thomas, E. D.: Bone marrow transplantation: A review of delayed complications. Br. J. Haematol. 57:185-208, 1984.
61. Reisner, Y., Kapoor, N., Pollack, S., Friedrich, W., Kirkpatrick, D., Shank, B., Csurny, R., Pollack, M. S., Dupont, B., Good, R. A., and O'Reilly, R. J.: Use of lectins in bone marrow transplantation. In: Gale, R. P., ed., Recent Advances in Bone Marrow Transplantation, New York: Alan R. Liss Inc., 1983, pp. 355-387.
62. Filipovich, A. H., Vallera, D. A., Youle, R. J., Quinones, R. R., Neville, D. M., Jr., and Kersey, J. H.: Ex-vivo treatment of donor bone marrow with anti-T-cell immunotoxins for prevention of graft-versus-host disease. Lancet 1: 469-472, 1984.
63. Remlinger, K., Martin, P. J., Hansen, J. A., Doney, K. C., Smith, A., Deeg, H. J., Sullivan, K., Storb, R., and Thomas, E. D.: Murine monoclonal anti-T cell antibodies for treatment of steroid-resistant acute graft-versus-host disease. Hum. Immunol. 9:21-35, 1984.
64. Gratama, J. W., Jansen, J., Lipovich, R. A., Tanke, H. J., Goldstein, G., and Zwaan, F. E.: Treatment of acute graft-versus-host disease with monoclonal antibody OKT3. Transplantation 38:469-474, 1984.
65. Sullivan, K. M., Shulman, H. M., Storb, R., Weiden, P. L., Witherspoon, R. P.,

McDonald, G. B., Schubert, M. M., Atkinson, K., and Thomas, E. D.: Chronic graft-versus-host disease in 52 patients: Adverse natural course and successful tratement with combination immunosuppression. Blood 57:267-276, 1981.

66. Storb, R., Prentice, R. L., Sullivan, K. M., Shulman, H. M., Deeg, H. J., Doney, K. C., Buckner, C. D., Clift, R. A., Witherspoon, R. P., Appelbaum, F. R., Sanders, J. E., Stewart, P. S., and Thomas, E. D.: Predictive factors in chronic graft-versus-host disease in patients with aplastic anemia treated by marrow transplantation from HLA-identical siblings. Ann. Intern. Med. 98:461-466, 1983.
67. Atkinson, K., Biggs, J. C., Ting, A., Concannon, A. J., Dodds, A. J., and Pun, A.: Cyclosporin A is associated with faster engraftment and less mucositis than methotrexate after allogeneic bone marrow transplantation. Br. J. Haematol. 53:265-270, 1983.
68. McDonald, G. B., Sharma, P., Matthews, D. E., Shulman, H. M., and Thomas, E. D.: Venocclusive disease of the liver after bone marrow transplantation: Diagnosis, incidence, and predisposing factors. Hepatology 4:116-122, 1984.
69. Schaller, R. T., Jr., and Schaller, J. F.: The acute abdomen in the immunologically compromised child. J. Pediatr. Surg. 18:937-944, 1983.
70. Springmeyer, S. C., Flournoy, N., Sullivan, K. M., Storb, R., and Thomas, E. D.: Pulmonary function changes in long-term survivors of allogeneic marrow transplantation. In: Gale, R. P., ed., Recent Advances in Bone Marrow Transplantation, New York: Alan R. Liss, Inc., 1983, pp. 343-353.
71. Atkinson, K., Bryant, D., Biggs, J., Concannon, A., and Dodds, A.: Obstructive airways disease: A rare but serious manifestation of chronic graft-versus-host disease after allogeneic marrow transplantation in humans. Transplant. Proc. 16:1030-1033, 1984.
72. Atkinson, K., Biggs, J. C., Hayes, J., Ralston, M., Dodds, A. J., Concannon, A. J., and Naidoo, D.: Cyclosporin A associated nephrotoxicity in the first 100 days after allogeneic bone marrow transplantation: Three distinct syndromes. Br. J. Haematol. 54:59-67, 1983.
73. Shulman, H., Striker, G., Deeg, H. J., Kennedy, M., Storb, R., and Thomas, E. D.: Nephrotoxicity of cyclosporin A after allogeneic marrow transplantation: Glomerular thromboses and tubular injury. N. Engl. J. Med. 305:1392-1395, 1981.
74. Myers, B. D., Ross, J., Newton, L., Luetscher, J., and Perlroth, M.: Cyclosporine-associated chronic nephropathy. N. Engl. J. Med. 311:699-705, 1984.
75. Atkinson, K., Biggs, J., Darveniza, P., Boland, J., Concannon, A., and Dodds, A.: Cyclosporine associated central nervous system toxicity after allogeneic bone marrow transplantation. Transplantation 38:34-37, 1984.
76. Thompson, C. B., June. C. H., Sullivan, K. M., and Thomas, E. D.: Association between cyclosporine neurotoxicity and hypomagnesemia. Lancet 2: 1116-1120, 1984.
77. Sklar, C. A., Kim, T. H., and Ramsay, N. K.: Thyroid dysfunction among long term survivors of bone marrow transplantation. Am. J. Med. 73:688-694, 1982.

78. Sanders, J. E., Buckner, C. D., Leonard, J. M., Sullivan, K. M., Witherspoon, R. P., Deeg, H. J., Storb, R., and Thomas, E. D.: Late effects on gonadal function of cyclophosphamide, total-body irradiation, and marrow transplantation. Transplantation 36:252-255, 1983.
79. Deeg, H. J., Flournoy, N., Sullivan, K. M., Sheehan, K., Buckner, C. D., Sanders, J. E., Storb, R., Witherspoon, R. P., and Thomas, E. D.: Cataracts after total body irradiation and marrow transplantation: A sparing effect of dose fractionation. Int. J. Radiat. Oncol. Biol. Phys. 10:957-964, 1984.
80. Bensinger, W. I., Baker, D. A., Buckner, C. D., Clift, R. A., and Thomas, E. D.: Immunoadsorption for removal of A and B blood-group antibodies. N. Engl. J. Med. 304:160-162, 1981.
81. Buckner, C. D., Clift, R. A., Sanders, J. E., Williams, B., Gray, M., Storb, R., and Thomas, E. D.: ABO-incompatible marrow transplants. Transplantation 26:233-238, 1978.
82. Lasky, L. C., Warkentin, P. I., Kersey, J. H., Ramsay, N. K. C., McClave, P. B., and McCullough, J.: Hemotherapy in patients undergoing blood group incompatible bone marrow transplantation. Transfusion 23:277-285, 1983.
83. Hansen, J. A., Clift, R. A., Thomas, E. D., Buckner, C. D., Storb, R., and Giblett, E. R.: Transplantation of marrow from an unrelated donor to a patient with acute leukemia. N. Engl. J. Med. 303:565-567, 1980.
84. Hansen, J. A., Clift, R. A., Beatty, P. G., Mickelson, E. M., Nisperos, B., Martin, P. J., and Thomas, E. D.: Marrow transplantation from donors other than HLA genotypically identical siblings. In: Gale, R. P., ed., Recent Advances in Bone Marrow Transplantation, New York: Alan R. Liss, Inc., 1983, pp. 739-756.
85. Thomas, E. D., Clift, R. A., Fefer, A., et al.: Marrow transplantation for the treatment of chronic myelogenous leukemia. Ann. Intern. Med. 104:155-163, 1986.
86. Locksley, R. M., Fluornay, N., Sullivan, K. M., and Meyers, J. D.: Varicella-zoster virus infection after marrow transplantation. J. Infect. Dis., in press.
87. Bowden, R. A., Sayers, M., Fluornoy, N., Newton, B., Banaji, M., Thomas, E. D., and Meyers, J. D.: Cytomegalovirus infection after marrow transplantation. N. Engl. J. Med. 314:1006-1010, 1986.

Appendix

Potential Complications Associated with the Most Frequently Used Immunosuppressive Drugs

Immunosuppressive drug	Complications
Azathioprine	Leukopenia and/or thrombocytopenia; nausea, vomiting, hepatotoxicity, skin rashes, alopecia, fever, diarrhea, steatorrhea, negative nitrogen balance
Steroids	Sodium retention, fluid retention, congestive heart failure in susceptible patients, potassium loss, hypokalemic alkalosis, hypertension
	Muscle weakness, steroid myopathy, loss of muscle mass, osteoporosis, vertebral compression fractures, asceptic necrosis of femoral and humeral heads, pathologic fracture of long bones
	Peptic ulcer with possible perforation and hemorrhage, pancreatitis, abdominal distention, ulcerative esophagitis
	Impaired wound healing, thin fragile skin, petechiae and ecchymoses, facial erythema, increased sweating, may suppress reactions to skin tests
	Increased intracranial pressure with papilledema, usually after treatment, convulsions, vertigo, headache

(continued)

Immunosuppressive drug	Complications
Steroids (continued)	Development of cushingoid state, suppression of growth in children, secondary adrenocortical and pituitary unresponsiveness, particularly in times of stress, as in trauma, surgery, or illness, menstrual irregularities, decreased carbohydrate tolerance, manifestations of latent diabetes mellitus, increased requirements for insulin or oral hypoglycemic agents in diabetics
	Posterior subcapsular cataracts, increased intraocular pressure, glaucoma, exophthalmos
	Negative nitrogen balance due to protein catabolism
ALG/ATG	Fever, chills, leukopenia, thrombocytopenia
	Rash, pruritus, urticaria, wheal and flare
	Arthralgia, chest or back pain, diarrhea, dyspnea, headache, hypotension, nausea, vomiting, night sweats, pain at infusion site, peripheral thrombophlebitis, stomatitis
	Anaphylaxis, dizziness, weakness or faintness, edema, herpes simplex reactivation
Cyclosporine	Renal dysfunction, tremor, hirsutism, hypertension, and gum hyperplasia
	Cramps, acne, convulsions, headache, diarrhea, nausea and vomiting, hepatotoxicity, abdominal discomfort, paresthesia, flushing, leukopenia, lymphoma, sinusitis, gynecomastia
Monoclonal antibodies	Pyrexia, chills, dyspnea, chest pain, vomiting, wheezing, nausea, diarrhea, tremor, severe pulmonary edema, infection, development of antimurine antibodies

Index